Psychiatry

ESSENTIALS OF CLINICAL PRACTICE

Psychiatry

ESSENTIALS OF CLINICAL PRACTICE

WITH EXAMINATION QUESTIONS, ANSWERS, AND COMMENTS

IAN GREGORY, M.D., F.R.C.P.(C), F.R.C.Psych.
Professor and Chairman, Department of Psychiatry,
Ohio State University College of Medicine,
Columbus

DONALD J. SMELTZER, M.A.
Assistant Professor, Department of Psychiatry,
Ohio State University College of Medicine,
Columbus

LITTLE, BROWN AND COMPANY   BOSTON

Library of Congress Catalog Card No. 77-70463

ISBN 0-316-32781-6 (C)
ISBN 0-316-32780-8 (P)

Printed in the United States of America

Contributing Authors

L. Eugene Arnold, M.D.
Associate Professor and Director of Child Psychiatry,
Departments of Psychiatry and Pediatrics, Ohio
State University College of Medicine, Columbus

Malcolm Gardner, Ph.D.
Associate Professor, Departments of Psychiatry
and Psychology, Ohio State University, Columbus

Walter Knopp, M.D.
Professor, Department of Psychiatry, Ohio State
University College of Medicine, Columbus

Preface

This book is the outcome of a highly successful *personalized study program* (PSP) that we initiated for our medical students in 1974. A two-month, full-time clinical clerkship in psychiatry has been required at Ohio State University since 1966. Although our clinical teaching has been successful, we have found an increasing need for supplementation of patient care experiences with up-to-date information from appropriate readings. This requires easy access to a concise yet comprehensive summary of psychiatric concepts and techniques that are essential to the clinical practice of all physicians.

The principal components of our personalized teaching are as follows:

1. Structured reading assignments (study units) organized around specific topics
2. A private meeting with an assigned tutor (resident or faculty member) after studying each unit
3. Completion of a practice quiz consisting of multiple-choice questions related to the study topics (although not necessarily derived specifically from the reading assignment)
4. Immediate remedial feedback from the tutor, with identification and discussion of problem areas of the individual student, but no grade given on the basis of the quiz results
5. Self-pacing progress based on mastery of assigned study units
6. Optional use of audiovisual aids and attendance at lectures
7. Satisfactory performance on a written final examination at the completion of the clerkship.

Our two graduating classes that were taught by this program obtained mean psychiatry scores on the National Board Examination that were substantially above the national candidate mean and very significantly increased over our previous classes. Without overemphasizing the importance of test scores, it may be noted that this is the only criterion of success readily available. Equally gratifying, our students have shown increased interest in psychiatry and have given very complimentary reports on their learning experience.

The present volume is the logical adaptation of our program to a self-study format. It contains a careful selection of up-to-date material that is relevant to students of psychiatry at all levels, from the medical student taking his first course (or clinical clerkship), to the busy physician preparing for an examination or in need of a ready reference for his clinical practice, to the experienced specialist who wishes to update his knowledge in those areas outside his day-to-day endeavors. We have tried to be selective rather than encyclopedic but have included with each chapter an eclectic list of references to which the reader may turn for more detailed information when he wishes.

Chapters 1 through 10 contain general information in a sequence based partly on the urgency with which it is required. Chapters 11 through 20 contain more specific information on various psychiatric syndromes, organized in the same sequence as the third revision of the *Diagnostic and Statistical Manual of Mental Disorders* (or *DSM-III*, currently in preparation by the American Psychiatric Association). The latter reflects the recent rapid growth in scientific understanding of mental health and mental disorders.

At the end of each chapter is a selection of sample questions similar to those asked in standardized examinations. Maximum benefit will be obtained by first reading the material in the chapter, then attempting to answer the questions, and only thereafter consulting the answer key and remedial feedback (contained in a separate section at the end of the book). Where possible, page references to the text have been included in the feedback; however, the questions and feedback alone cannot possibly cover all the material included in the text itself, and we recommend that students avoid the temptation to refer to the questions and answers prematurely. As in our personalized instruction program, we have viewed the practice quizzes as simply an additional study tool and have therefore felt free to supplement the presentation in the text by introducing additional concepts in the question sets.

It takes a great deal of time and effort to condense or distill the accumulated wisdom from a knowledge explosion that is still continuing. In this venture we are most fortunate to have had capable assistance from a number of colleagues, three of whom also contributed directly to the text itself. Malcolm Gardner and Walter Knopp worked with us closely in developing and implementing our PSP program for medical students and have also contributed much of Chapter 18 (Sexual Response, Dysfunction, and Deviation). L. Eugene Arnold has been responsible for all of our educational programs in child and adolescent psychiatry for the past two years, and he contributed Chapter 19.

It is also a great pleasure to acknowledge the efforts of others who have helped to make our task easier. We are most grateful to Ms. Gretchen Hammond and Ms. Andrea Ardito for their invaluable secretarial assistance. We are indebted to Dr. Aaron Beck for his kind permission to reproduce the revised version of his depression inventory. It is also a pleasure to thank our many students who helped us recognize what needed to be done and how best to do it.

I. G.
D. J. S.

Contents

Psychiatry

ESSENTIALS OF CLINICAL PRACTICE

1. Development and Dynamics

A man will sometimes rage at his wife when in reality his mistress has offended him, and a lady complains of the cruelty of her husband when she has no other enemy than bad cards.
Samuel Johnson

PSYCHIATRY AND PSYCHOANALYSIS

Psychiatry

This term, derived from Greek roots meaning "mind-healing," refers to the medical science that deals with the origin, diagnosis, treatment, and prevention of *mental disorders.* These disorders may affect persons of all ages, and may involve either intellectual or emotional processes, verbal or nonverbal behavior. They may result from disturbances in biological function, or from the adverse influence of psychological or sociocultural factors.

A *psychiatrist* is a licensed physician specializing in psychiatry. In the United States his or her education usually includes three or four years in an approved residency following graduation from medical school. Additional training is necessary for certain subspecialties such as child psychiatry and psychoanalysis.

All medical schools in the United States currently include psychiatry as a standard part of the curriculum, usually in the form of a required clinical rotation. It is also one of the major subjects in the examinations of the National Board of Medical Examiners and of the Federated Licensing Examinations Board (FLEX).

Psychotherapy

This is a generic term used for treatments that are based mainly on communication (verbal or nonverbal) between therapist and patient or client. The American Psychiatric Association defines *medical psychotherapy* as a procedure carried out by a physician trained in psychiatric medicine to treat mental, emotional, and psychosomatic illness.

This is usually accomplished through a relationship with the patient in an individual, group, or family setting. It assumes that psychological illness and physical illness are inseparable, entails continuing medical diagnosis and responsibility, and may be carried out with concurrent pharmacologic or other medical treatments.

Psychoanalysis

This is the branch of science developed by Sigmund Freud and his followers and devoted to the study of human psychological functioning and behavior. Three applications of psychoanalysis are usually distinguished as follows: (1) a method of investigation or research into mental processes; (2) the development of a systematized body of knowledge and theory concerning human behavior and development; and (3) a method of treatment (psychotherapy) for psychological or emotional illness. Psychoanalysis involves *free association* and the analysis of dreams, fantasies, thought processes, and behaviors in relation to emotion (*affect*). A limited return to earlier methods of reacting (*regression*) is encouraged, so that derivatives of forbidden wishes and repressed memories may find expression in current ideas and feelings. Hitherto unconscious conflicts, associated with earlier traumatic experiences, are made conscious through *interpretation,* which involves the analysis and elimination of defenses and resistances. Psychoanalysis and other psychotherapies derived from it have been considered most effective in the treatment of some neuroses, and have also found increasing application in attempts to modify character disorders.

Psychodynamics

Literally interpreted, this is the study of mental forces in action. Current usage of the term focuses on intrapsychic processes (rather than interpersonal relationships) and involves the role of unconscious motivation in human behavior. The current psychoanalytic view of psychodynamics is based on Freud's *structural theory,* according to which there are three major divisions (structures) of the psychic apparatus: the *id* (representing instinctual drives); the *ego* (representing executive and inhibiting functions); and the *superego* (representing the influences of conscience and the need to strive toward an idealistic goal). Each of the mental structures is assumed to involve interaction between innate and environmental factors. Psychodynamics is concerned with both the genesis and the development of current mental processes and behavior.

Psychopathology

This is a broad term referring to the study of significant causes and processes responsible for the development of mental disorders, as well as to the various manifestations of these disorders. Psychodynamics should therefore be regarded as a subset of the larger field of psychopathology, which may be viewed as concerned with description, dynamics, development, and causation (etiology).

Psychology

This term refers to an academic discipline, a profession, and a science dealing with the study of mental processes and behavior in man and animals. The minimum standard for election to full membership in the American Psychological Association is a doctoral degree (usually in philosophy or in psychology). A number of subspecialties are recognized, including clinical psychology, which is concerned traditionally with the diagnosis and evaluation of mental disorders, and in more recent years with psychotherapy. One aspect of the training of clinical psychologists is *psychometry,* defined as the science of testing and measuring mental and psychological ability, efficiency, potential, and functioning. Test administration is sometimes performed by a *psychometrist* with a bachelor's or master's degree, although interpretation of test results remains the responsibility of professionals with more advanced training.

HISTORY OF DYNAMIC PSYCHIATRY

During the latter part of the nineteenth century, an English neurologist named *John Hughlings Jackson* (1835–1911) formulated some important principles concerning the *dissolution of function* within the nervous system, with consequent regres-

sion to earlier developmental levels. He viewed the nervous system as being organized in hierarchical fashion, with the most complex functions (associated with the cerebral cortex) as the most recently acquired from an evolutionary point of view and also the ones most vulnerable to dissolution under conditions of lesion, trauma, or stress. Jackson noted a regression of neural function to lower and more primitive levels under adverse conditions, and recognized that higher centers may be concerned with inhibiting the function of lower centers; the latter would then act unopposed if the functions of higher centers were disrupted. In analyzing the effects of brain damage, he therefore distinguished between *negative* symptoms due to loss of function (loss of "government") and *positive* symptoms due to release from inhibition, which he characterized as "the anarchy of the now uncontrolled people." For every mental state there was a corresponding physical state in the brain, and the observable symptoms and signs of neurological and psychiatric disorder consisted of a combination of positive and negative symptoms. Jackson's principle of the dissolution of complex functions and his concepts of dynamic interaction within the nervous system not only are relevant to the manifestations of organic brain syndromes, but also were employed by Freud in his formulations on unconscious intrapsychic dynamic processes.

At about the same time, many neurologists were becoming aware that there were some patients whose bodily symptoms could not be attributed to anatomical lesions in the nervous system. Such patients (with *conversion hysteria* and other neuroses) appeared relatively intact in intellectual, emotional, and behavioral function—and were frequently seen as clinic outpatients or general hospital patients rather than as residents of mental hospitals. The main stimulus to psychological treatment and understanding of such patients came from the therapeutic application of *hypnosis.*

Franz Anton Mesmer (c. 1733–1815) was a German physician who claimed to be able to cure all illnesses by the touch of a rod, thereby equalizing a magnetic field that was assumed to fill the universe. Disease was attributed to the uneven distribution of animal magnetism. However, Mesmer's views were criticized by the French Academy of Sciences, and he was forced to retire from his fashionable practice in Paris. A British surgeon, *James Braid* (1795–1860), rejected Mesmer's theories but became interested in his technique, which he termed hypnosis ("nervous sleep"). The French physician *Ambrose Liébeault* (1823–1904) became interested in hypnotism after listening to a report of Braid's work before the French Academy of Sciences, and applied the technique in the treatment of hysterical patients at Nancy.

In 1883 *Hippolyte Bernheim* (1840–1919), the physician in charge of the Nancy Asylum, referred a patient suffering from sciatica to Liébeault and was amazed to find the patient subsequently cured. Bernheim in turn became an exponent of hypnotism, which he regarded as merely an exaggerated form of *suggestion* and only quantitatively different from the phenomena of normal mental function. He also investigated posthypnotic suggestion, or "latent memory," by "implanting" suggestions during the hypnotic trance that the patient later carried out without any recollection of the suggestion or its source. Bernheim was among the first to use the term *psychoneurosis,* but did not consider that suggestibility and posthypnotic amnesia were restricted to neurotic patients.

By contrast, the more famous French physician *Jean-Martin Charcot* (1825–1893) regarded hypnotic phenomena as unique to hysteria patients. Charcot took charge of La Salpêtrière in 1866, and attracted many students who witnessed his dramatic demonstrations. One of his students, *Pierre Janet* (1859–1947), studied many other neurotic manifestations including phobias, anxiety, obsessions, various abnormal impulses, and tics. He is best remembered for his report (1899) that some neurotic patients recalled traumatic memories under hypnosis and became well after such ideas were consciously expressed. While he corroborated Freud's early findings on the clinical significance of unconscious processes and the therapeutic effects of emotional catharsis, Janet's methods of treatment were directed more toward conscious and emotional reeducation.

The man destined to become the best-known student of Charcot and Bernheim was *Sigmund Freud* (1856–1939), who was born in Freiberg, a small town in Moravia, which was then part of Austria. His father was a Jewish merchant who moved his family to Vienna when Freud was a child, and Freud continued to live there until 1938, when the political situation forced him to take refuge in London. He died there the following year. Freud was a brilliant student and experienced some conflict between his theoretical interests or scientific curiosity and the practical necessity of earning a living as a physician. For six years he worked in Ernst Brucke's physiological laboratory and studied the histology of the nervous system. He graduated from medical school in 1881, and one year later he transferred to the general hospital where he continued studying the anatomy of the brain and organic diseases of the nervous system. In 1885 he went to Paris to study for a year under Charcot. The following year he married, and opened a neurological practice in Vienna.

The neurological practice involved many neurotic patients, and Freud was dissatisfied with the then current techniques of hydrotherapy, electrotherapy, massage, rest, and diet. From Charcot he had learned that hysteria could occur in men as well as in women and that hypnosis could produce hysterical symptoms as well as remove them. From Bernheim he had learned that private patients could not be hypnotized as readily as could charity patients in the clinic, and that suggestion alone (in the waking state) might be as effective as suggestion performed while the patient was under hypnosis.

After his visit to Bernheim in 1889, Freud collaborated with *Josef Breuer,* who had previously used hypnosis in the prolonged treatment of a hysterical girl (from 1880 to 1882). Under hypnosis this patient (Anna O.) had recalled previously forgotten and highly emotional experiences, from which specific symptoms could be dated. After talking over these emotional experiences with Breuer under hypnosis, she had been relieved of the symptoms that had stemmed from the experiences. Freud confirmed these observations, and he and Breuer published their results in *Studies on Hysteria* (1893–1895). They postulated that ideas and memories having unpleasant emotional significance are banished from accessibility by an involuntary and automatic mental force that they called *repression;* that repressed material may be recalled under hypnosis; and that some detail of a repressed traumatic experience may be shown to have identity with some aspect of a hysterical symptom. They termed the transformation of emotional impulse into an abnormal bodily function *conversion,* their method of treatment *emotional catharsis,* and the emotional release that took place *abreaction.*

FREUDIAN PSYCHOANALYSIS

Freud encountered various problems in the application of hypnosis and suggestion to patients. Not all patients could be hypnotized, and symptoms removed during hypnosis were apt to be replaced by other symptoms before long. Moreover, hypnosis had no effect on the repressive forces responsible for excluding traumatic memories from consciousness. However, he found that repressed material could sometimes be recalled with difficulty in the waking state by the use of a process called *free association,* involving uninhibited verbal reporting of all conscious thought regardless of apparent irrelevancy. He realized that these free associations were not really free, and concluded that they were determined by unconscious material that had to be analyzed and interpreted. He therefore termed his new technique psychoanalysis (1896).

He also noted that when patients free-associated, dreams of the night before or of many years previously might occur to them. Free associations to fragments of dreams often led more quickly to the disclosure of unconscious memories and fantasies than free associations to other subjects, and he concluded that dreams represented symbolic or disguised forms of *wish fulfillment.* He termed the image recalled on awakening the *manifest content* and the true underlying motive the *latent content.* He postulated that the symbols represented in

dreams are derived not only from the experiences of the individual, but also from a widespread tendency of people in a given culture to represent certain unconscious thoughts (particularly sexual ones) by characteristic symbols. Thus the human body might be represented by a house; the male genitalia by snakes, sticks, weapons, or trees; and the female genitalia by boxes, caves, other containers, or doorways.

For a while Freud believed that a neurosis originated in some isolated emotional shock that the patient had undergone. He used the methods of free association and *dream analysis* to help patients recall repressed emotional experiences, and this process was frequently accompanied by relief from the neurotic symptoms. However, some patients returned after a short time with somewhat different symptoms. Freud's explanation for this was that he had not analyzed sufficiently far back in the patients' lives, and he began probing further back into childhood and even infancy.

Eventually he came to modify his theoretical formulation. A number of his female patients reported having been seduced or sexually attacked by fathers, brothers, or other relatives, but some of these reports were found to have no factual basis. Freud decided that these false memories represented fantasies of later childhood that arose from conflicts and unfulfilled wishes of early childhood. He further postulated that neurosis was the result of early childhood conflicts between drives and fears. Mediating between drives seeking discharge (especially the sexual drive) and the fear and guilt engendered by these drives, the developing ego had resolved the conflict by repressing the drives from awareness; since the drives were thereby rendered not inactive but merely unconscious, the result was the formation of neurotic symptoms.

Freud thus came to believe that a cure of neurosis might be accomplished by a revival of the emotional attitude of early childhood (regression) without the necessity of achieving full recall of actual events. As the patient reexperiences these repressed emotions, he unconsciously displaces onto the analyst the feelings, attitudes, and wishes originally associated with significant persons in his early life. The patient's positive or negative feelings toward the analyst thus constitute a symbolic reliving of the previous emotional experience. This phenomenon, which takes place to some extent in all kinds of psychotherapy and other significant interpersonal relationships, is called *transference.* The reciprocal phenomenon, in which the therapist develops illogical attitudes or feelings toward the patient as a result of his own old conflicts or inappropriate stereotyping, is called *countertransference.*

Partly because of his own discomfort, and partly because of the transference relationship with the analyst (whom the patient may at various times view as a punishing authority figure or as a benevolent parent whose acceptance is desired), the patient undergoing psychoanalysis experiences occasional inability or unwillingness to discuss certain topics. These episodes, which are usually but not always unconsciously motivated, are called *resistances.* The analysis of transference and resistance is the prime function of the psychoanalyst. At appropriate times during the analysis he comments to the patient about what is happening, or perhaps about what is not happening. This process is called *interpretation,* and is aimed at helping the patient have greater insight into his own needs and conflicts so that he can consider realistic solutions for them.

The three successive goals toward which Freud directed his efforts in psychoanalysis may now be summarized as follows: (1) understanding the patient's unconscious emotions or conflicts and *interpreting* them to the patient at the right time; (2) forcing the patient to confirm such interpretations through his own recall, by enabling the patient to understand the resistances that prevented their recall; and (3) enabling the patient to relive repressed emotional situations. The main theories arising out of these efforts to help patients may be divided into three broad groups: (1) *economic concepts;* (2) *dynamic concepts,* including the *libido theory*; and (3) *topographic concepts* and the *structural theory* of personality.

Economic Concepts

This area of Freud's theories concerned the fundamental modes of operation and the distribution of psychic energies. The term *libido* is a quantitative concept referring to the drive energy of the sexual instinct, which was eventually interpreted in the broader sense of all strivings toward pleasurable experience. Other major forces governing motivation were the *aggressive* drive and the *self-preserving* interests of the individual. (The latter are sometimes called the ego instincts.) Freud conceived of dammed-up psychic energy as causing pain and tension, and the release of energy as producing pleasure. The basic tendency to seek pleasure and avoid pain was termed the *pleasure principle,* which is modified during the course of development by the *reality principle,* bringing about the postponement of impulse gratification in accordance with the demands of the environment. An even more basic tendency than the pleasure principle was termed by Freud the *repetition compulsion,* which consisted of the tendency to repeat emotional situations and experiences regardless of their apparent pleasurable or painful consequences.

Dynamic Concepts

These dealt with the interaction of forces leading to conflict or overt behavior. Originally he divided all instincts into the sex drive (serving the pleasure principle) and the self-preservative drives (serving the reality principle). Subsequently he combined both of these into the concept of *eros,* which he now considered opposed by *thanatos,* consisting of the aggressive drives toward death, destruction, and dissolution. Freud's concept of the death instinct is his most controversial one and has been severely criticized both within and outside of the psychoanalytic field. Most analysts, however, retain and use the concepts of the libidinal and aggressive instinctual drives.

Libido Theory

This includes a theoretical description of a characteristic maturational sequence of libidinal or psychosexual phases in development from birth to mature adulthood. The drive organization is subject to *progression, regression,* and *fixation,* determined in part by the extent to which the individual encounters normal, frustrated, or excessive gratification.

The *oral phase* is the earliest stage of development, and is associated with behavior appropriate to the first year of life, particularly extreme *dependency.* Fixation at or regression to this level of development is considered typical of schizophrenia, manic-depressive psychoses, alcoholism, and other drug dependence.

Society chooses the second year of life as an appropriate time for toilet training, and the child derives conscious pleasure from his excretory functions and his ability to control them. This *anal phase* of development implies the ability to give or withhold, and involves the child's learning to make compromises between his primitive wishes and the rewards obtained by conforming with the demands and expectations of significant adults responsible for his care. "Anal" traits persisting in adults include excessive orderliness, miserliness, and obstinacy. If present to an excessive degree, they may be associated with the development of an obsessive-compulsive neurosis.

The next period of psychosexual development lasts from the age of about 2½ to 6 years and is known as the *phallic phase,* since children may at this time display considerable sexual interest and curiosity focused on the penis or the clitoris. The observed difference between male and female genitalia may lead to the childhood fantasy that female genitalia result from the loss of a penis. According to psychoanalytic theory, the boy then develops a *castration complex,* fearing castration at the hands of his father. The reasoning here is that he wishes to replace his father in his mother's affections and is experiencing envious and aggressive wishes toward his father (the *Oedipus complex*). At the same age a girl is assumed to have a similar Oedipus (or Electra) complex over her forbidden longings to replace her mother in the affections of her father. Much of the girl's behavior at this age has been referred to as *penis envy,* which may be generalized or persist as a female wish for male attri-

butes, positions, or advantages. Various forms of sexual deviation and dysfunction in both sexes are considered to have their origins at this phase of development.

The next phase described in the libido theory lasts from the age of about 6 years until puberty and is regarded as one of *sexual latency.* The Oedipus complex has usually been resolved (to be reactivated at least temporarily at the time of puberty), and the child has made a decisive identification with the appropriate parent (or surrogate) and formed an effective superego (conscience and ego-ideal). The intrafamilial relationships of the preschool years constitute the nucleus of his knowledge of the human race, which is now expanded in school and play activities, in relationships with adults outside the family, and in collaborative or competitive activities with his peers. Old techniques of adaptation will be repeated and reinforced, or extinguished and replaced by newer techniques that are found more rewarding. Maladaptive patterns of behavior, however, may well be perpetuated by continuation of the conditions under which they developed, or lack of motivation for change.

The *genital phase* is initiated by puberty and leads to a reawakening of sexual interest that is now conscious, verbalized, and acted on in accordance with the mores of the peer group. During this period there is increasing desire to be freed from infantile dependency and to achieve adult status. This desire results in rejection of the standards and validity of the demands imposed by parents and other adults, with a tendency for uncritical acceptance of the philosophy of the peer group. In this process there is often partial identification with others of the same sex who are just a little older than the individual, and who are admired by his peer group. Ideally, the gradual emancipation from parental controls is accompanied by increasing responsibility and mature genitality based on mutual respect.

Topographic Concepts
These concepts, originally set forth in Freud's *The Interpretation of Dreams* (1900), constituted

his early attempts to map the mind and its activities. He described the mind as divided into three regions that were distinguished from each other by the accessibility of their contents and the nature of their functions. The *conscious* portion, which may be compared with the small visible tip of an iceberg, was regarded by Freud as a kind of sense organ of attention serving the function of awareness. It can accept external input from sensory perceptions of environmental stimuli and internal input from the *preconscious* portion of the mind. The latter contains wishes, ideas, memories, and feelings that are accessible to the conscious by an act of attention. The mental activities of the conscious and preconscious are called *secondary process thinking,* and are characterized by systematic organization, respect for logical connections and low tolerance for inconsistencies, a tendency to delay instinctual discharge, and attempts to conform to the demands of external reality and the individual's moral values. It is closely governed by the reality principle and is responsible for logical thought and action in adult life.

The *unconscious* portion of the mind contains material that cannot be made conscious by focusing attention. It contains repressed ideas, wishes, and affects that can become conscious only by first entering the preconscious, which censors them and attempts to keep them unconscious. Repressed material may reach consciousness when the censor is relaxed (as in dreams), is overpowered (as in neurotic symptom formation), or is fooled (as in jokes). Mental activity of the unconscious is called *primary process thinking* and is characterized by lack of organization, disregard for logical connections and acceptance of contradictions, absence of a time concept and a tendency to seek immediate gratification of instinctual drives, and attempts to obtain wish fulfillment with no regard for the demands of external reality. It is closely governed by the pleasure principle, and makes frequent use of *symbolization* (in which one object or idea takes over the significance of another, which it resembles in some way), *condensation* (in which several concepts become fused and replaced by a single symbol), and *displacement* (in which the affective component of an unacceptable idea is transferred to a symbolic substitute). Primary-process thinking is characteristic of very young children, of normal dreaming at all ages, and of severe psychosis or mental retardation.

Freud was soon dissatisfied with the topographical theory and eventually replaced it with his structural theory of personality. The more useful concepts of the first theory were carried over into the second, including the division of mental activity into primary and secondary process and the concept of a dynamic unconscious.

Structural Theory

Advanced by Freud in 1923, this theory views the psychic apparatus as divided into three structures called the id, the ego, and the superego, and differentiated on the basis of function. The *id* represents the unorganized source of primitive instinctual impulses, as summarized in the sentence *"It wants."* The *ego* was initially viewed as the seat of the conscious, intellectual, and self-preservative functions, as summarized in the sentence *"I will, or I will not."* The *superego* develops from the ego, and fulfills such functions as those summarized in the imperatives *"You shall (must), or you shall (must) not."* Two aspects of the superego are distinguished: (1) the *conscience,* developed through *internalization* (introjection) and automatization of the many prohibitions of early childhood; and (2) the *ego-ideal,* developed through *identification* with the attributes of those who are admired or envied. The superego has also been characterized as the part of the personality that is "soluble in alcohol."

In current psychoanalytic theory the ego is regarded as the integrative and executive portion of the personality, adapting constantly to the forces and pressures exerted by the id, the superego, and external reality. The defense mechanisms discussed below are therefore viewed as maneuvers by the ego in its efforts to maintain the integrity of the individual, and take place whether this individual is currently considered normal, neurotic, or psychotic. Any given defense mechanism may involve varying degrees of reality distortion, may meet with varying success in assisting the overall efforts of the individual toward adaptation, and may be used with varying frequency by different persons. It is these latter factors that determine the extent to which a given defense mechanism should be regarded as abnormal or maladaptive.

DEFENSE MECHANISMS AGAINST CONFLICT AND ANXIETY

Mental mechanism is a generic term for a variety of psychic processes that are functions of the ego and primarily operate unconsciously (i.e., without requiring an initiating act of attention); included are perception, memory, logical thinking, and the *defense mechanisms.* The latter are defined as unconscious psychic processes that attempt to alleviate anxiety and eliminate conflict. Conscious efforts are frequently made for the same reason, but true defense mechanisms operate unconsciously. Following is a subset of defense mechanisms discussed in current references. Some of the mechanisms serve other purposes in addition to defensive ones.

Repression

This is the common denominator and precursor of all other defense mechanisms. It involves the involuntary relegation of unbearable ideas and impulses into the unconscious, whence they are not ordinarily subject to voluntary recall, but may reemerge in disguised form through the operation of other mental mechanisms. Repression may involve keeping out of conscious awareness information or impulses that have never been conscious, or, alternatively, may involve a form of purposeful (although unconsciously mediated) forgetting. Pathological loss of memory (amnesia) may, of course, result from organic brain disease as well as from emotional conflict, but even organic damage to the brain may result in some selective amnesia associated with the repression of painful thoughts or impulses. Repression needs to be distinguished from *suppression*, which is not an unconscious defense, but a conscious effort to control and conceal or postpone dealing with unacceptable impulses, thoughts, feelings, or acts.

Denial

In early psychoanalytic theory this term was used to refer to the denial of intolerable external reality. This mechanism may be likened to the ostrich burying its head in the sand, with the implication that what cannot be perceived does not exist and cannot therefore be painful. For example, a patient dying of cancer may deny his impending death and make elaborate plans for his future; he may even be a physician who has been informed of the nature of his disease and is well aware of the consensus regarding his life expectancy. Similarly, the loss or death of a loved person may be denied, so that the individual believes and acts as though the lost loved one were still present or will soon return. Such convictions and behavior may in extreme cases involve psychotic distortion of reality. In milder degrees there may be excessive preoccupation with inner fantasy, which is at least temporarily more satisfying than the painful external reality.

In modern usage, denial may also describe the disavowal of intolerable thoughts, feelings, or wishes. Neurotic patients frequently deny the reality of sexual or hostile impulses in themselves or others. The hysterical woman may thus act in a seductive and provocative manner without consciously recognizing the implications of her behavior, and may then be surprised and hurt when her boyfriend reacts by making sexual advances. The denial of dysphoric affect may be observed in a patient who becomes euphoric or even manic following the loss of a loved person, or in other circumstances that would normally result in grief.

Reaction Formation

This is a process in which attitudes and behavior are adopted that are the opposites of the impulses to which the individual is reacting. The mother who unconsciously hates an unwanted child may react toward this child by overprotection and overindulgence ("smother love"). The individual with strong unconscious hostility toward other human beings may react against this by extreme concern for the welfare of animals and lead an antivivisection campaign. A person with strongly repressed sexual impulses may deplore the ready availability of salacious literature, and take an active part in a campaign for censorship of reading materials or movies, perhaps even assuming the role of one of the censors, so that he is exposed to the material from which others are to be "protected."

Overcompensation

This term, whose use has sometimes been ascribed to the mechanism of reaction formation, is more often applied to any conscious or unconscious process in which a real or fancied physical or psychological deficit inspires exaggerated correction. Congenital or acquired bodily defects sometimes lead to prodigious efforts to overcome them, a few such handicapped individuals having become world-renowned athletes. Similarly, the stutterer may succeed in becoming a fluent speaker or the shy introvert may strive to become adept in social situations.

Counterphobic Behavior

This is said to occur when the individual deals with fears by approach rather than avoidance, such as the acrophobic person who becomes a sky diver.

Rationalization

Unconscious efforts through which an individual justifies and makes consciously tolerable those feelings, behaviors, and motives that would otherwise be intolerable to him are involved here. Hostile, punitive, and sadistic behavior toward children may be rationalized as having been provoked by them, or as motivated by concern for their welfare ("spare the rod and spoil the child"). The unacceptable tendencies remain repressed and hidden from the individual concerned, although not necessarily from those around him. A special example of this mechanism is the "sour grapes" maneuver, whereby failure becomes less painful through disparagement of the goal. Similarly, the "sweet lemon" maneuver permits the individual to convince himself that an unsatisfactory reality is not only tolerable but even pleasant.

Intellectualization

This is a mechanism closely related to rationalization, referring to the excessive use of intellectual processes and logical arguments as a means of avoiding stressful emotional experiences. The intellectualizer controls his conflicts and impulses by thinking about them, and thereby avoids experiencing the emotions they engender.

Projection

In this defense mechanism emotions, motivation, and behaviors that are viewed as unacceptable, repugnant, or inconsistent with one's personality (ego-alien or ego-dystonic) are not only denied but also attributed to (projected onto) other individuals. While this process may be considered relatively normal in the infant or young child, in adults it is apt to involve profound distortions of reality, resulting in paranoid delusions. In place of an intolerable impulse toward sexual relations with a man other than her husband, a paranoid woman may attribute to her husband the infidelity she rejects in herself. Or she may project onto another man the wish to have sexual relations with her. Similarly, a man with unacceptable latent homosexual feelings toward another man may first deny love while admitting hate, and then project this hate onto the other man who is then perceived as a persecutor.

Identification

In this unconscious process an individual models his behavior and attitudes after those of another person. It is viewed as one of the most important mechanisms involved in personality development, with respect both to psychosexual development and to the development of the superego, or internal control system. This form of identification has also been spoken of as *internalization,* since it involves taking into oneself the instructions, prohibitions, and attitudes of the individual with whom the identification is made. The term *introjection* has also been applied to the symbolic taking into oneself of other individuals, but it has been discarded as inaccurate and unsatisfactory by some analysts. Similarly, the concept of *incorporation* refers mainly to the infant's taking certain attributes of another person into his own body through his mouth, and does not refer to the more mature process of identification described above. The latter is not restricted to personality development, however, and may become a defensive measure when an individual identifies with an aggressor or a powerful enemy.

Displacement of Affect (Emotion)

This is a process whereby a feeling is displaced or redirected from the original object or person onto a more acceptable or less dangerous substitute. It is a mechanism of great importance in daily living, in personality development, in understanding the manifestations of psychiatric disorder, and in the treatment of psychiatric patients. Its daily significance may be observed in the transfer of dangerous hostility, such as may be aroused by an employer or business associates, onto members of the individual's family, opponents in sporting events, minority social groups (scapegoats), or people in foreign countries who are perceived as enemies. (See the quotation at the beginning of this chapter.) The developmental significance involves sexual or hostile feelings toward parents, deeply ingrained through childhood experiences repeated over many years, that are displaced onto others of the same sex as the parent or onto representatives of authority encountered throughout adult life. Examples of displacement in the development of psychiatric symptoms may be seen in the deviation of sexual impulses from forbidden persons of the opposite sex onto various less dangerous substitutes, or in the redirection of fear resulting in the development of phobias. During psychiatric treatment, the unconscious displacement of affect constitutes the basis of *transference,* the patient's irrational feelings and behavior toward his therapist based on earlier interpersonal relationships, and also of *countertransference,* consisting of the therapist's unconscious and illogical emotional reaction toward his patient.

Substitution

Similar to displacement, but involving a more acceptable form of activity than displacing the emotion onto another individual, this mechanism may replace a murderous impulse with a minor aggression or release it in some impersonal destructive act such as chopping wood or striking a punch-ing bag. Such substitutive activity is sometimes considered to have therapeutic as well as dynamic significance.

Sublimation

This is the defense considered most important to society as a whole, since it consists of diverting unacceptable instinctual drives (particularly sexual and aggressive drives) into personally and socially acceptable channels, such as various forms of creative activity. Since the unacceptable drive is permitted expression (satisfying the demands of the id), although in a disguised form (meeting the requirements of the superego), intrapsychic conflict is resolved in a manner ordinarily viewed as healthy, and symptom formation does not occur. This concept should *not* be applied to platonic love, from which the sensual element has been excluded, and which was referred to by Freud as aim-inhibited love.

Turning Feelings Toward Oneself

Sometimes known as *retroflexion,* this is another defense against intolerable impulses such as hostility. In this instance, the consequence is lowered self-esteem, self-accusation, and depression, but there are other forms this defense may take, such as turning sexual feelings back upon the self, resulting in narcissism.

Regression

The actual or symbolic reversion under stress to patterns of behavior and gratification that are more typical of a developmental stage previously successfully completed is called regression. It is implied by the turning inward of sexual feelings and the return to self-love, to which reference has just been made, but it may also involve many other forms of immature behavior. It occurs under a wide variety of circumstances such as during normal sleep, play activities, severe physical illness, and in neurotic or psychotic disorders. Regression under conditions of stress or frustration should be distinguished from *fixation.* The latter is a premature arrest in development generally considered to be due either to excessive frustration or to excessive gratification at some specific stage of development.

Conversion

The mechanism by which unconscious conflicts are given symbolic external expression in the form of various bodily symptoms, such as loss of sensation, loss of movement, or involuntary movements, but which has no underlying organic pathology, is called conversion. It is one of the main mechanisms used in hysterical neuroses, the other being *dissociation,* which involves a psychological separation or splitting off of a mental function or group of functions from the rest of the personality. The latter results in a variety of manifestations such as loss of memory, fugue (loss of memory with physical flight), somnambulism (sleepwalking), and multiple personality.

Isolation

This is a process that is largely restricted to obsessive-compulsive neuroses, in which an unacceptable impulse, idea, or act is separated from its original memory source. The isolated impulse then becomes the basis of compulsive rituals such as touching or repeated washing. These rituals may also constitute forms of *undoing,* whereby an attempt is made to alleviate guilt for unacceptable past behavior by actions of symbolic atonement. Thus, repeated washing of the hands may be a symbolic atonement for various activities (real or imagined) such as masturbation, theft, or murder.

Acting Out

The behavioral expression of unconscious emotional conflicts or feelings of hostility or love in actions not consciously recognized as related to such conflicts or feelings is called acting out. One interpretation of delinquent behavior is that it represents a defense against conscious anxiety through the acting out of such unconscious conflicts or impulses. Sexually promiscuous behavior on the part of a teenager may be unconsciously motivated by hostile feelings toward a parent or other authority figure.

INTERPERSONAL RELATIONSHIPS AND COMMUNICATION

Many orthodox psychoanalysts have disagreed with Freud on certain points of theory, such as the polarity of the life and death instincts. A large number, however, have preferred to differentiate their theories and therapeutic techniques quite clearly from those proposed by Freud, and are referred to as *neo-freudians.* About a dozen such groups are commonly recognized and are distinguished as follows:

Use of active analytic techniques (e.g., Sandor Ferenczi, Wilhelm Stekel, Franz Alexander, and Thomas French)
Use of analytic play therapy (Anna Freud and Melanie Klein)
Analytic psychology (Carl Jung)
Character analysis and orgone therapy (Wilhelm Reich)
Cognitive development (Jean Piaget)
Developmental analysis (Erik Erikson)
Ego psychology (e.g., Paul Federn, Edoardo Weiss, Heinz Hartmann, Ernst Kris, and Rudolph Loewenstein)
Existential analysis (Ludwig Binswanger)
Holistic analysis (Karen Horney)
Individual psychology (Alfred Adler)
Transactional analysis (Eric Berne)
The Washington cultural school (Harry Stack Sullivan, Erich Fromm, et al).

The preceding groups differ from one another, but there has been increasing emphasis on social relationships rather than biological factors, on ego functions rather than id and superego functions, on the striving for self-actualization rather than the sex instinct, and on the present situation as an outcome of early experiences. *Erich Fromm* argued that man is primarily a social being, and pointed out that the rivalry frequently seen between father and son was not found in societies that lacked strong patriarchal authority. He regarded both the Oedipus complex and the neuroses as expressions of a conflict of man's legitimate strivings for freedom, self-fulfillment, happiness, and independence, versus those social arrangements that frustrated these strivings.

Harry Stack Sullivan (1892–1949) defined psychiatry as the study of interpersonal relations, and applied modified analytic techniques to the treatment of young hospitalized schizophrenic patients. His concern with communication processes has had a major impact on American psychiatry, although many others have made significant contributions in this area, and some relevant observations were made before Sullivan's time.

Nonverbal Communications

A former mental hospital superintendent told of a visit he had had many years ago from a member of his board of trustees who wanted to meet "a real live mental patient." Wishing neither to shock his visitor nor to open his administration to criticism, the superintendent selected a hypomanic patient who was recovering and would soon be leaving the hospital. The patient proved to be genial and talkative during the interview, until the guest rose and turned to leave. At that point the patient yelled loudly, leaped on the man's back, wrestled him to the floor, put his hands around the man's throat, and started to squeeze. He was restrained without much difficulty, and the trustee departed hurriedly. The superintendent then took the patient to task for his unexpected violent behavior, and asked him what on earth had prompted these actions. To this the patient calmly replied, "Well, he so obviously *expected* something like that, I hated to disappoint him."

Nonverbal communication may be the language of both love and hate, and this music may contradict the words that it accompanies. Among the important information conveyed nonverbally are *affect* (joy or sorrow, fear or anger) and *role expectation* (how we expect another to act). To attack is to provoke retaliation. To repress is to incite rebellion. To run away is to invite pursuit. To walk around with a chip on one's shoulder is to ask that someone knock it off. To expect the worst of others results in the communication of mistrust and invites rejection that leads to *self-fulfilling prophesies* (behavior that is typical of a paranoid individual).

To act like a doormat is to invite others to wipe their feet. To wear a sign on one's back that says "Don't kick me" might well lead to just that type of consequence. To behave in a flirtatious or seductive manner is to encourage sexual advances, whether they will be consciously recognized and welcomed or rejected (sometimes with surprise, as in the denial that is typical of hysterical patients).

The signals transmitted or received are to some extent specific to the social groups to which the participants originally belonged or are currently members of. The analysis of *transactional sequences* in terms of *ego-states (Parent, Child,* or *Adult)* and frequently observed interactions constituted the basis for Eric Berne's best-seller *Games People Play* (1964). In a subsequent volume, *What Do You Say After You Say Hello?* (1972), Berne elaborated on the therapeutic analysis of *life scripts,* to which we shall refer again in Chapter 6.

REVIEW QUESTIONS

1. A mental mechanism commonly used by well-adjusted adults and tending to produce socially beneficial behavior is:
   (A) intellectualization
   (B) displacement
   (C) identification
   (D) sublimation
   (E) isolation

2. Common to all defense mechanisms and all neurotic symptoms is the phenomenon of:
   (A) repression
   (B) conversion
   (C) displacement
   (D) narcissism
   (E) identification

3. The mental mechanism characteristic of normal ego development is:
   (A) condensation
   (B) regression
   (C) identification
   (D) repression
   (E) projection

4. In Freud's model of normal psychosexual development, object relations:
   (A) are present at birth

    (B) first appear during the oral phase
    (C) first appear during the anal phase
    (D) first appear during latency
    (E) do not appear until adolescence

5. In its final form, Freud's drive theory stated that the two drives that are central to human behavior are the sexual drive and:
    (A) aggression
    (B) self-preservation
    (C) curiosity
    (D) pleasure
    (E) hunger

6. Freud's interpretation of paranoia involved:
    (A) latent homosexuality
    (B) repression
    (C) denial
    (D) projection
    (E) all the above

7. All the following processes are involved in normal superego development *except*:
    (A) internalization
    (B) identification
    (C) incorporation
    (D) introjection
    (E) isolation

8. A physician who believes that cigarette smoking is beneficial because it helps control weight is probably using the mechanism of:
    (A) derealization
    (B) dissociation
    (C) intellectualization
    (D) rationalization
    (E) reaction formation

9. An example of primary process thinking by a mentally healthy adult is:
    (A) logical problem-solving
    (B) reflex action
    (C) intuition
    (D) learning
    (E) nocturnal dreaming

10. In psychoanalytic therapy, the term *abreaction* refers to:
    (A) irrational feelings of the patient toward the therapist
    (B) irrational feelings of the therapist toward the patient

    (C) conscious or unconscious efforts by the patient to avoid recalling repressed material
    (D) temporary worsening of symptoms during the course of therapy
    (E) recalling and reliving of repressed experiences with release of appropriate affect

11. The mental structure that mediates conflicts between unconscious impulses and external reality is the:
    (A) id
    (B) ego
    (C) superego
    (D) ego-ideal
    (E) preconscious

12. A patient undergoing psychoanalytic therapy tends to displace his feelings, attitudes, and wishes from the important life figures with whom they are actually associated onto the therapist. This unconscious process is called:
    (A) projection
    (B) identification
    (C) free association
    (D) transference
    (E) countertransference

13. The much-loved wife of a middle-aged executive was rushed to a hospital emergency room late one evening after complaining of chest pains. Despite rapid delivery by the ambulance and excellent emergency medical care, she died a short while later. Her husband responded to the news by loud expressions of anger and threats of a malpractice lawsuit directed toward the intern in the emergency room. This hostile behavior probably results from the defense mechanism of:
    (A) projection
    (B) undoing
    (C) regression
    (D) over-compensation
    (E) displacement

14. On the following morning, this grieving widower went to his office to take care of vital business. By means of a conscious effort to avoid thinking about his loss, he was able to manage his affairs efficiently and leave a

few hours later. His employees remarked about his apparent lack of emotional display. The man's ability to function as he did can be attributed to his use of:

(A) suppression
(B) sublimation
(C) denial
(D) reaction formation
(E) counterphobic behavior

Summary of Directions

A	B	C	D	E
1, 2, 3 only	1, 3 only	2, 4 only	4 only	All are correct

---

15. Characteristics of the id include:
    (1) locus of inborn instinctual drives
    (2) inability to delay gratification
    (3) disregard for reality
    (4) secondary process thinking
16. Nonverbal communication is:
    (1) usually unconsciously mediated
    (2) learned very early in life
    (3) often related to affects or role expectations
    (4) relatively unimportant to verbally fluent adults
17. Intrapsychic defense mechanisms are:
    (1) functions of the ego
    (2) infrequently used by well-adjusted persons
    (3) intended to resolve conflicts and alleviate painful affect
    (4) sometimes consciously initiated
18. Character traits in adults that are viewed as originating in experiences during the anal phase of development include:
    (1) stubbornness
    (2) excessive neatness
    (3) stinginess
    (4) low frustration tolerance
19. The mechanism of displacement is responsible for:
    (1) transference and countertransference in therapy

(2) paranoid ideation
(3) phobias
(4) compulsive rituals

20. Psychoanalytic theories of psychosis include the following:
    (1) Depressive psychosis represents retroflexed hostility.
    (2) Psychoses are characterized by incapacity for normal emotional interest in other persons and things.
    (3) Mania involves reaction formation against overwhelming depression.
    (4) Conflicts associated with psychotic adaptations occur primarily between the person and his environment.

SELECTED REFERENCES

1. American Psychiatric Association (1975). *A Psychiatric Glossary* (4th Ed.). Washington, D.C.: American Psychiatric Association.
2. American Psychoanalytic Association (1968). *A Glossary of Psychoanalytic Terms and Concepts* (2nd Ed.), edited by B.E. Moore and B.D. Fine. New York: American Psychoanalytic Association.
3. Arieti, S. [Ed.] (1974). *American Handbook of Psychiatry* (2nd Ed.). New York: Basic Books.
4. Freedman, A.M., Kaplan, H.I., and Sadock, B.J. [Eds.] (1975). *Comprehensive Textbook of Psychiatry/II.* Baltimore: Williams & Wilkins Company.
5. Freud, Anna (1937). *The Ego and the Mechanisms of Defense* (reprinted 1946). New York: International Universities Press.
6. Freud, S. (1920). *A General Introduction to Psychoanalysis* (reprinted 1953). New York: Perma Books.
7. Nemiah, J.C. (1973). *Foundations of Psychopathology.* New York: Oxford University Press, Inc.
8. White, R.B., and Gilliland, R.M. (1975). *Elements of Psychopathology: The Mechanisms of Defense.* New York: Grune & Stratton.

2. Description and Classification

"When I use a word," Humpty Dumpty said in rather a scornful tone, *"it means just what I choose it to mean — neither more nor less."*
Lewis Carroll, Through the Looking-Glass

The present chapter is concerned with defining the symptoms of psychiatric disorder, and includes a summary of the most widely accepted classification of psychiatric disorders and syndromes. The latter is based in part on what is currently known concerning their etiology, but very similar manifestations (symptoms or syndromes) may result from different complex interactions between biological, psychological, and sociocultural determinants. The relative contribution of one or another group of factors may vary from individual to individual, and the definition of abnormality itself may be influenced by cultural perspective as well as the observer's judgment of whether the behavior is disproportionate in degree or duration to any recognizable stimulus or provocation.

There is no universal agreement on logical grouping or sequence for defining psychiatric symptoms. We will present them in four major groups, according to their main impact: (1) the *sensorium*, which is generally considered to be synonymous with *consciousness* and includes perception, orientation, and memory; (2) *cognition*, which refers to data analysis, and involves processes such as comprehension, judgment, reasoning, and intelligence; (3) *affect*, or emotional tone and response; and (4) *conation*, concerned with motivation and motor behavior. Although it may be helpful to group mental processes in this manner, they should *not* be viewed as flowing logically and unidirectionally from perception through analysis and affect to action. On the contrary, the many functions are interdependent, and a disorder arising at any point in the network (e.g., affect) may profoundly influence many other functions such as perception, memory, and motor behavior.

DISTURBANCES IN SENSORIUM

Consciousness may be viewed as a continuum in the level of arousal from extreme overstimulation (such as that due to amphetamines or LSD), through normal wakefulness, to the other extreme of coma. *Clearness* or *intactness* of sensorium implies that the person is correctly oriented, has a reasonably accurate memory, and is well aware of the nature of his surroundings. Intermediate states between this condition and sleep or coma may be referred to as *clouded* consciousness. More specific terms include *confusion* (disturbed orientation) and *stupor* (real or apparent lack of awareness of surroundings with failure to respond to stimuli).

Disorientation involves loss of awareness of the self in relation to time, place, or other persons. Precise awareness of time is the aspect of orientation most vulnerable to toxic or other organic intellectual impairment. Disorientation for time tends to precede and last longer than disorientation for place, which in turn tends to precede and last longer than loss of the ability to recognize other persons. In severe brain syndromes, however, patients may be unable to recognize persons with whom they have been living for years.

Memory consists of three essential processes: (1) *registration*, involving the recording of an experience in the brain; (2) *retention*, involving the persistence of a registered experience; and (3) *recall*, involving the ability to recover and consciously recognize a previously retained memory trace. The last is the most essential process in the evaluation of memory.

Amnesia is pathological loss of memory, in which certain experiences are forgotten and become inaccessible to conscious recall. Amnesia may be due to organic brain syndromes or emotional disorders or a combination of both. Memory for recent events is usually most vulnerable in organic brain syndromes (like orientation for time). Loss of memory is apt to be much more circumscribed and selective in the case of hysterical dissociative reactions. Amnesia may be *anterograde* (forward in time) or *retrograde* (backward in time) from a given event of physical or emotional trauma (e.g., head injury or fright).

Paramnesia consists of a distortion of recall that usually involves inclusion of false details or wrong relationships in time or confusion of memory with fantasy. In *retrospective falsification* there is an unconscious distortion of real past experiences to conform to present emotional needs. In *confabulation* there is spontaneous and unconscious fabrication of responses about experiences that cannot be recalled. This term should not be used to describe delusional beliefs or conscious lying. It is generally associated with the Korsakoff triad (amnesia, confabulation, and polyneuritis) but is not infrequent in other organic brain syndromes. A simple test for confabulation is to ask the patient a question like What did you do last night?

Other forms of paramnesia include *déja vu,* a subjective feeling that an experience occurring for the first time has actually happened before, and *déja entendu,* the feeling that a new auditory perception has been experienced before.

Disturbances in perception are often seen in hysterical conversion reactions or in other illnesses such as schizophrenia and organic brain syndromes, which may include hysterical features. Patients with physiologically intact nervous systems may experience partial or complete blindness, deafness, glove or stocking anesthesia, or genital anesthesia associated with frigidity. Various forms of diminished sensitivity to tactile stimuli are referred to as *hypesthesia.* The reverse would be extreme sensitivity to touch or pain, *hyperalgesia.* Other visual misperceptions sometimes found in hysteria include *macropsia,* in which objects appear larger than they really are, and *micropsia,* in which objects appear smaller than they are. Complete failure to perceive a stimulus is sometimes called a *negative hallucination.*

Illusions are misinterpretations of real external sensory experiences. They may involve any of the senses and are therefore referred to as visual, auditory, olfactory, gustatory, or tactile (the latter sometimes being known as *haptic*).

Hallucinations are false sensory perceptions in the absence of any external stimulus. Like illu-sions, they may affect any of the senses, and occur in both organic brain syndromes and functional psychoses. However, auditory hallucinations are most typical of the schizophrenias, whereas visual and haptic (tactile) hallucinations are more characteristic of acute (reversible) organic brain syndromes, including those caused by such psychotomimetic drugs as LSD and mescaline. Haptic hallucinations include *formication* (the feeling that insects are crawling in or on the skin), which is most typical of alcoholic delirium tremens, cocainism, or amphetamine psychosis. Hallucinations of smell and taste may occur in convulsive disorders (uncinate fits). *Hypnagogic* hallucinations occur in the semiconscious state immediately preceding sleep, and are usually of no pathological significance. A psychotic state in which hallucinations are experienced by a person having a clear sensorium is called *hallucinosis.*

DISTURBANCES IN THINKING AND INTELLIGENCE

Form of Thinking

The form that thinking takes may be concrete or abstract; logical or dereistic; autistic or overinclusive. *Concrete,* or *literal, thinking* predominates in normal early childhood, in the mentally retarded, and in some patients with organic brain syndromes or with schizophrenia. *Abstract thinking* is a prevailing mode for healthy, intelligent adults. The term *dereistic* emphasizes the unrealistic and illogical quality of associations typical in schizophrenics, while the term *autistic* emphasizes the process of inner fantasy within the self; however, the two terms are often used interchangeably. *Overinclusive thinking* implies an inability to exclude irrelevant, extraneous material from the associations and response.

The difference between these forms of thinking may be illustrated by the responses of persons asked to interpret simple proverbs. When one asks what is usually meant by the saying "A stitch in time saves nine," the following concrete, or literal, response might be obtained: "If you had a tear in your clothing, and sewed it up right away, you'd be saving time." Two autistic responses given by schizophrenic patients to the same question are as follows: "If I would take a stitch ahead of time, I would know nine times better how to do another stitch"; and from another patient, "I could do something and it would help everyone else." An overinclusive response to the same brief question may consist of half a dozen sentences of varying degrees of irrelevancy.

Stream of Thought

Thinking expressed through *speech* may show various forms of associative abnormality. *Emotional blocking* results in interruption of the train of thought or speech. Severe blocking may result in complete *mutism,* which is found in retarded, depressive, or schizophrenic psychoses. (Voluntary refusal to talk, usually for emotional reasons, is called elective mutism.)

The opposite state of affairs consists of *logorrhea* (excessive normal speech) or *pressured speech* that has a compulsive quality and is difficult to interrupt. Impairment in the goal-directedness of thought and speech is termed *circumstantiality* or *tangentiality*; the former implies frequent irrelevancies and digressions but eventual reaching of the desired goal, while the latter implies that the goal is never reached. *Flight of ideas* is an almost continuous high-speed flow of speech that becomes increasingly fragmented or illogical as it becomes more rapid. This is most typical of acute manic states, in which tangential associations may give way to rhyming, punning, and *clang associations,* in which new directions for thought and speech originate in the sounds of words rather than their meanings.

Neologisms are idiosyncratic words not readily understood by the listener and usually formed by the condensation of two or more concepts, as in the poem "Jabberwocky" by Lewis Carroll. (" 'Twas brillig, and the slithy toves did gyre and gimble in the wabe: All mimsy were the borogroves, and the mome raths outgrabe. . .") In the absence of some humorous or other logical intent, neologisms are strongly suggestive of schizophrenia and secondarily of organic brain disorders.

Verbigeration consists of the stereotyped meaningless repetition of words or sentences, and is also most often seen in schizophrenia. The same is true of *word salad,* which is a jumble of neologisms or incoherent syllables, words, and phrases that lack any logical meaning or sequence.

Perseveration is the morbid, stereotyped repetition of the same response (verbal or nonverbal) to several unrelated questions or stimuli. It is most typical of organic brain syndromes. *Aphasia* is a more general term for all disturbances of language and communication due to organic brain syndromes. In *motor* (or *expressive*) *aphasia,* comprehension remains intact but speech is lost. In *sensory* (or *receptive*) aphasia, comprehension is also lost.

Content of Thought

This may be distorted in a variety of ways, some of which occur within normal limits in well-adjusted persons of all ages. The most common of these phenomena is *fantasy,* an imagined sequence of events or mental images that are recognized as unreal but are either expected or hoped for. Fantasy can serve the creative purpose of planning future action, and is also used as a refuge for unfulfilled wishes (daydreaming). The latter aspect of fantasy becomes pathological when it occupies a major portion of the person's mental behavior so as to impair his capacity for normal relationships and behavior, as in the autism that is characteristic of schizophrenia.

An *obsession* is a persistent and unwanted idea or impulse that cannot be eliminated by logic or reasoning. Obsessions are usually associated with *compulsions,* which are repetitive, unwanted urges to perform specific stereotyped acts. Usually these acts serve to alleviate the anxiety caused by the obsessions but are contrary to the person's usual wishes or standards. These symptoms may be associated with *magical thinking,* involving an unrealistic belief that certain thoughts, words, or actions can lead to the fulfillment of wishes or the warding off of evil consequences. While this form of thinking may occur as a normal phenomenon in children, in members of primitive cultures, or in obsessive-compulsive neurotic patients, it may also reach delusional intensity in schizophrenic patients.

Phobias are obsessive and unrealistic but intense fears of specific external objects or situations. According to psychoanalytic theory, the phobia arises through displacement of fear originating in internal (unconscious) conflict onto an external object symbolically related to the conflict. A large number of specific names for different varieties of phobia have been derived from Greek roots (e.g., acrophobia, a fear of heights; agoraphobia, a fear of open spaces; and claustrophobia, a fear of closed spaces), but these terms are much less commonly used now than formerly. The term *phobia* should be reserved for specific, focused, unrealistic fears and not used as a synonym for all kinds of fear.

DELUSIONS. Delusions are the most extreme deviation in thought content, and are pathognomonic of psychosis. They are defined as fixed, false beliefs that are maintained despite objective evidence and logical argument to the contrary. Furthermore, the belief is not one ordinarily shared by others who have similar educational and sociocultural backgrounds (e.g., common superstitions and political or religious convictions). Delusions may be associated with disturbances of perception (illusions and hallucinations), impairment of memory, or disturbances of affect. The main varieties of delusion are as follows:

Delusions of reference involve the incorrect belief that coincidental or unrelated events (usually the innocent remarks or behavior of other people) have particular reference, meaning, or application to the individual concerned.

Delusions of control or influence are unrealistic beliefs about magical ("telepathic") communication and control of a person's thoughts or behavior by another. In delusions of *active* control the patient has the grandiose notion that he can control other people or objects in this manner; in delusions of *passive* control he believes his own thoughts and behavior are attributable to an external agent.

Delusions of persecution are false beliefs that others are hostile and single one out for unwel-

come attention or persecution. Delusions of reference, control, and persecution involve the mental mechanisms of denial and projection, and are prominent manifestations of paranoid psychoses.

Delusions of grandeur consist of unrealistic beliefs in one's importance, identity, wealth, fame, power, or knowledge. They are characteristic of manic psychoses (with a mood of euphoria or exaltation), but are also relatively malignant symptoms of various paranoid psychoses, including schizophrenia and those psychoses associated with organic brain syndromes.

Delusions of guilt, self-accusation, worthlessness, hopelessness, or *poverty* are characteristic of patients with depressive psychoses.

Somatic delusions are any fixed, false beliefs concerning the structure or function of one's own body, and are commonly associated with depressive or schizophrenic psychoses. *Nihilistic delusions* are a special variety of somatic delusion in which the patient believes that a part or all of himself is nonexistent. They are considered most typical of severe involutional melancholia.

Disturbances of Intellectual Functions

Intelligence has been defined as the capacity to learn and to utilize appropriately what one has learned. This definition is deceptively simple, since learning also implies comprehension, memory, integration, and mobilization of information to solve new problems. Nevertheless, considerable progress has been made in studying the development and measurement of various intellectual functions. These functions increase progressively during childhood and adolescence up to the age of about sixteen years, by which time maximum intellectual function for the individual has been attained. IQ and other concepts related to the measurement of intelligence are discussed in Chapter 4.

The *intellectual capacity* of a person may be regarded as his theoretical maximum potential, determined at the time of conception and attainable only under optimal circumstances. His *intellectual function* at any given time is what is measured by intelligence tests, and usually shows considerable stability throughout life, except when impaired by various forms of psychiatric disorder. When the intellectual function is consistently much lower than the average for persons of his age group (from early childhood onward), there is *mental retardation* (also known at various times as *mental deficiency, intellectual subnormality, amentia,* or *oligophrenia).* These terms are all associated with diminished potential for understanding, learning, remembering, and problem-solving.

Intellectual impairment consists of a reduction in various intellectual abilities commencing at any time after birth, and sometimes not until old age. Such impairment of intellectual function may result from a wide variety of acute (reversible) or chronic (irreversible) brain disorders or, alternatively, from psychoses such as schizophrenia or severe depression.

DISTURBANCES IN AFFECT

Affect is defined as emotional feeling tone, and is usually regarded as synonymous with *emotion.* In the newborn infant emotional responses are undifferentiated, but the excitement resulting from strong stimulation is soon distinguishable as either *distress* or *delight.* The latter constitutes the basis for one of the *four primary emotions* (i.e., joy), whereas distress becomes differentiated into the remaining three primary *dysphoric* emotions (anger, sorrow, and fear).

Normal Joy
Normal joy results from gratification through the approach and attainment of a desired goal. In *euphoria* there is an exaggerated feeling of well-being, with diminished perception of physical pain and diminished control by the superego, so that there may be impulsive and reckless behavior, with disregard of future consequences. The elevated mood is out of proportion to any objective evidence of goal attainment, and may even sometimes represent a paradoxical reaction (reaction formation) to circumstances that would normally provoke sorrow (e.g., loss of health or bereavement). *Elation* is usually regarded as a second level in the

scale of pleasurable affects, exceeded by *exaltation* or *ecstasy.* However, any elevation of mood may also be accompanied by *lability* of affect, which involves erratic and unpredictable variations in mood, with temporary episodes of misery, anger, or violence.

Normal Anger
Normal anger is the usual outcome of frustration, with blocking of goal attainment. Three general categories of frustration have been distinguished: (1) *environmental* frustration, due to external obstacles, such as those imposed by parents during early childhood; (2) *personal* frustration, due to inability to attain desired goals because they are beyond the reach of the individual's abilities, as is often the case with educational and occupational strivings of adolescence and early adult life; and (3) *conflict* between motives, one of which cannot be satisfied without frustrating another. The latter in turn may be divided into three major categories: (1) *approach-approach* conflict (two equally attractive goals); (2) *avoidance-avoidance* conflict (two painful consequences resulting in immobilization and withdrawal); and (3) *approach-avoidance* conflict, in which the individual is simultaneously attracted and repelled by the same goal, since this goal involves both reward and punishment. The approach-avoidance conflict may be the most difficult to resolve, and may result in marked vacillation, since the avoidance gradient may be steeper than the approach gradient, with fear becoming predominant as the individual gets closer to the source of conflict.

Mild frustration may be an important stimulus to problem-solving, and normal personality development implies learning to tolerate a reasonable amount of frustration. However, excessive frustration may have adverse consequences, such as feelings of helplessness, impotent rage, depression, regressive behavior, or fixation in development.

Normal Sorrow or Grief
The loss of a loved object (e.g., a person, property, health, or self-esteem) or feelings of futility and helplessness associated with overwhelming frustra-

tion are implied in defining normal sorrow or grief.

In *pathological depression* there is morbid sadness, dejection, and misery, together with an exaggerated perception of physical pain and of conscience with inappropriate feelings of guilt and remorse. Persons vulnerable to depression often react with impotent and retroflexed rage under conditions of frustration that would lead others to respond with externally directed anger and aggression or retaliation.

Fear

Fear involves the perception of impending danger or disaster, with consequent motivation toward avoidance and escape. Fear is focused on a consciously recognized external threat or danger, although in *phobias* the fear is irrational and focused on some object other than the original source (through displacement). In *anxiety,* however, there is apprehension, tension, or uneasiness associated with the anticipation of danger or future disaster, the nature of which is still largely unrecognized (i.e., vague, nonspecific, objectless, or "free-floating"). In patients, anxiety often appears to represent fear of impulses, emotions, and behaviors that are socially unacceptable and consciously intolerable to the patient, such as sexual and aggressive impulses. *Panic* is a state of acute overwhelming anxiety accompanied by disorganization of personality and functioning.

Ambivalence refers to the coexistence of two opposing emotions toward the same object (person or goal), either or both of which may remain largely unconscious, e.g., coexisting love and hate toward the same person.

In addition to the preceding manifestations of prevailing mood or emotional tone, there may be increased or decreased *variability of emotional reaction or response.* This excessive variability of affect, often associated with prevailing euphoria or neurotic anxiety, is termed *lability.* In psychotic depression, by contrast, there is usually diminished variation in emotional response, as is also true in *apathy* (in which mood is neither elevated nor depressed but shallow or flattened). Apathy may be observed in some patients with organic

brain syndromes or chronic schizophrenia, where it tends to be associated with a relatively poor prognosis.

An *inappropriate* emotional response consists of a display of affect that is qualitatively different from the response that would be experienced by most people under similar circumstances, e.g., hysterical laughter in a context in which grief or anger would be more appropriate. An inappropriate response represents one form of incongruity between ideation, emotion, and behavior that is most characteristic of schizophrenic patients.

DISTURBANCES IN MOTOR BEHAVIOR

Motor behavior may be disturbed in various subtle ways among persons with personality disorders or neuroses. In some the behavior may be socially unacceptable, while in others it may inconvenience the patient more than other persons around him. Thus the person with a *compulsion* must repeatedly carry out some stereotyped act or ritual (such as continually washing his hands) that is frequently related to a recurrent obsessional thought or phobia, the compulsive behavior representing a symbolic form of undoing or atonement and serving to alleviate the anxiety associated with the obsession.

Apart from such disturbances of behavior in otherwise well-integrated persons, there are various forms of regressive or grossly abnormal behavior that are associated with severe disorders of cognition and affect. There may be generalized *retardation of movement,* sometimes amounting to stupor; or extreme motor restlessness, agitation, or excitement. Either may occur in organic brain syndromes, in schizophrenias, or in major affective psychoses.

The term *cataplexy* refers to a sudden transient attack of muscle weakness and loss of tonus; it is often associated with narcolepsy (see Chap. 7). By contrast, *catalepsy* refers to an increase in tonus with rigidity of posture, and may be associated with severe hysterical or schizophrenic states or organic brain syndromes. Catalepsy is sometimes seen in the form of *waxy flexibility (cerea flexibilitas)* in which the patient will, with resistance, allow his limbs to be moved, and then maintain them in whatever position they are placed, regardless of awkwardness or discomfort. This rather dramatic symptom is most commonly associated with the catatonic stupor of schizophrenia.

Automatisms are mechanical, repetitive, apparently undirected behaviors that may occur in fugue states (hysterical or epileptic) or in schizophrenias. Various other forms of unusual behavior usually associated with a diagnosis of schizophrenia include prolonged *posturing,* stereotyped repetitions of certain movements (e.g., facial grimaces or bodily mannerisms), *negativism* (doing the opposite of what is requested), or *echopraxia* (imitating the movements of another person). The latter is similar to *echolalia,* which involves immediate repetition of another's words or phrases (usually encountered in schizophrenia or organic brain syndrome).

Having reviewed the major symptoms found in various psychiatric disorders, we shall now present a summary of the diagnostic nomenclature accepted by the American Psychiatric Association. This is compatible with the *International Classification of Diseases* approved by the World Health Organization. The Arabic numerals in the following section represent the first three digits of the four- or five-digit diagnostic code.

SUMMARY OF PSYCHIATRIC NOMEN-CLATURE ADAPTED FROM DIAGNOSTIC AND STATISTICAL MANUAL OF MENTAL DISORDERS, 2ND EDITION, AMERICAN PSYCHIATRIC ASSOCIATION, 1968

I. Mental Retardation (310–315)

Subnormal general intellectual functioning, originating during the developmental period, and associated with impairment of either learning and social adjustment, or maturation, or both. Classified according to degrees of retardation (ranges of intelligence quotient, each corresponding with one standard deviation of the normal distribution curve of intelligence).

310. **Borderline:** IQ 68 to 83 (1 to 2 standard deviations below mean).

311. **Mild:** IQ 52 to 67 (2 to 3 s.d. below mean).
312. **Moderate:** IQ 36 to 51 (3 to 4 s.d. below mean).
313. **Severe:** IQ 20 to 35 (4 to 5 s.d. below mean).
314. **Profound:** IQ under 20 (more than 5 s.d. below mean).
315. **Unspecified:** IQ not determined.

Each of the preceding degrees of retardation is subclassified as following or associated with: infection or intoxication; trauma or physical agent; disorders of metabolism, growth, or nutrition; gross brain disease (postnatal); unknown prenatal influence; chromosomal abnormality; prematurity; major psychiatric disorder; psychosocial (environmental) deprivation; or other condition.

II. Organic Brain Syndromes (290–294 and 309)

Disorders caused by or associated with impairment of brain tissue function. Impairment may affect all intellectual functions, memory, orientation, and judgment, and be accompanied by lability and shallowness of affect. May be *acute* and temporary, due to *reversible* changes in brain cell functions; or *chronic* and permanent, with *irreversible* damage to brain structure or metabolism.

290. **Senile and presenile dementias**
E.g., Alzheimer's disease and Pick's disease

291. **Alcoholic psychoses**
Delirium tremens, Korsakoff's psychosis, other alcoholic hallucinosis, alcoholic paranoid state, etc.

292. **Psychosis associated with intracranial infection**
General paralysis; syphilis of the CNS; epidemic encephalitis; etc.

293. **Psychosis associated with other cerebral condition**
Cerebral arteriosclerosis, other cerebrovascular disturbance, epilepsy, intracranial neoplasm (tumor), degenerative disease of the CNS, brain trauma (head injury), etc.

294. **Psychosis associated with other physical condition**
Endocrine disorder, metabolic or nutritional disorder, systemic infection, drug or poison intoxication (other than alcohol), childbirth, etc.

III. Psychoses Not Attributed to Physical Conditions Listed Previously (295–298)

Mental functioning is sufficiently impaired to interfere grossly with the individual's capacity to meet the ordinary demands of life appropriate to attained developmental level. The impairment may involve marked distortion of socially accepted interpretations of reality. Frequently accompanied by severe distortions of perception, intellectual functioning, affect, motivation, and behavior, and by personality decompensation and regression. Patients usually lack insight into the nature and severity of the disturbance, and formerly admission to a hospital was accomplished by involuntary commitment.

295. **Schizophrenia (formerly known as dementia praecox)**
A group of psychotic disorders manifested by characteristic disturbances of thinking, mood, and behavior. Mental status is attributable primarily to a thought disorder, frequently associated with misinterpretations of reality and sometimes with delusions and hallucinations.

Simple type – apathy, lack of initiative, and social withdrawal, but without conspicuous hallucinations, delusions, or intellectual impairment.

Hebephrenic type – shallow and inappropriate affect with hallucinations, delusions, mannerisms, and silly and regressive behavior.

Catatonic type – marked disturbance in motor behavior, with either excessive activity and excitement (excited subtype) or alternatively with generalized inhibition, withdrawal, and stupor (withdrawn subtype), or both.

Paranoid type – poorly systematized delusions, usually accompanied by hallucinations and hostility, and sometimes by aggressive behavior.

Acute schizophrenic episode – sudden onset of schizophrenic symptoms that may resolve rapidly or may develop into another definable type.

Latent type – disorders sometimes designated as incipient, prepsychotic, pseudoneurotic, pseudopsychopathic, or borderline schizophrenia.

Residual type – signs of schizophrenia in a patient who was formerly but is no longer psychotic.

Schizo-affective type – mixture of schizophrenic symptoms with pronounced elation or depression.

Childhood type – schizophrenic symptoms appearing before puberty.

Chronic undifferentiated type – schizophrenic symptoms of prolonged duration, not predominantly those of any other type.

296. **Major affective disorders (affective psychoses)**
A group of psychoses characterized by a single disorder of mood, either extreme depression or elation, that dominates the mental life of a patient.

Involutional melancholia – severe depression during the involutional period, with no history of previous psychosis, and not attributable to some life experience.

Manic-depressive illness – severe mood swings with a tendency to remission and recurrence.

Manic type – consists exclusively of manic episodes.
Depressed type – consists exclusively of depressive episodes.

Circular type — patient has had at least one depressive episode and at least one manic episode.

297. Paranoid states
Psychotic disorders in which a delusion, generally persecutory or grandiose, is the essential abnormality.

Paranoia — logical elaboration of a single delusion (monomania).

Involutional paranoid state (involutional paraphrenia) — delusion formation with onset in the involutional period.

Other paranoid state — intermediate between paranoid schizophrenia and true paranoia.

298. Other psychoses
Psychotic depressive reaction (reactive depressive psychosis). Severe depression attributable to some life experience.

IV. Neuroses (300)
300.
The chief characteristic is anxiety that may be consciously experienced or unconsciously controlled by means of various psychological defense mechanisms. There is no gross distortion of reality testing nor disorganization of personality. Such persons usually seek help voluntarily as outpatients.

Anxiety neurosis — diffuse, or "free-floating," anxiety and apprehension, often accompanied by overactivity of sympathetic nervous system, in the absence of realistically dangerous situations.

Hysterical neurosis — involuntary psychogenic loss or disorder of function.

Conversion type — loss of sensory or voluntary motor function (i.e., anesthesia or paralysis) or, alternatively, sensory hyperacuity or motor hyperactivity (tic, tremor, or epilepticlike seizures). Autonomic function is not impaired.

Dissociative type — alterations in consciousness or identity, such as amnesia, fugue, sleep-walking, or multiple personality.

Phobic neurosis — intense fear of an object or situation that the patient consciously recognizes to be no real danger to him.

Obsessive-compulsive neurosis — persistent, unwanted obsessional thoughts and/or compulsions to perform repetitive actions.

Depressive neurosis — an excessive reaction of depression due to internal conflict or an identifiable event such as loss of a love object.

Neurasthenic neurosis — chronic weakness, easy fatigability, and sometimes exhaustion.

Depersonalization neurosis — feelings of unreality and of estrangement from the self, body, or surroundings.

Hypochondriacal neurosis — preoccupation with the body and with fear of presumed diseases of various organs.

V. Personality Disorders and Certain Other Non-Psychotic Mental Disorders (301–304)
301. Personality disorders
— characterized by deeply ingrained maladaptive patterns of behavior that are perceptibly different in quality from psychotic and neurotic symptoms. The patterns are usually life-long and are often recognizable by the time of adolescence: Paranoid personality, cyclothymic (affective) personality, schizoid personality, explosive (epileptoid) personality, obsessive-compulsive (anankastic) personality, hysterical (histrionic) personality, asthenic personality, antisocial (psychopathic or sociopathic) personality, passive-aggressive personality, inadequate personality.

302. Sexual deviations
— sexual interests directed primarily toward objects other than people of the opposite sex, toward sexual acts not

usually associated with coitus, or toward coitus performed under bizarre circumstances: fetishism, pedophilia, transvestism, exhibitionism, voyeurism, sadism, masochism, etc.

303. **Alcoholism** — alcohol intake sufficient to damage physical health or personal or social functioning, or necessary for normal functioning: episodic excessive drinking, habitual excessive drinking, alcohol addiction.

304. **Drug dependence** — addiction to or dependency on drugs other than alcohol, tobacco, and caffeine-containing beverages: opium, opium alkaloids, and their derivatives, synthetic analgesics with morphinelike effects, barbiturates, other hypnotics and sedatives or "tranquilizers," cocaine, *Cannabis sativa* (hashish or marihuana), other psychostimulants (amphetamines, etc.), hallucinogens, etc.

VI. Psychophysiological Disorders (305)

305. A group of disorders characterized by physical symptoms that are caused by emotional factors and involve a single organ system, usually under autonomic nervous system innervation. Physiological changes are those that normally accompany certain states, but the changes are more intense and sustained.

Skin disorder — e.g., neurodermatosis, pruritus, atopic dermatitis, and hyperhydrosis.

Musculoskeletal disorder — e.g., backache, muscle cramps, and tension headaches.

Respiratory disorder — e.g., asthma, hyperventilation syndromes, etc., in which emotional factors play a causative role.

Cardiovascular disorder — e.g., paroxysmal tachycardia, hypertension, and migraine, in which emotional factors play a causative role.

Gastrointestinal disorder — e.g., pylorospasm, peptic ulcer, ulcerative or mucous colitis, constipation, etc., in which emotional factors play a causative role.

Genitourinary disorder — e.g., disturbance in menstruation or micturition, dyspareunia, and impotence.

Endocrine disorder — e.g., hyperthyroidism.

Disorder of organ of special sense — e.g., disorder of the eye or ear in which emotional factors play a causative role. Conversion reactions are excluded.

VII. Special Symptoms (306)

306. A category for the occasional patient whose psychopathology is manifested by a single specific symptom: speech disturbance, specific learning disturbance, tic, other psychomotor disorder, disorder of sleep, feeding disturbance, enuresis, encopresis, cephalalgia, etc.

VIII. Transient Situational Disturbances (307)

307. More or less transient disorders of any severity, occurring in individuals without any apparent underlying mental disorders, and representing an acute reaction to overwhelming environmental stress:

Adjustment reaction of infancy — e.g., grief due to separation from mother.

Adjustment reaction of childhood — e.g., jealousy due to birth of a younger sibling.

Adjustment reaction of adolescence — e.g., irritability and depression due to school failure.

Adjustment reaction of adult life — e.g., reaction to unwanted pregnancy, military combat, prison sentence.

Adjustment reaction of late life — e.g., reaction to forced retirement.

IX. Behavior Disorders of Childhood and Adolescence (308)

308. Disorders occurring in childhood and adolescence that are more stable, internalized, and resistant to treatment than transient situa-

tional disturbances, but less so than psychoses, neuroses, and personality disorders: hyperkinetic reaction, withdrawing reaction, overanxious reaction, runaway reaction, unsocialized aggressive reaction, group delinquent reaction, etc.

X. Conditions without Manifest Psychiatric Disorder and Nonspecific Conditions (316–318)

316. **Social maladjustments** without manifest psychiatric disorder: e.g., marital maladjustment, social maladjustment, occupational maladjustment, dyssocial behavior.

317. **Nonspecific conditions**

318. **No mental disorder**

XI. Nondiagnostic Terms for Administrative Use (319)

319. Diagnosis deferred, boarder, experiment only, etc.

REVIEW QUESTIONS

21. An elderly and slightly confused man was brought by his son for a physical examination. At the beginning of the examination, the patient complained of "bowel trouble." He then continued to repeat the same words about "bowel trouble" in response to all subsequent questions or requests by the physician. This is an example of:
    (A) echolalia
    (B) coprolalia
    (C) coprophilia
    (D) perseveration
    (E) fixation

22. An 8-year-old child, confined to bed with a fever, became first excited and then upset on seeing his bedroom curtains moving slightly in a draft. He told his mother that he thought he had seen his father (who was currently on a business trip many miles away). This situation most likely represents:
    (A) an illusion
    (B) a hallucination
    (C) a delusion

(D) *fausse reconnaissance*
(E) agnosia

23. A 30-year-old man consulted his family physician for help after experiencing impotence during several recent attempts to have intercourse with his wife. He appeared to be extremely anxious, and he told the physician that the problem was urgent, since strangers who passed him on the street had begun smiling at him. He was sure that their smiles were meant to mock him because of his impotence. This patient's misinterpretations of the innocent actions of strangers is best described as:
    (A) an illusion
    (B) a delusion of reference
    (C) projection
    (D) a fantasy
    (E) xenophobia

24. A 55-year-old male patient was referred by his cardiologist for psychiatric evaluation. The patient said that his cardiac pacemaker, which he had had for years, was now controlling his thoughts and actions. He was quite fearful, and expressed the belief that refusal to act as the pacemaker directed would result in the pacemaker causing his heart to stop beating. He insisted that the pacemaker be removed at once despite the cardiologist's strong advice to the contrary. This patient's irrational belief about his pacemaker is best called:
    (A) hypochondriasis
    (B) a phobia
    (C) a delusion of influence
    (D) an obsession
    (E) a preoccupation

25. An amphetamine addict began picking at his skin with needles in an attempt to remove "small worms crawling under my skin and itching like the devil." The patient was experiencing:
    (A) akathisia
    (B) hypochondriasis
    (C) micropsia
    (D) somatic delusions
    (E) formication

26. A mental phenomenon characterized by a feeling of unreality and strangeness about oneself is called:
    (A) free-floating anxiety
    (B) depersonalization
    (C) fugue
    (D) agnosia
    (E) clouding of consciousness

27. *La belle indifférence* is an emotional state typically associated with:
    (A) antisocial personality disorder
    (B) hysterical neurosis
    (C) chronic schizophrenia
    (D) organic brain syndromes
    (E) mental retardation

28. *Anaclitic depression* refers to a type of affective disturbance that occurs during:
    (A) infancy
    (B) psychoanalysis
    (C) terminal illness
    (D) middle age
    (E) organic brain syndromes

29. Rapid succession of thoughts without logical connection is called:
    (A) pressure of speech
    (B) flight of ideas
    (C) logorrhea
    (D) word salad
    (E) bulimia

30. Functional amnesia is usually due to:
    (A) dissociation
    (B) minor head trauma
    (C) Korsakoff's psychosis
    (D) sleep deprivation
    (E) schizophrenia

31. According to the American Psychiatric Association's *Diagnostic and Statistical Manual of Mental Disorders,* second edition (DSM-II), the major classification of diagnoses of mental retardation is based on:
    (A) time of onset
    (B) etiology
    (C) pathological findings
    (D) nature of symptoms
    (E) estimated IQ

32. Delusions are *least* likely to be found in:
    (A) organic brain syndromes
    (B) psychotic depression
    (C) acute mania
    (D) paranoid personality disorder
    (E) hebephrenic schizophrenia

33. The best definition of *blocking* is:
    (A) inability to follow simple logical ideas
    (B) rejection of the ideas of others
    (C) sudden interruption in the sequence of thought
    (D) amnesia involving selected affectively charged experiences
    (E) sudden illogical change in the sequence of thought

34. When asked his wife's name, a manic patient replied: "My wife is Heather, tough as leather but light as a feather. Isn't this great weather we're having, doc? . . . " This quotation contains an example of:
    (A) word salad
    (B) neologisms
    (C) perseveration
    (D) echolalia
    (E) clang associations

35. The types of delusions *least* likely to be seen in a depressive psychosis are:
    (A) delusions of poverty
    (B) delusions of guilt
    (C) somatic delusions
    (D) nihilistic delusions
    (E) delusions of reference

Summary of Directions

A	B	C	D	E
1, 2, 3 only	1, 3 only	2, 4 only	4 only	All are correct

---

36. Disturbances of affect include:
    (1) panic
    (2) apathy
    (3) phobias
    (4) obsessions

37. Terms that are roughly synonymous with

"mental retardation" include:
(1) amentia
(2) dementia praecox
(3) oligophrenia
(4) dementia
38. Magical thinking is frequent in schizophrenia and in:
(1) anxiety neurosis
(2) obsessive-compulsive neurosis
(3) hysterical neurosis
(4) normal preschool childhood

SELECTED REFERENCES

1. American Psychiatric Association (1968). *DSM-II: Diagnostic and Statistical Manual of Mental Disorders* (2nd ed.). Washington, D.C.: American Psychiatric Association.
2. American Psychiatric Association (1975). *A Psychiatric Glossary* (4th ed.). Washington, D.C.: American Psychiatric Association.
3. Hamilton, M. [Ed.] (1974). *Fish's Clinical Psychopathology: Signs and Symptoms in Psychiatry.* Bristol: John Wright and Sons, Ltd.

3. Psychiatric Evaluation

A friend is a person with whom I may be sincere.
Before him, I may think aloud.
Ralph Waldo Emerson

THE INITIAL PSYCHIATRIC INTERVIEW

There are varying attitudes toward what should be accomplished in an initial psychiatric interview. In some situations the emphasis has been on standardized questioning and recording of a combined mental examination and psychiatric history for purposes of diagnostic evaluation. In other situations *the first psychiatric interview is correctly viewed as the first therapeutic interview,* which requires a much greater degree of flexibility on the part of the interviewer. The latter approach is more consistent with the perceived needs of the patient, and is increasingly favored by those responsible for teaching psychiatric evaluation. We shall therefore emphasize certain aspects of the interpersonal relationship before proceeding to the standardized recording of any information that may be obtained. The physician must be particularly aware of the nonverbal communications (of affect and role expectation) by himself toward the patient, as well as by the patient toward the physician.

The patient may approach this new situation with fear or mistrust, and with expectations that he will be criticized, ignored, deceived, or rejected. It is up to the physician to convey to the patient an attitude of respect and warm acceptance, on which a relationship of trust may be developed. This may be easier for the physician if he recognizes that such negative feelings as the patient may have toward him are largely the result of *transference* (displacement) resulting from the patient's previous experiences and relationships with parents and others in authority. The patient may also view the physician as in league with hostile relatives or others who have lowered his self-esteem by suggesting or arranging the interview. The patient's first impression of the physician may either confirm his fears or lead to their

modification and eventual abandonment. The interviewer must therefore show interest, understanding, and acceptance of the patient and his feelings — although not necessarily approval of his behavior. The patient should be interviewed alone, in quiet and comfortable surroundings. The interview should be for an adequate period of time, usually forty-five or fifty minutes, and should be uninterrupted, as for example by telephone calls, or by the physician referring to his watch.

Effective interviewing involves catalysing and maximizing the patient's ability to communicate both verbally and nonverbally. Complete lack of structure in the interview situation and uncertainty about what is required of him may provoke excessive anxiety in the patient. Long periods of silence should be avoided. On the other hand, the physician should not block the patient's communications about significant problems by too-frequent questions that turn the interview into an interrogation.

Initially, the physician should encourage the patient to tell his own story as freely as possible and should listen without interrupting. It may be desirable to stimulate the patient by asking such questions as What led to your coming to see me? or, Whose idea was it that you should come here? followed by Why do you think he felt it would be a good idea? When the patient stops spontaneously, he can often be encouraged to proceed or elaborate if the interviewer nods, changes position (e.g., leans forward in his chair), or offers minimal verbal cues, such as "yes," or "and then . . . ," or "go on . . . ," or repetition of the last few words in the patient's narrative. When the time comes for the physician to ask questions, they should be as general as possible — for example, How did you feel about that? or, How do you feel most of the time? rather than specific questions that may be answered briefly. Questions that can simply be answered yes or no should be avoided initially, as should all leading questions suggesting a definite answer — for example, Do you feel unhappy?

Certain kinds of information may be required that, if sought by direct questioning early in the interview, might make the patient feel threatened.

It is necessary for the physician to establish whether there is any danger of suicidal or homicidal behavior and to form some estimate of such matters as intelligence, evidence of organic brain disease, the presence of hallucinations or delusional beliefs, sexual behavior, and relationships with various members of the family. It is frequently possible to obtain some of this information without direct questioning by simply encouraging the patient to elaborate on some of his spontaneous statements.

It may be appropriate to ask direct questions about factual information (such as his age at the time his father died), but there are certain techniques that may be helpful when dealing with more sensitive information: (1) *Narrowing* involves asking a sequence of questions proceeding from general areas to specific issues; (2) *progression* involves arranging a sequence of questions to progress from less intimate to more intimate matters; (3) *embedding* involves concealing a significant question in the middle of a sequence of questions that appear routine and affectively neutral; (4) *leading questions* are based on an assumption that has not been previously admitted — for example, What do you usually do when you get angry with your wife?; (5) *holdover questions* involve ignoring emotionally charged material about which a patient blocks early in the interview, and asking about it later on in another context; and (6) *projective questions* involve general attitudes or values — for example, If you could rub a magic lamp, and have three wishes all come true, what would they be?

Recording of Information

During interviews recording of information presents certain problems, and it is easy to agree with Menninger that a great deal of nonsense has been written and spoken about taking notes. Some written notes may be desired by the physician for a number of reasons: so that he may refresh his memory about what transpired before he next sees the patient; so that he may review his basis for evaluation and therapeutic formulations; or so that he may prepare systematic records of the psychiatric history and mental examination for administrative, legal, educational, or possible research purposes. With such goals in mind, it may be desirable to record a number of the patient's statements (and even the interviewer's comments) verbatim. Most patients will in fact accept the physician's need to make some written notes, and their acceptance will be enhanced by the physician's confidence in the belief that some note-taking is reasonable.

On the other hand, detailed and compulsive recording of notes will become obtrusive in the interview situation and will interfere with spontaneous communication by both the patient and the physician. To eliminate the need to take some written notes, and to analyze the interaction between patient and physician in more detail subsequently, increasing use has been made of tape recordings. However, this should not be done without the knowledge and consent of the patient. It should also be remembered that interviews in the presence of a tape recorder, one-way observation window, or television or movie camera may lead to quite different interactions between patient and physician than communication with each other in complete privacy.

Three Successive Phases of the Initial Interview

The *opening phase* includes the ordinary rituals and greetings of a first meeting, the expert and unobtrusive observation of the patient, and the introduction of the theme for the meeting by certain initial statements. The *middle phase* is a free-wheeling and unhurried inquiry to which most of the interview is devoted, and is a time for conscious clarification rather than for the interpretation of unconscious dynamic processes. The *end phase* of the first interview involves a casual inventory of what has been communicated, and the making of proper arrangements for the next step, whether or not it will be a second interview with the patient. Before the end of the initial interview, the physician should have reached an opinion about whether there is any likelihood of the patient harming himself or others, what further information is necessary or desirable, and whether further evaluation or treatment should be carried out in the community or in the hospital. If the patient is in good contact with reality, such future plans should be discussed with him fully. An effort should also be made to be explicit about the cost of the recommended evaluation and treatment, what alternatives are available, the physician's opinion about possible consequences if treatment is not undertaken, and the basic obligations of the patient and the therapist.

The initial psychiatric interview may sometimes also be the last, and it is always possible to use a single interview as the basis for recording a *psychiatric examination* (also known as a *mental status* or *psychological examination*). On the basis of a single interview, it is sometimes necessary to express a summary opinion regarding the patient — for example, that he is mentally retarded or suffering from an organic brain syndrome; that he shows psychotic distortion of reality or requires involuntary admission to a hospital; or that he is or is not competent to handle his financial affairs, to make a will, to stand trial, or to care for his children.

More frequently, however, such opinions or plans for treatment are *not* formulated on the basis of a single cross-sectional view of the patient, but on a longitudinal developmental account of his life history and patterns of adaptation. This history may be given primarily by the patient, or supplemented extensively by interviews with other persons, and the comprehensive evaluation of the patient also often involves physical examination, indicated laboratory investigations, and appropriate psychological tests. We shall now consider the organization of data frequently followed in recording the patient's psychiatric history and examination.

RECORDING THE PSYCHIATRIC HISTORY

The psychiatric case history differs from the medical case history in a number of ways. One difference concerns the multiplicity of sources from which psychiatric information may be obtained. Some of this information may be available before the patient is interviewed, and its nature will depend on the source of referral and the reasons for psychiatric evaluation. Patients referred by general physicians have usually had recent extensive physical examinations; those referred by social agencies may be accompanied by reports containing detailed information about their family and interpersonal relationships; those referred by courts of law may have considerable documentation of the circumstances leading up to the referral; those who have already been committed to mental hospitals will have had written statements made about the reasons for their admission.

Once the physician has access to the patient, however, it is preferable to interview him before interviewing any relatives, friends, or other informants who may be available. In many instances, it will also be desirable to interview significant relatives and even involve them in therapy, but this should always be done with the full knowledge and consent of the patient unless he is a young child or is grossly irrational. Psychoanalysts and other therapists engaged in long-term intensive psychotherapy generally interview relatives only in the presence of the patient, and will not communicate with other persons about the patient without his consent and complete knowledge of the content of such communications.

The need for information obtained from others is likely to be greatest when the patient is a young child, is mentally retarded, has an organic brain syndrome or a functional psychosis, or has a personality disorder characterized by antisocial behavior. Some therapists prefer to make a separate record of all historical information obtained from persons other than the patient. This is not the usual practice, however, and it is customary for the psychiatric history to be a composite record obtained from various sources, with specific mention of the informants' names and opinions when their accounts conflict with one another. In general this history begins with identifying data about the patient, a summary of the presenting problem, and a history of the present illness. This is followed by a family history, the developmental life history of the patient, and his own comments about his adult patterns of adjustment.

Identifying Data

Identifying data include the patient's name, his or her clinic or hospital file number, the date of his or her initial interview or admission, and such other items as address, telephone number, sex, age at last birthday, date of birth, place of birth, race, religion, education completed, occupation, marital status, and next of kin.

The Presenting Problem

The presenting problem may be perceived differently by the patient, by his family, by his referring physician or other source of referral, and by the physician undertaking the psychiatric evaluation. These varied perceptions of the situation should all be recorded, with inclusion of verbatim statements when possible.

Present Illness

The description of the present illness should be a chronological and well-organized account of onset and development, of all changes noted in the patient's behavior and conversation, and of all changes in his physical health or environmental situation that may have precipitated or contributed to his present difficulties.

Answers should be obtained to such questions as the following: Have there been any recent changes in intellectual performance or memory, in mood or activity level, in sleeping habits, in eating habits or weight, in elimination, menstruation, or sexual behavior? Has there been any evidence of hallucinations or delusions, of suicidal or homicidal preoccupation? Do the patient's symptoms vary from one time to another, and are such changes regular (e.g., according to the time of day) or related to contact with certain other persons? What changes have taken place in the patient's relationships with other members of his family, with his employer, fellow employees, or friends? In what ways have his performance at work and interest in other activities been affected?

In addition to information about possible *precipitating factors* or *perpetuating factors* such as secondary gains from his illness, there should be a statement regarding *any treatment* the patient has recently received for a psychiatric disorder. This should include the name of the therapist, the type of treatment, and the amounts of any medications being taken. If the patient has been undergoing psychotherapy or has been hospitalized on a psy-

chiatric service, the dates should be noted and his written permission requested to obtain a transcript of his records.

Family History

Data concerning both the patient's family of origin (close blood relatives) and his family of orientation (those with whom he lived most of his childhood) may provide information about his hereditary endowment, the interpersonal relationships of childhood, and the sociocultural milieu in which he developed. From all these points of view, it is much more important to have data concerning close relatives, whether they be biological parents and siblings, or stepparents, adoptive or foster parents and siblings, than it is to have data concerning more remote connections such as grandparents, aunts, uncles, and cousins (although gross abnormalities in the latter group may also be significant).

The most relevant objective data to obtain concerning parents and siblings — biological or social — are sex, age, educational and occupational status, history of major bodily illness, and any evidence of psychopathology (such as mental retardation, organic brain syndromes, suicide, psychosis, neurosis, delinquency, or alcoholism). It may also be desirable to record miscarriages and stillbirths, and any consanguinity in the parents (the exact relationship being specified). The deaths of any of these close relatives should also be recorded, noting at what age and from what cause, together with the age of the patient at the time, and the apparent impact on the patient of this event in his life. Details concerning separation and divorce of the parents are also significant, and again the age of the patient at that time and his reaction to such parental loss should be recorded. The details of the patient's relationships with parents and siblings may be elaborated on here or in succeeding sections of the history.

The religious orientation in the patient's childhood home should also be investigated. Were the parents of the same religion, and was religious observance important to them? How did the patient come to feel about religious observance, and how is this reflected in his adult behavior?

Developmental History

Developmental history is frequently recorded in chronological sequence under such headings as birth, infancy, early childhood, school days and later childhood, the adolescent period, and adult adjustment patterns. This approach emphasizes age-appropriate and inappropriate behaviors, but sometimes results in fragments of related information being widely separated in the format of the history. Some clinicians prefer to organize data along several developmental sequences, each of which proceeds from early childhood into adult life — for example, intellectual maturation, school and occupational history, religion and relationships with authority, social interaction with peers, sexual and marital history. The latter approach, however, also tends to result in some fragmentation of information that is related in time. Therefore, it appears desirable to encourage flexibility in recording developmental data, as well as in securing such information from the patient or others.

Details of the mother's health during pregnancy are relevant to the patient's intrauterine development, and any history of toxicity or difficult delivery should be noted. Although there is often considerable retrospective falsification, it may be useful to inquire about whether the patient's birth was wanted and planned, whether he was fed by breast or bottle, whether he experienced colic or early feeding difficulties, the course of bowel and bladder training, and at what ages the patient first sat up, crawled, walked, and talked. Any history of convulsions and other physical illnesses should be noted, as well as any early admission to hospital or other institutions. Details of any early problem behavior such as temper tantrums, excessive masturbation, enuresis, night terrors, or stuttering should be explored.

Opportunities for social interaction with peers may be provided or prevented by parents. It may be significant to note whether the patient brought friends to his own home or visited other children in their homes, whether he had birthday parties or was invited to other children's birthday parties, whether he was deprived in comparison with siblings or other children in the neighborhood, whether he had friends to stay in his home overnight or was invited and permitted to stay in their homes overnight, whether there were prolonged periods of separation from parents (e.g., sickness, vacations, summer camp, or being away at school) and at what ages such separations occurred.

Early interactions with the patient's parents may be mirrored in subsequent relationships with teachers, employers, the police, and other authority figures. The adjustment of the patient during his school years should include information on the numbers and locations of different schools attended, with reasons for any transfers, regularity of attendance (including accounts of absences due to physical illness, emotional problems, or truancy), academic progress (advancing through grades, repeating grades, and class standing), extracurricular activities (athletic and social), and interpersonal relationships with teachers and other students. The subsequent occupational history should include information about the nature of employment, the nature and location of jobs, approximate income and reasons for changing employment, and relationships with employers and co-workers. Details of military service should include reasons for enlistment or rejection, duties performed, rank and nature of discharge, and particulars of any periods in hospital or of any conflict with military authorities. Appearances in court, contacts with social agencies and the police, and reformatory or jail sentences should also be noted.

Information should gradually become available from the patient concerning the nature and sources of *sexual information,* his recollection of childhood fantasies and explorations, the reaction of parents and others toward his sexual curiosity and experimentation, preparation of the patient for and his or her reaction to the onset of ejaculation or menstruation, any formal sexual instruction received, sexual feelings aroused by persons of either sex or other sources of gratification, and overt sexual behavior, including masturbation and homosexual and/or heterosexual activities. There should be some attempt to evaluate the main characteristics of sexual partners, and the nature, extent, and variety of premarital, marital, and extramarital relationships. Information may include conscious reasons for marriage, probable unconscious factors influencing the selection of a mate, the personality characteristics of the mate, significant aspects of marital interaction, communication and compatibility, decisions about family planning and contraceptive measures employed, the ages and characteristics of the patient's children, his attitudes toward them, family problems and conflicts, and reasons for any separation or divorce.

Medical History

Medical history should include a chronological record of all significant illnesses, accidents, and operations, noting their severity, the duration of disability, and any lasting sequelae. Under certain circumstances it may be necessary to make special inquiries about a history of convulsions, encephalitis, head injury, or venereal disease. Other significant information may include the patient's use of alcohol, cigarettes, barbiturates, other sedatives, narcotics, or patent medicines. His exposure to various occupational toxins such as lead, arsenic, and mercury should also be investigated.

Adult Personality Traits and Psychopathology

These factors may have become evident in summarizing the present illness or some of the longitudinal trends in the developmental history, but they will usually require further elaboration. What have been the patient's predominant mood, activity level, interests, degree of social participation? What are his greatest sources of satisfaction and dissatisfaction? What have been his main personality characteristics, his intrapsychic dynamics and defenses, and his significant adult interpersonal relationships? What have been his main attitudes toward himself, his attitudes toward others, and his aspirations for the future? What evidence is there of previous maladaptation — intellectual, emotional, or behavioral? Is there any history of previous psychiatric evaluation, treatment, or hospitalization that has not already been reviewed under the history of the present illness? In the latter event it will frequently be desirable to obtain

further information from those who were responsible for the patient's treatment, and the patient's signed consent to obtain this information should be requested.

RECORD OF PSYCHIATRIC EXAMINATION (MENTAL STATUS)

The topics and questions itemized in the preceding section do *not* constitute an exhaustive list of all relevant factors in personality development, and need *not* be asked or answered for each separate patient, particularly not in any rigid sequence. Similarly, the current trend is toward flexibility in recording data relevant to the psychiatric examination. While the latter may always be written on the basis of a single interview, observations made during several interviews with the patient are often combined into a portrait of his current adaptations over a period of several days or even weeks.

Information relevant to the psychiatric examination has already been presented in parts of Chapters 1 and 2, and may be organized and presented in a similar manner in the record of the mental status examination; for example, under such headings as perception, intellectual function, affect, motivation, behavior, conversation, dreams, fantasy life, and dynamics (intrapsychic and interpersonal). More frequently, however, clinical interaction with the patient results in information being obtained in a different sequence from that described above, and it is often recorded in the sequence in which it is obtained, which proceeds from relatively objective observational data to more subjective interpretations based on inference.

Appearance and Behavior

This category includes a general statement of such characteristics as the patient's height, weight, posture, clothing, and facial expression. Does the patient appear well groomed and neatly dressed, or does he seem careless of his appearance, disheveled, or inappropriately dressed? Does his appearance suggest that he is older, younger, or about equal to his actual age? Does he appear composed, relaxed, and at ease, or is he tense, uncomfortable, apprehensive, fearful, restless, or agitated? Is he alert and responsive, or somnolent, withdrawn, disinterested, or dejected? Is there increased or decreased motor activity, or does he show any unusual involuntary movements, peculiar mannerisms, bizarre gestures, or repetitive stereotyped movement? Is there any aggressive, violent, or destructive behavior? Is his facial expression mobile or unchanging, bland or miserable, angry or fearful? Does the patient make and maintain eye contact with the examiner, or does he avoid looking at him directly, particularly at certain times in the interview? Does the patient laugh, smile, weep, or blush?

Conversation or Verbal Behavior

Verbal behavior often corresponds to the level of motor activity, and may be either increased or decreased. Speech may be clear and animated, or the voice may be quiet and monotonous. The patient may converse spontaneously, or only in response to questions, or not at all. Questions may be answered readily or reluctantly, promptly or after considerable delay, relevantly, circumstantially, or irrelevantly. The predominant thought content may be revealed by spontaneous productions or digressions in response to questions, and may indicate preoccupation with a wide variety of interpersonal or intrapsychic problems. These responses may reveal disorders of mood (e.g., euphoria or depression), perception (e.g., illusions or hallucinations), and ideation (e.g., delusions). Disordered thought processes may also be indicated by poverty of ideas, flight of ideas, loose associations, concrete (literal) or overinclusive thinking, or neologisms.

Samples of conversation may be recorded verbatim, and may include the patient's initial statements or other spontaneous remarks, evidence of predominant thought content, evidence of unusual ideation, and significant responses to questions, including mention of any time lag before such questions are answered.

Emotional Tone

Emotional tone should be noted — for example, anxiety, fear, anger, euphoria, depression, or apathy. This should be distinguished from the *emotional responsiveness or reactivity,* which may be characterized by the amount of overall variability (either lability or shallowness) and by the degree of appropriateness to the situation and thought content (see Chap. 2).

Disorders of Perception

These disorders may involve any of the five senses. Such disturbances may sometimes be inferred from the patient's behavior — for example, if he appears to be picking imaginary objects out of the air, or holding a one-sided conversation when he is in a room by himself. Alternatively, distortions of perception may be reported in response to a general question such as Have you had any unusual or strange experiences lately?, but it may be necessary to make more specific inquiries regarding unusual smells, a strange taste in the food, unusual sensations in certain parts of the body, hearing voices when there is no one in the immediate vicinity, or seeing things that other people do not seem able to recognize. The nature of any such experiences should be explored, and also the patient's interpretations of what is causing them. It may be helpful to ask if he thinks many people have such experiences, and why they should happen to him, or why he feels he was chosen to have such experiences.

Disorders of Ideation

Disorders of ideation (such as delusions), which are intimately related to disorders of perception, may include auditory hallucinations interpreted as messages from God, or as the voices of imagined persecutors. Frequently, however, delusions occur in the absence of hallucinations or illusions, and appear more related to the prevailing emotional tone. Various types of delusions were described in Chapter 2, and if present they may or may not be evident in an initial interview. Unrealistic ideas of grandeur (of wealth, power, and prestige) or of self-accusation, worthlessness, and hopelessness, are more likely to be apparent than delusions of reference, active or passive influence, or persecution. These may be deliberately concealed because the patient recognizes that other persons disbelieve his own convictions. Sometimes the latter may be revealed by asking general questions such as Have any other people been showing an unusual interest in you? or alternatively, Has anyone been interfering in your life, or deliberately making life difficult for you? It may also be necessary to ask more specific questions as to whether other people appear to have access to private information about the patient, whether they watch him, talk about him, spread information about him, try to control his thoughts or actions, exploit him, hold him back, or discriminate against him in other ways. The evidence on which he bases any such beliefs should be explored, and also the reasons why he thinks he is being subjected to such experiences.

Fantasies, Dreams, and Dynamics

The same key will not open the locks of all doors, and the physician must accumulate a variety of "skeleton keys," each of which may be helpful in gaining access to the patient's trust and willingness to discuss his innermost feelings and fantasies. Some patients will reveal considerable inner fantasy in response to simple questions about the nature and frequency of their daydreams. Others unwittingly reveal a great deal more, albeit in symbolic and distorted form, in their reports of the nighttime dreams that they recall after awakening. The analysis and interpretation of such dreams constitutes one of the tasks of analytically oriented psychotherapy, but unconscious dynamic defense mechanisms may be evident to the physician in a variety of behaviors that the patient demonstrates in his daily living and interaction with others. Such mechanisms of adaptation should be recorded in the mental examination, as well as summarized in connection with subsequent diagnostic formulations and plans for treatment.

Intellectual Function

Both optimal and current intellectual functions may be estimated by means of psychological tests that will be outlined in the next chapter. Nevertheless, the physician should be alert for clues regarding the patient's current level of intellectual function in comparison with other persons of the same age, and also with the optimal level at which the patient has ever functioned. In children and adolescents up to the age of sixteen years, the intelligence quotient (IQ) may be expressed as a ratio of the mental age (in comparison with the average member of the general population) divided by the chronological age, then multiplied by 100. A 12-year-old child functioning at the intellectual level of the average 9-year-old child would have an IQ of approximately 75. Any adult patient functioning at the intellectual level of the average 8-year-old child would have an IQ of approximately 50 (i.e., 8 divided by 16, times 100).

Direct questions intended to measure intellectual function may be considered insulting by the patient when they are asked during a clinical interview. It is therefore generally preferable to estimate intellectual capacity (or maximum potential) from the patient's previous education, current vocabulary, comprehension, and general information. Under some circumstances, it may be appropriate to ask a few such general questions as What is the population of the United States, and of the state or town or city in which he lives; What is the distance from his current location to certain well-known cities? One might also ask him for information about well-known places or persons. Persons of similar intelligence may vary in their accumulation of such general information, and accurate answers may not be as significant as the nature of each response and the incompatibility between responses — for example, that the population of the United States is "about twenty billion," while the population of one of its constituent states is given as "about twenty-four billion." Such questions, as well as simple arithmetical calculations, can be presented within the context of what the patient remembers from the time he was in school. However, for most patients such questions will be unnecessary and may be perceived as insulting, thus damaging to the relationship with the physician.

Memory and Orientation

Impairment of intellectual functions generally includes some degree of memory impairment and disorientation. Remote memory concerning such events as date and place of birth, schools attended, employment, marriage, and children is usually better preserved than memory for recent events. The latter may be tested by asking the patient to count to 42 and then stop, to recall three objects after several minutes, to recall the name of the physician or other person on the ward, to recall when he was admitted to the hospital or what he ate at recent meals, etc. Similarly, orientation as to person and place is usually better preserved than orientation as to time (day of the week, date of the month, and even the month or year). Here again, some questions can be introduced much more readily than others, as by the physician's remarking, "Let's see now, what's the date today?" (without waiting a lengthy period for a reply), or asking the patient's date of birth, date of marriage, or date of admission to the hospital. However, assessment of memory and orientation by indirect means during the clinical interview is generally preferable to direct questioning.

Conscience, Judgment, and Insight

Superego functions, conscience, aspirations, and internal controls are not static, but may vary with mood and other factors such as the ingestion of alcohol or other drugs. It should be recalled that actions speak louder than words, and a reliable history of past behavior provides the best information concerning former ethical standards and motivation. However, some estimate of present superego functions may be revealed by the patient's currently verbalized attitudes toward past behavior (e.g., regrets, guilt, and remorse), and his ideals and plans for the future. An evaluation should also be made of other aspects of the patient's judgment and of his insight into the nature of his current problems. Some patients may be entirely lacking in insight and may either repudiate forcefully the notion that they have a psychiatric problem or be unable to understand the reason for their referral. Others may partially recognize the presence of a problem, while a few may have a much more thorough understanding of the origin, nature, and dynamics of their personali-

ties and psychopathology. A patient who has such detailed knowledge, but is unable to modify maladaptive behavior, is sometimes described as having intellectual insight, whereas such knowledge associated with modification or abandonment of maladaptive behavior may be described as emotional insight. Analytically oriented psychotherapy was formerly focused on interpretation of unconscious dynamics leading to intellectual insight, but has become increasingly concerned with the "corrective emotional experiences" that may lead to emotional insight and the abandonment of maladaptive behavior.

FURTHER EVALUATION, DIAGNOSIS, TREATMENT PLANNING, AND OUTCOME

We have so far considered three aspects of the patient's evaluation — the initial psychiatric interview or consultation, the subsequent elaboration and recording of a more comprehensive psychiatric history, and the main areas of concern in recording a mental-status or psychiatric examination. There are three further broad categories of information that may be sought by the physician before he formulates a diagnosis and plan for treatment. The extent to which the physician utilizes these additional techniques of evaluation may vary greatly according to the problems presented by the individual patient, the training of the physician, and the type of situation in which he is practicing. Before considering diagnosis and treatment, we shall review the types of information that may be obtained through the use of hypnosis or drugs, the administration of standardized psychological tests, and the application of the physical examinations in which every physician has been trained.

Psychiatric Examination under Hypnosis or Drugs

Sometimes pertinent information remains inaccessible during psychiatric interview. This may be because the patient is mute, shows marked emotional blocking, or has amnesia for a certain period of time. Under such circumstances, he may become much more communicative through *hypnosis,* or the administration during an interview of any of a variety of sedative, tranquilizing, or stimulant drugs. The therapeutic benefits of such procedures, however, are often of questionable value or very short-lived. By contrast, the judicious use of antipsychotic, antidepressant, or antianxiety drugs over more extended periods of time is commonly regarded as a means of increasing accessibility to psychotherapy.

Since the time of the ancient Romans it has been known that alcohol tends to decrease inhibition and increase conversation about emotionally charged subjects, as reflected in the dictum "in vino veritas." During World War II, intravenous barbiturates such as sodium amytal or sodium pentothal were widely used in the treatment of combat fatigue, and were subsequently popularly misrepresented as truth serums. There is in fact no guarantee that a patient will tell all or even a significant part of the truth when under the influence of such drugs. However, intravenous narcosis with these agents may greatly facilitate conversation, and sometimes the increased verbalization will be dramatic. A marked increase in speech and emotional response may also occur after the intravenous injection of a stimulant such as methamphetamine (Desoxyn), or after inhalation of such drugs as nitrous oxide, carbon dioxide, or ether. Less dramatic but quite effective increases in communication may be accomplished by the oral administration of sedative or tranquilizing drugs, without the undesirable side effects of overstimulation (prolonged agitation, insomnia, or fragmentation of thinking).

The use of hypnosis and drugs in psychiatric evaluation has diminished progressively since the years immediately following World War II. In the event that any such adjuncts are used in psychiatric evaluation, however, the dates and details of such diagnostic interviews should be recorded separately. It should also be borne in mind that the mental state of the patient is *not* the same when he is under the influence of these adjuncts as it is at other times.

The Administration of Standardized Psychological Tests

The extent to which standardized psychological tests are employed in psychiatric evaluation and treatment planning depends on a number of factors. These include the training and theoretical orientation of the physician and the availability of competent clinical psychologists. Psychological tests in common usage include those for measurement of intelligence and intellectual impairment, objective behavioral or subjective personality (self-report) inventories, projective techniques (such as sentence completions, the Rorschach ink blots, the Thematic Apperception Test, and House-Tree-Person drawings), and tests of vocational interests, preferences, or aptitudes. In a number of clinic and hospital settings, it has been customary to routinely administer several standard psychological tests, to be supplemented by additional testing in specific areas when indicated.

The training of a psychiatrist usually includes some formal instruction and considerable clinical familiarization with the practical applications of selected psychological tests. Many other physicians now also receive some basic instruction and experience in the application of psychological tests while in medical school. Increasing numbers of nonpsychiatric physicians are making use of such knowledge and requesting psychological tests for their patients, without necessarily referring the patient for psychiatric evaluation. The next chapter contains summary information on a number of psychological tests in widespread use.

Medical Assessment

Physical examination, including a brief or detailed neurological examination as indicated, should be performed and recorded as soon after the initial psychiatric interview or admission to hospital as possible. This is considered desirable for two general reasons: (1) that a variety of psychopathology may be precipitated or perpetuated by neurological or other somatic illness, and (2) that the psychiatric patient with somatic complaints may need evidence that the latter have been investigated thoroughly before he is ready to accept the idea that his bodily complaints may have a psychological etiology and to respond to psychiatric treatment.

Due to their training and to their interest in conducting long-term intensive individual psychotherapy, many psychiatrists prefer *not* to perform physical examinations on their patients, and over a period of time may lose their original competence to do so. Such psychiatrists prefer to be regarded as "talking" rather than "touching" doctors, and this preference may be reflected in their rejection of the physician's white coat, stethoscope, and other equipment of the profession. Since patients referred to psychiatrists by other physicians have generally had recent (and sometimes extensive) somatic investigations, it may indeed be unnecessary or undesirable to repeat these after the patient's referral. If, on the other hand, the patient has had no such somatic investigations, the psychiatrist may refer the patient to a general physician or to a neurologist for necessary physical examination and laboratory investigations.

Repeated somatic investigations with equivocal or negative results, concerning which the patient is not informed, may strongly reinforce the patient's belief in a somatic etiology. Even more reinforcing of such a conviction is the patient's being subjected to a number of medical treatments or surgical procedures prior to his referral for psychiatric evaluation. On the other hand, there is a need for prompt investigation (whether by the therapist or by another physician) of somatic complaints appearing for the first time during psychotherapy. This may be a problem when the patient has previously "cried wolf" on a number of occasions through numerous bodily complaints for which no organic basis was found. It is necessary to bear in mind, however, that a hypochondriacal or hysterical patient may still develop organic disease, and the latter should be evaluated by a physician.

In addition to a general examination and a reasonably comprehensive neurological examination, a number of routine laboratory investigations may be included in the initial evaluation, such as a complete blood count and differential, a serological test for syphilis, a urinalysis, and a chest x-ray. Some psychiatrists have also recommended routine tests of thyroid function or electroencephalography. Positive findings on physical examination or laboratory investigations may or may not be causally related to the patient's presenting psychopathology, but they should always be summarized in the overall diagnostic evaluation.

Diagnostic Formulation and Treatment Planning
Psychiatric diagnosis is generally summarized under several headings, the first of which may be termed the *descriptive* (or *clinical*) *diagnosis,* based on the standard nomenclature of psychiatric syndromes that was summarized in Chapter 2. A second general heading is the *dynamic diagnosis,* which includes predominant intrapsychic defense mechanisms, significant current interpersonal relationships, precipitating and perpetuating stress, and deprivation. A third heading consists of the *developmental* (or *genetic*) *diagnosis,* which constitutes a summary of adverse factors perceived as significant in personality development and in determining predisposition to psychopathology. A fourth heading consists of the *somatic diagnosis,* and the probable relationship of the latter to the presenting psychiatric problems.

Comprehensive *plans for psychiatric treatment* may also be summarized under several headings, and should include the nature and frequency of proposed psychotherapy (individual, family, or group); the proposed social and milieu therapy in a hospital setting; social casework to be undertaken with relatives or other key persons in the patient's environment; pharmacological agents to be administered; any proposal for electroshock or other somatic treatment of the psychopathology; and any somatic treatment indicated for organic bodily illness.

Various forms of psychiatric treatment will be outlined in later chapters. In recording the psychiatric evaluation, however, it may also be desirable to attempt to *predict the outcome* of whatever treatments are recommended, taking into account the nature of the patient's problems, his age, intelligence, and personality resources (or ego strength), as well as his family and socioeconomic circumstances (external reality situation).

Progress Notes and Final Summaries
The frequency and content of *progress notes* will depend on the nature of the evaluation and treatment, and the setting in which it is undertaken. Many psychotherapists make some written notes of communications by their patients and themselves (verbal or nonverbal) during the course of

each interview, and do not attempt to elaborate or summarize these notes until the time of termination. Others interview the patient without taking any notes, and write a summary statement after each interview. This may consist of one sentence or a brief paragraph. A number of institutions require progress notes at specified intervals – for example, daily during the first week or month after the patient's admission, or at intervals of one week, one month, or even one year in some state hospitals. In the opinion of many psychiatrists, there should be flexibility in both the frequency and content of such progress notes, but a written note is recommended each time the patient is seen, no matter how brief the note may be.

Final summaries are also required in many settings, and may range from half a page to many pages in length. The content usually includes identifying data, presenting problems, a summary of the initial interview and evaluation, a history of the present illness and personality development, a summary of the psychiatric examination and psychological tests, any positive findings in the physical examination and laboratory investigations, psychosocial and somatic treatment procedures, the progress of the patient during therapy, and an evaluation of the patient's reality situation and adaptational resources at the time of termination. This type of summary, written while the information is still fresh in mind, may prove most valuable to the therapist in the event that the patient returns for further consultation or therapy after a lapse of time, and it can always be supplemented by brief progress notes in the event of any such further interviews or written communications.

REVIEW QUESTIONS

39. A 60-year-old man with Parkinson's disease poorly controlled by medication has shown increasing signs of depression. A nonpsychiatric physician treating him should:
    (A) avoid talking about death or suicide with him
    (B) suggest that a rest in the hospital might be helpful
    (C) refer him to a psychiatrist

(D) reassure him that things will get better
(E) ask him, Do you ever wonder if it's worth going on?

40. During her first interview with a male physician, a young unmarried woman suddenly says, "I don't know why I'm talking to you – all men are bastards!" She has not previously mentioned any difficulties with men. A good response by the physician at this point would be:
    (A) You must have had some very unhappy experiences with men.
    (B) I understand how you feel.
    (C) What makes you feel this way?
    (D) This attitude must be a great hindrance to you.
    (E) Would you like me to refer you to some other doctor?

41. A 33-year-old woman, recently married, is consulting a physician because of repeated anxiety attacks. She admits that she is anxious when at home alone, but initially is evasive about the reason. Toward the end of the interview she suddenly blurts out, "I'm afraid a man might break into the house." She then quickly adds, "I don't see anything abnormal about that. Lots of women are afraid to be alone at night." A good response by the physician would be:
    (A) No, that isn't abnormal.
    (B) But your fear is not very realistic.
    (C) Why not invite someone to stay with you when your husband is away?
    (D) You shouldn't let this fear limit your life.
    (E) Even if they're not abnormal, let's try to understand your feelings.

42. A 20-year-old man who has been unemployed for several months is brought to a hospital emergency room by two friends. They report that he has been talking and behaving very strangely for the past week and apparently not eating or sleeping. During a brief interview he is preoccupied with abstruse religious and philosophical topics. The interviewer has difficulty communicating with him due to his use of many strange words and the lack of logical

coherence to his sentences. The most important thing to accomplish during the rest of the interview is to:

(A) persuade him to begin taking antipsychotic medication immediately
(B) inquire about his history of drug use
(C) get him to agree to consult a psychiatrist as soon as possible
(D) inquire about disturbing experiences during the past few weeks
(E) arrange for admission to a psychiatric unit

43. A 25-year-old man has just been admitted for the third time to a psychiatric hospital. His previous discharge diagnosis was paranoid schizophrenia. Although the patient is very suspicious and hostile, the resident conducting the intake interview succeeds in establishing good rapport. At the end of the interview, the patient spontaneously says, "You're not like the other doctors — I can trust you." He then surreptitiously shows the resident a switchblade knife concealed in his clothing, explaining that he needs it for protection. The resident should take the following action:

(A) Keep the matter confidential and not risk damaging the patient's trust. Plan to make this a basis for future therapy.
(B) Suggest that the patient give him the knife, but not make an issue of the matter if he refuses. Then act as in (A).
(C) Tell the patient that knives are totally forbidden on the unit, and give him 24 hours to decide whether to dispose of the knife or request discharge.
(D) Insist that the patient hand over the knife, and call for all necessary assistance if he refuses.
(E) Say nothing, then quietly tell the nursing staff so that they can later "discover" the knife and take it away from him.

SELECTED REFERENCES

1. Bernstein, L., and Dana, R.H. (1970). *Interviewing and the Health Professions.* New York: Appleton-Century-Crofts.
2. Bird, B. (1973). *Talking With Patients.* Philadelphia: J. B. Lippincott Co.
3. Gill, M.M., Newman, R., and Redlich, F.C. (1954). *The Initial Interview in Psychiatric Practice.* New York: International Universities Press.
4. MacKinnon, R.A., and Michels, R. (1971). *The Psychiatric Interview in Clinical Practice.* Philadelphia: W. B. Saunders Co.
5. Menninger, K.A. (1962). *A Manual for Psychiatric Case Study* (2nd Ed.). (The Menninger Clinic Monograph Series, No. 8) New York: Grune & Stratton.
6. Stevenson, I. (1960). *Medical History-Taking.* New York: Hoeber.
7. Sullivan, H.S. (1954). *The Psychiatric Interview.* New York: W. W. Norton Co.

4. Psychological Tests

For now we see through a glass, darkly; but then face to face: Now I know in part; but then shall I know even as also I am known.
First Epistle of Paul to the Corinthians, Chapter 13, Verse 12

A psychological test is an instrument for obtaining a sample of controlled observations of a person's behavior in a standard situation, so that such behavior may then be evaluated uniformly. Since the beginning of the present century, at least 2,000 test procedures have been designed to assess various aspects of psychological function. These include tests that assess intelligence or problem-solving ability; impairment of intellectual functions (e.g., perception, memory, or reasoning); personality and dynamics; interpersonal relationships and psychopathology; and vocational interests and aptitudes.

The main advantages of the use of tests are that the data are collected in a relatively uniform manner; that the evaluation of findings from tests is more objective than of those from clinical interviews; that data permit comparisons within and between individuals; that observations made during psychological testing are usually easier to record than those made in clinical interviews; that data may be obtained without the patient's awareness (or verbal participation); and that a broad sample of the subject's behavior may be obtained in a short time. The main limitations of psychological tests involve their relative lack of flexibility; the artificiality of a test situation; and the limited aspects of personality or dynamics revealed by any single test. However, a more comprehensive evaluation of intelligence and personality may be obtained when several selected psychological tests are interpreted in relation to each other and to other data obtained during the course of psychiatric evaluation.

Two important characteristics of psychological tests are their reliability and their validity. **Reliability** refers to replicability, or the extent to which

results remain consistent or reproducible under identical conditions. The term **validity** refers to the extent to which a test can be shown to actually measure any particular attribute or quality that it claims to measure. One of the advantages of the Minnesota Multiphasic Personality Inventory (to be described in a later section) is that it includes several validity indices that reveal the test-taking attitudes of the subject, and hence suggest how much confidence may be placed in the inferences drawn from other scales.

Standardized psychological testing of individuals or groups should involve **uniformity of examination procedure,** and those administering tests should try to acquire identical habits in their administration. The test environment should be quiet and comfortable. With some tests it may be necessary to establish rapport and attempt to maintain the subject's motivation and interest. Directions regarding test procedures should be standardized, as should the recording of test data. The subject's verbal responses to projective tests should be recorded verbatim, and objective criteria for scoring applied wherever possible.

The following selected psychological tests will now be considered briefly: (1) tests of intelligence, (2) tests for organic brain damage, (3) projective tests, and (4) the Minnesota Multiphasic Personality Inventory.

TESTS OF INTELLIGENCE

The first test of intelligence was designed by two Frenchmen, Alfred Binet and Theophile Simon, who were investigating the problem of mental retardation in school children. Their test was published in 1905, and consisted of 30 items arranged in order of increasing difficulty. These included following a moving object with the eyes, recognizing food and simple objects in a picture, comparing two lines of different lengths, repeating spoken sentences, memorizing objects in a picture, finding rhymes for a given word, completing sentences, and defining abstract terms. In 1908 Binet published a revised scale and introduced the concept of *mental age.* Questions of increasing complexity were assigned empirically to various ages from 3 to

11 years, and mental age was determined by the level up to which the child was able to complete all or most of the appropriate tests successfully.

Lewis M. Terman of Stanford University modified the Binet test further, and spent several years standardizing and validating it on 2,000 school children prior to publishing his results in 1916. He selected six tests for each year of life (so that each correct item would correspond to two months in mental age) and added items that extended the mental age score upward. The **Stanford-Binet test** was later extended down to the 2-year-old level and expanded to include many more items at upper levels. It remains a valuable measure of intelligence and development in children and in mentally retarded adults.

The concept of *intelligence quotient* (IQ) was introduced by Wilhelm Stern in 1912. He suggested that the ratio between the child's mental age (MA) and chronological age (CA) would remain relatively constant during childhood. Since intelligence is assumed to be fully developed by the age of 16 years, this figure is used as the upper limit of mental age and of chronological age in computing IQ from the formula:

$$IQ = \frac{MA}{CA} \times 100$$

If a 12-year-old child (CA = 12) has the mental age of an average 9-year-old (MA = 9), this would mean that his IQ is 75 (borderline mental retardation). On the other hand, an 8-year-old child with the mental ability of an average 12-year-old would be found to have an IQ of 150 (very superior). It is also easy to estimate the mental age of mentally retarded adults from their IQ using a maximum chronological age of 16. Hence, an adult with an IQ of 50 would be found to have the mental age of an average 8-year-old, or an adult with an IQ of 25 would be found to have the mental age of the average 4-year-old.

The *frequency distribution of intelligence* in the general population (excluding persons with brain damage) approximates that of the normal (Gaussian, or bell-shaped) curve. More than two-thirds

of all observations fall between the values at one standard deviation above and one standard deviation below the mean. More than 95 percent of all observations fall between the values at two standard deviations above and two standard deviations below the mean. The mean intelligence quotient is 100, and the standard deviation for IQ is approximately 16, as shown in Figure 4-1.

The *percentile rank* of a person's IQ in the population is the cumulative relative frequency of all persons having *lower* IQs than his. This means that the corresponding percentile rank for each IQ level shown in the above diagram would be obtained by adding all the frequencies *to the left* of the appropriate IQ. The percentile rank corresponding with each IQ shown in the diagram would therefore be as follows:

Intelligence Quotient	Percentile Rank
68	2.3
84	15.9
100	50.0
116	84.1
132	97.7

The **Wechsler Adult Intelligence Scale** (WAIS) derives an overall estimate of intelligence from eleven subtests, six of which measure *verbal* aptitude (information, comprehension, digit span, arithmetic, similarities, and vocabulary) and five of which measure *performance* (picture arrangement, picture completion, block design, object assembly, and digit symbol). The raw scores on each of the eleven subtests are converted into equivalent weighted scores (standardized according to the age group of the subject) from which the verbal, performance, and full-scale intelligence quotients are determined. The **Wechsler Intelligence Scale for Children** (WISC) also combines several verbal and performance subtests, and has been well standardized for children in the age range of 5 through 15 years.

The **Shipley-Hartford** is a brief test consisting of only two parts, vocabulary (40 items) and abstract reasoning (20 items). It may be administered to groups, and yields a reasonable approxi-

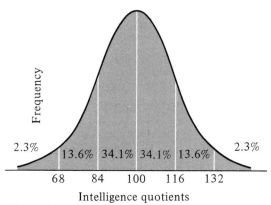

2.3%   13.6% 34.1% 34.1% 13.6%   2.3%

68   84   100   116   132

Intelligence quotients

Figure 4-1.

mation to the IQ scores obtained on the WAIS in the range of about 75 to 125. The Shipley-Hartford test was first introduced in 1939 as a test for organic brain damage, since the latter may result in severe impairment of some intellectual functions (particularly abstract reasoning), while other intellectual functions may remain well preserved (particularly vocabulary). The ratio obtained by dividing the abstract reasoning score by the vocabulary score and then multiplying by 100 is termed the *conceptual quotient*. This quotient should remain close to the norm of 100 in persons without intellectual impairment, but is often below 70 in those whose abstract reasoning is moderately impaired by either organic brain damage or functional psychopathology such as schizophrenia or severe depression.

TESTS FOR ORGANIC BRAIN DAMAGE

Mild or moderate organic brain damage tends to produce selective impairment of various intellectual functions. This may result in far more than the usual degree of variation in scores (scatter) among various subtests of the WAIS. Vocabulary and general information may be better preserved than other verbal tasks or performance subtests, which require both recent memory (recall) and perceptual motor control. Another test that is often sensitive to such impairment uses the **Porteus Mazes**, which increase in complexity and are scaled according to the mental age at which they can usually be completed.

A third numerical index of possible organic brain damage is the **memory quotient (MQ)** derived from the **Wechsler Memory Scale**, which contains seven subtests involving personal and current information, orientation, mental control, recall of items from short stories, recall of digits, visual reproduction, and associative learning. Persons without brain damage tend to have memory quotients that correspond roughly to their intelligence quotients, while those with organic brain syndromes tend to have MQ scores lower than their IQ scores.

The **Bender-Gestalt test** consists of nine geometric designs that are presented one at a time to the subject, who is asked to copy each design in turn. This is one of the most widely used tests for organic brain damage, which often results in recognizable patterns of faulty reproduction of the designs. However, the Bender test is also used as a projective test that may reveal ego function and personality conflicts, particularly in children.

The **Graham-Kendall Memory for Designs** measures both visual-motor control (like the Bender test) and also immediate visual memory. The subject is shown a series of fifteen cards, each containing a single design that he is asked to memorize and reproduce immediately. Mistakes in accuracy of reproduction are scored numerically (from 0 to 3 per design), and persons without brain damage are expected to attain a total test score of less than 6 (out of a possible maximum of 45). The range of 6 to 11 is considered borderline, and any higher score is strongly suggestive of organic brain damage.

There are many other specialized tests for organic brain damage, but a description of these is beyond the scope of the present brief review.

PROJECTIVE TESTS

Projective tests consist of unstructured tasks that elicit responses which reveal the subject's underlying feelings, personality, and psychopathology. The tasks are simple and require imagination, such as drawing pictures, making up sentences, finding shapes in ink blots, or telling stories about stimulus situations. The subject is not aware of any social norms and should therefore be unable to falsify his responses to conform with some pattern that he thinks is expected of him. The tests, however, have been administered to large numbers of persons with and without psychiatric disorders, and the clinician is able to interpret the subject's responses in accordance with this empirical information.

The **House-Tree-Person (HTP) drawing test** is an unstructured projective test in which the subject is presented with four sheets of plain white paper (8½ by 11 inches) and a medium-soft pencil. He is first asked to draw a house, and when this is completed he is asked to draw a tree (on a separate sheet). He is then asked to draw a person (if he asks which sex, he is told to draw whichever sex he prefers), and finally he is asked to draw a person of the sex opposite to the one he has already drawn. After the drawings have been completed, the examiner may inquire about various characteristics of the objects and persons drawn. Related projective techniques include drawing a family or animals, using pencil, colored crayons, or paints. Such drawings often yield information about the subject's self-concept, significant interactions with other persons, affects, motivation, and conflict.

Sentence completion tests are a form of projective technique that is somewhat more structured than the drawing tests. Most of these tests consist of about fifty to seventy-five opening phrases that the subject is asked to develop into complete sentences. Areas of interest include the subject's attitudes toward members of his family (particularly parents and spouse), his past frustrations and failures, and his future goals and desires. Such information often speeds up the process of evaluation as well as the early stages of therapy. Significant responses include the expression of intense feelings, contradictions, omission of responses to specific phrases, and lengthy elaborations on others.

The **Rorschach test** was introduced in 1921 and consists of 10 quasisymmetrical ink blots that are used as stimulus material. Five of these are dark gray (with many different shadings), two are dark gray and red, and the last three are multicolored. The 10 cards are presented to the subject in standard sequence, and the examiner notes the reactions of the subject, the way in which he turns the cards, the time taken before responding, and the exact verbal content of all responses. After the responses to all cards have been completed, they are again presented in sequence to find out what part of the blot was used for each response, what determinants entered into the response (form, color, shading, etc.) and how far the subject can specify or elaborate the concepts involved. Each response is *scored* with respect to the following characteristics:

1. *Location:* use of the whole blot (W), large detail (D), small detail (d), or response to white space (S).

2. *Determinants:* human movement (M), animal movement (FM), inanimate movement (m), shading as diffusion (K), shading suggesting three dimensions or vista (FK), contour or form alone (F), surface shading (Fc), shading as texture (c), white or black used as a color (C'), colored object with form (FC), color with indefinite form (CF), and color only, with form disregarded (C).

3. *Content:* human (H), animal (A), human anatomy (At), man-made objects (Obj), and nature (N).

4. *Form level:* scored plus or minus, depending on how well the response corresponds to the contour of the blot area used.

5. *Popularity-originality:* depending on whether the response is one of the ten most frequently given (popular), or whether it is found less often than once in a hundred records (original).

Other significant factors in scoring the Rorschach test are the *total responses* (R), which usually number between 15 and 30, and the *reaction time* before the first response on each card, which is usually about 30 seconds. Prolonged reaction time, a sudden drop in form level, or total rejection of certain cards may be described as shading shock or color shock and may indicate emotional disturbance resulting from concepts aroused by these stimuli. The *psychogram* indicates the frequency distribution of the responses according to their determinants (movement, form, shading, and color). Interpretation is not based on a single response or category of responses, but on their distribution in the complete record. Significant statistical differences may be found between groups of persons with various forms of psychiatric disorders, but individual diagnoses cannot be made as reliably as by means of other tests such as the MMPI. On the other hand, interpersonal dynamics are more likely to be revealed by projective techniques such as the following.

The **Thematic Apperception Test (TAT)**, developed by Henry Murray in 1935, consists of thirty pictures and one blank card. The pictures show persons of various age and sex groups in ambiguous but potentially dramatic situations. The subject is asked to make up a story about each picture, telling how the situation came about, the relationships between the persons in the picture, what has been happening to them, how they feel, and what will be the outcome. The subject tends to identify with one of the characters in each picture, and projects an image of himself and of his relationships with the significant persons in his life. Like dreams, the subject's stories may be used as points of departure for free associations, and the test may provide fruitful areas for further exploration in the early stages of therapy.

The **Children's Apperception Test (CAT)** was introduced by Leopold Bellak in 1949 for use with children between the ages of 3 and 10 years. It involves animals rather than humans as the central characters, but may also give helpful information about self-concept and interpersonal relationships, relevant both to psychopathology and therapy.

MINNESOTA MULTIPHASIC PERSONALITY INVENTORY (MMPI)

The Minnesota Multiphasic Personality Inventory (MMPI) was developed by Starke Hathaway and Charnley McKinley in 1940, and has become the most widely used objective personality test in the world, with translations into more than a dozen different languages. It is a standardized self-report consisting of responses to 566 true-false questions. The MMPI questions are provided in booklet, card-sorting, and audio-tape forms. The test may be used with subjects as young as 12 years of age, as long as the reading level is sixth grade or higher.

The time usually required to answer all questions varies from about forty-five to ninety minutes.

Subsets of the subject's responses are counted to yield scores on four validity scales and ten clinical scales. The counted responses for each validity scale or clinical scale are next plotted graphically in the form of T-scores (see Fig. 4-2), which approximate the normal (Gaussian) frequency distribution (see Fig. 4-1) in the general population. Each scale is plotted along a separate *vertical* line and has a mean T-score of 50, and a standard deviation of 10. Hence, one standard deviation above the population mean corresponds with a T-score of 60, two standard deviations above the mean with a T-score of 70, and so on.

This means that about half the population will exceed a T-score of 50 on any *single* scale; 15.9 percent will exceed a T-score of 60; and about 2.3 percent will obtain a T-score higher than 70 on any single scale. However, the combined probability of obtaining a T-score higher than 70 on *at least one scale* (i.e., one or more scales) is much higher. Since elevations on the scales are *not* mutually exclusive, about 15 to 20 percent of normal persons are found to have a T-score above 70 on at least 1 of the 10 clinical MMPI scales. In a sample of psychiatric inpatients, however, about 75 percent of those cooperating with testing soon after admission were found to have at least one T-score over 70.

Responses on the four *validity scales* of the MMPI (scales ?, L, F, and K) indicate the subject's test-taking attitude. The first of these scales (?) represents questions left unanswered, which are usually few in number and can be ignored (or scored twice, in both a deviant and a normal direction, to give two boundary profiles, the space between which would include all possibilities). Marked elevations on the F (frequency) scale suggest *overstatement* of emotional problems, which may occur for various reasons, including confusion, lack of comprehension, or a deliberate "faking sick." Elevations on a number of clinical scales are likely to be exaggerated when the F scale is high enough to render the profile invalid. Elevations of scale L (lie) and K (correction) tend to

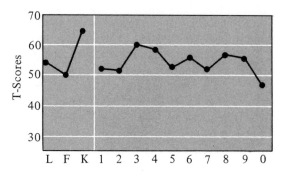

Figure 4-2.

indicate *understatement* of emotional problems, or a tendency to conceal psychopathology, as in Figure 4-2.

In this profile, the elevations on L and K scales indicate an extremely guarded and defensive test-taking attitude. This person is only admitting to socially acceptable attitudes, is minimizing emotional problems, and is denying painful reality or unpleasant feelings or motives. Although all ten clinical scales are well within normal limits, the marked defensiveness indicates that the profile is probably invalid.

The ten *clinical scales* of the MMPI were derived from the responses of persons with deviant character traits or specific forms of psychiatric disorder. Marked elevations on these scales are associated with the following traits or diagnoses: hypochondriasis (Hs or 1); depression (D or 2); hysteria (Hy or 3) — more frequently conversion than dissociation; psychopathic deviation (Pd or 4) — antisocial personality; masculinity-femininity (Mf or 5) — elevation indicates attributes more typical for the opposite sex; paranoid state (Pa or 6); psychasthenic *neurosis* (Pt or 7) — anxiety and obsessive-compulsive traits; schizophrenic *psychosis* (Sc or 8); mania (Ma or 9); social introversion (Si or 0). Before reading the interpretation beneath the following profile, it may be helpful for you to try to make your own interpretation.

This profile (Fig. 4-3) appears to be technically valid, but shows marked elevations on depression (2) and other *neurotic* scales (7 and 3), with social introversion or withdrawal (0), and somatic complaints in excess of organic dis-

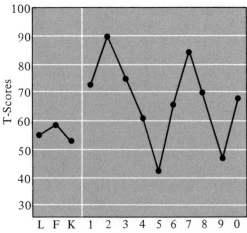

Figure 4-3.

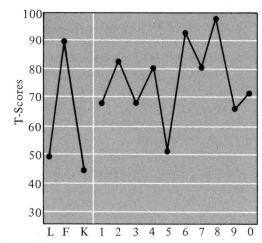

Figure 4-4.

ease (1). Combined elevations of several scales are more frequent than isolated elevations of a single scale. The three scales most often elevated in neurotic patients are 2 (D), 3 (Hy), and 7 (Pt). The four scales most often elevated in *psychotic* patients or those with antisocial personality disorders are scales 4 (Pd), 6 (Pa), 8 (Sc), and 9 (Ma). The following is another relatively frequent profile among recently admitted psychiatric inpatients.

The marked elevation on scale F (Fig. 4-4) renders the profile of doubtful validity due to overstatement, but if intellectual function is within normal limits (i.e., an IQ of more than 80), one

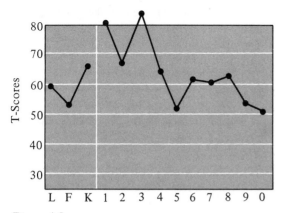

Figure 4-5.

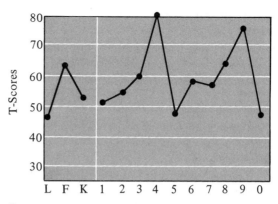

Figure 4-6.

could conclude that the subject was not too confused to respond to MMPI test questions. This patient is reporting grossly psychotic — schizophrenic (8) and paranoid (6) — symptoms, with accompanying depression (2), social alienation or impulsive behavior (4), anxiety (7), and social withdrawal (0). He or she may be psychotic or deliberately faking psychosis.

Now let us turn to the profile of an adult female patient who is likely to be under the care of an internist or a neurologist.

This profile (Fig. 4-5) is of doubtful validity due to defensive and guarded test-taking attitudes. There is a strong tendency to minimize emotional problems. The most prominent characteristics are somatic complaints without an adequate organic basis (scale 1), together with probable hysterical manifestations (scale 3). This person is likely to be viewed by others as having an exaggerated need for affection, demanding sympathy, and getting appreciable secondary gain from symptoms. There is a strong tendency toward denial of unpleasant reality, painful emotions, or unacceptable motives in the self or others. By contrast, let us turn to one further illustrative MMPI profile with a pattern that is more likely to be found in an adolescent or young adult male.

This profile (Fig. 4-6) appears to be valid, with no tendency to exaggerate or minimize problems at this time. The most prominent characteristics are likely to be the uninhibited acting out of sexual

and aggressive impulses. There is a probable history of behavior problems since early childhood, with long-standing underachievement, impulsiveness, and a strong tendency to manipulate and blame others. This person is likely to impress others as having insufficient self-control, and as being egocentric and self-indulgent. There is resentment of authority figures with frequent resistance or rebellion, and a strong possibility of excessive use of or dependency on alcohol or other drugs. Employment history is likely to be erratic, with an even stronger probability of poor marital adjustment, leading to frequent separation and divorce. The most likely diagnosis would be antisocial personality, but a significant minority may show manic or other psychotic disorders.

We should be careful not to use psychological tests to provide diagnostic labels that become self-fulfilling prophecies. Test results themselves may change as subjects change during therapy. However, psychological tests may help to lead us to the most effective therapy in the shortest possible time.

REVIEW QUESTIONS

44. The Wechsler Adult Intelligence Scale (WAIS):
    (A) measures the innate intellectual ability of the subject
    (B) includes both verbal and performance subtests
    (C) provides little help in differentiating organic from functional pathology

(D) all of the above
(E) none of the above

45. When repeated applications of a psychological test produce similar results in similar circumstances, the test may be described as:
    (A) valid
    (B) objective
    (C) culture-free
    (D) biased
    (E) reliable

46. A major reason for the widespread use of the MMPI is:
    (A) administration and scoring require little special skill
    (B) it is relatively unaffected by the subject's *current* mental status
    (C) it has high validity even when the subject is poorly motivated
    (D) it provides more information on dynamics than do projective tests
    (E) it has high validity for discriminating between organic and functional pathology

47. Each of the following is useful for investigating the hidden motives and fantasies of preadolescent children *except:*
    (A) MMPI
    (B) modeling clay
    (C) finger painting
    (D) Children's Apperception Test (CAT)
    (E) Draw-A-Person Test (DAP)

48. The intellectual functioning of a 32-year-old mentally retarded man whose estimated IQ is 25 is comparable to that achieved by the average person whose chronological age is:
    (A) 2 years
    (B) 4 years
    (C) 8 years
    (D) 16 years
    (E) 25 years

49. A 20-year-old woman has an IQ of 130. Her intellectual functioning can be described as:
    (A) equal to that of the average person of age 26
    (B) unimpaired at the time of testing
    (C) in the upper 3 percent of the population
    (D) all of the above
    (E) none of the above

50. Approximately 50 percent of the general population have IQ scores in the range of:
    (A) 70 to 100
    (B) 84 to 116
    (C) 90 to 110
    (D) 68 to 132
    (E) 90 and above

51. A T-score of 80 on the F scale of the MMPI is *least* likely to indicate:
    (A) malingering
    (B) comprehension difficulty
    (C) random responding
    (D) severe psychopathology
    (E) denial of psychopathology

Summary of Directions

A	B	C	D	E
1, 2, 3 only	1, 3 only	2, 4 only	4 only	All are correct

---

52. The Shipley-Hartford Test:
    (1) provides a numerical estimate of IQ
    (2) is helpful in detecting organic intellectual impairment
    (3) measures both verbal and abstract thinking
    (4) is used as a projective test

53. The Bender-Gestalt Test:
    (1) provides a numerical estimate of IQ
    (2) is helpful in detecting organic intellectual impairment
    (3) measures both verbal and abstract thinking
    (4) is used as a projective test

54. Factors which affect IQ scores include:
    (1) educational background
    (2) hereditary endowment
    (3) test-taking motivation
    (4) anxiety level

55. Projective psychological tests differ from objective tests by:
    (1) having definite right and wrong answers
    (2) greater dependence on indeterminate stimuli
    (3) being better standardized
    (4) requiring specialized training and greater experience for meaningful interpretation

SELECTED REFERENCES

1. Anastasi, A. (1968). *Psychological Testing.* New York: Macmillan.

2. Cronbach, L.J. (1970). *Essentials of Psychological Testing* (2nd Ed.). New York: Harper & Row.

3. Good, P.K., and Brantner, J.P. (1974). *A Practical Guide to the MMPI.* Minneapolis: University of Minnesota Press.

4. Horst, P. (1966). *Psychological Measurements and Prediction.* Belmont, California: Wadsworth Publishing Co.

5. Lachar, D. (1974). *The MMPI: Clinical Assessment and Automated Interpretation.* Los Angeles: Western Psychological Services.

6. Weiner, I.B. [Ed.] (1976). *Clinical Methods in Psychology.* New York: Wiley-Interscience.

5. Psychosocial Determinants of Behavior and Psychopathology

Men's natures are alike; it is their habits that carry them far apart.
Confucius

LEARNING AND UNLEARNING

It has been said that man differs from animals in that he drinks when he is not thirsty and mates all the year round. Many a true word is spoken in jest, and sexual behavior does illustrate an evolutionary progression in the relative significance of learning as contrasted with genetic programming.

Lower organisms may have complex reproductive rituals (courtship, mating, etc.) that are automatized by genetic coding and mediated by hormonal control. Male and female rats raised in isolation from infancy will mate successfully by instinct on attaining biological maturity. This will occur on the first occasion that they are placed together, provided the female is in the appropriate stage of the estrus cycle. Rhesus monkeys, by contrast, must learn how to interact socially and sexually if they are to mate successfully. In their extensive comparison of sexual behavior in many species of animals and in 190 human societies, Ford and Beach noted that the cerebral cortex has assumed a greater and greater degree of direction over all behavior, including that of a sexual nature. They concluded that human behavior is more variable and more easily affected by learning and social conditioning than is that of any other species.

Learning may be defined as any relatively permanent change in behavior that results from past experience. Not all learning involves improvement in behavior, and in fact some learning may be undesirable in its consequences. Moreover, some changes in behavior that take place with repetition are not the result of learning but of growth, fatigue, or physical damage.

One factor common to many situations in which learning takes place is *association,* which involves some connection in time and place between two events. Association is a basic process in learning; however, *motivation* is often an important prerequisite for learning to take place, or for the practical application of previous learning to the solution of new problems.

In Chapter 1 we focused on unconscious dynamic forces and mechanisms of adaptation, psychoanalytic concepts of personality development, and the interpersonal communication of affect and role expectation. In Chapter 2 we presented a description of psychopathology, and discussed the impact of loss, frustration, and conflict on affect and behavior. In the present chapter we shall consider further psychosocial determinants, beginning with the following major aspects of learning: respondent conditioning; operant conditioning; imitation; escape and avoidance learning; avoidable punishment; unpredictable and unavoidable punishment.

Respondent Conditioning (Classical or Pavlovian Conditioning)

Respondent conditioning refers to the type of learning studied in the classical experiments of the Russian physiologist Ivan P. Pavlov. The process involves a simple reflex response to a specific stimulus, which is paired with a hitherto neutral stimulus during the process of conditioning. Pavlov worked with dogs and measured their salivary secretion in response to various stimuli. Others have worked with various species, including man, and with other forms of reflex response to stimulation.

If a hungry animal is presented with food, it will salivate. In this situation food represents an *unconditioned stimulus* (UCS), and salivary secretion represents the corresponding *unconditioned response* (UCR). If now the presentation of food is repeatedly accompanied by the presentation of some hitherto neutral stimulus (e.g., buzzer, bell, or tuning fork) the latter becomes a *conditioned stimulus* (CS) capable of eliciting salivation, which is now a *conditioned response* (CR).

The development of a conditioned response takes place through *reinforcement* of the conditioned stimulus, by pairing it with the unconditioned stimulus (i.e., food). When the conditioned stimulus or signal is presented alone, without the unconditioned stimulus or food, the conditioned response is *nonreinforced*. When there is repeated presentation of the conditioned stimulus with nonreinforcement, the conditioned response will then tend to diminish in strength or to disappear completely through the process of *extinction*.

Complete extinction does *not* mean that a response has been permanently eliminated or unlearned, however. If the animal is subsequently returned to the laboratory after a period of rest, without any further reinforcement, the conditioned response is usually found to have reappeared (at less than its earlier strength) through *spontaneous recovery*. Moreover, it will tend once more to attain maximum strength with *less* reinforcement of the conditioned stimulus than was necessary in the original process of conditioning.

Classical conditioning is a process of *stimulus substitution,* in which a previously neutral stimulus acquires the power to evoke a response originally evoked only by some other specific stimulus. At first, however, there is a strong tendency to *stimulus generalization,* so that a dog conditioned to salivate at the sound of a tuning fork may also salivate at the sound of a buzzer or a bell, or almost any other noise that is made in the laboratory. The more similar the new stimulus is to the conditioned stimulus, the greater the tendency for the conditioned response to occur in the absence of reinforcement. However, if all stimuli with the exception of the specific conditioned stimulus go unreinforced, the animal will eventually learn perceptual *discrimination,* and the conditioned response will be elicited only by the appropriate stimulus — e.g., only one of many bells or a tuning fork with a specific frequency or tone.

Each of the situations previously outlined involves *primary reinforcement* of the conditioned stimulus by the specific unconditioned stimulus (i.e., food). Pavlov also found, however, that a conditioned stimulus (i.e., the signal alone, without food) would serve effectively as a form of *secondary reinforcement* for another, different

conditioned stimulus to produce the desired response. The strength of the latter response tends to be less than that of the original conditioned response, since secondary reinforcement is accompanied by gradual extinction of the response (which is no longer paired with the primary reinforcer). Pavlov was able to carry this higher-order conditioning one step further, and obtain weak responses to a third-order stimulus, but this was the limit of the process.

In much of the literature on classical conditioning, both the unconditioned and conditioned stimuli have been presented through the exteroceptive organs of sensation such as eyes and ears. However, there have also been many studies on interoceptive conditioning, involving internal bodily perception and reflexes in both animal and human subjects. The subject is more likely to be unaware of such interoceptive stimuli, and the process of conditioning tends to be slower in development, but more fixed and irreversible — i.e., less readily extinguished. It appears likely that early conditioning of this nature has a lasting impact on various physiological functions, and may be relevant to the development of psychophysiological disorders.

Operant Conditioning (Instrumental Learning)

Operant conditioning is a process in which a behavioral response is strengthened by subsequent reinforcement that is contingent on the response being made. One of the first attempts to study changes of behavior brought about by its consequences was reported by Edward Lee Thorndike in 1898. He placed a hungry cat in a box from which it could escape by unlatching the door and thereby get access to food outside the box. At first the animal exhibited various kinds of agitated behavior, and considerable time elapsed before it opened the door by accident. However, after the cat had been placed in the box repeatedly, the behavior leading to its escape occurred at progressively shorter intervals, until it could leave the cage immediately. Thorndike used the term *law of effect* to describe this form of learning. It subsequently became known as *operant* conditioning, since the behavior operates on the environment to attain a desirable result. It may also be known as *instrumental* learning, since the behavior is instrumental in generating reinforcing consequences.

The strength of operant learning may be measured by monitoring the *frequency* of a given response. B. F. Skinner designed a darkened sound-resistant box in which rats are able to obtain a pellet of food by pressing a lever. The lever is connected with a recording system that produces a graphic tracing of the *number of lever-pressings,* plotted against the *length of time* that the rat is in the box. The strength of learning under various conditions is shown by the rate of response (lever-pressing) during reinforcement, and by both the rate of response and total number of responses during nonreinforcement and extinction.

This type of learning has been studied in many species, including man, and is more relevant to the development of personality and psychopathology than is respondent conditioning. However, there are many similarities between the two processes, including the general laws of reinforcement, extinction, spontaneous recovery, generalization, and discrimination outlined in the previous section.

Reinforcement is necessary for the formation or maintenance of a conditioned response. Without reinforcement, the desired response is either not formed or extinguished. *Positive reinforcement* consists of the presentation of desirable consequences (e.g., food, water, or sexual contact). *Negative reinforcement* results from the removal of unpleasant stimuli (such as a loud noise, a very bright light, extreme cold or heat, or painful electric shock). Negative reinforcement (removal of aversive stimuli) should be contrasted with *punishment* — which involves either the presentation of a negative reinforcer (aversive stimulus) or removal of a positive reinforcer. Various aspects of punishment will be considered later, after a discussion of escape and avoidance learning.

Extinction requires that responses be made in the absence of reinforcement, and is generally a more effective way of reducing or eliminating such responses than either punishment or forgetting. In *forgetting,* the effect of conditioning wears off

gradually as time passes, but no nonreinforced responses are elicited during this time. Extinction of a response may occur quite rapidly, whereas forgetting is apt to be a slow process, and Skinner reported sizable extinction curves of as long as 6 years in pigeons (about half the life span of the pigeon) after the response had last been reinforced. The effectiveness of extinction in eliminating a response may be further increased by reinforcement of an incompatible response, resulting in competitive or reciprocal inhibition of the response that it is desired to eliminate.

As in the case of respondent conditioning, the satisfaction of any primary physiological drive (e.g., for food, water, or sexual contact) for purposes of learning is termed *primary reinforcement,* while the satisfaction of drives toward learned goals is termed *secondary reinforcement.* A secondary or conditioned reinforcer may provide generalized reinforcement (positive or negative) when it has been paired with more than one primary reinforcer. Several important generalized reinforcers arise when behavior is reinforced by other people. Thus behavior is reinforced when it secures the attention of others, is reinforced more strongly when it obtains their approval, and more strongly still when it results in manifestations of affection. Another example of learned or secondary reinforcement that is generalized is the rewarding of behavior with money.

In operant conditioning, new behavior may be acquired by differential reinforcement through successive approximations. This involves the reinforcement of those elements of available responses that resemble the final form of behavior that is desired, while component responses having little or no similarity to this behavior are left unrewarded and hence extinguished. By gradually raising the requirements for reinforcement in the direction of the final form that the behavior is to take, available responses can be shaped into patterns that did not previously exist in the repertoire of the organism.

Partial or intermittent reinforcement schedules result in behavioral responses that are more resistant to extinction than when they have been learned by reinforcement every time the response occurs. Simple types of intermittent reinforcement consist of *fixed-ratio* schedules (with reinforcement after a specified number of responses have occurred), or *fixed-interval* schedules (with reinforcement after a specified period of time has elapsed, if a response has occurred within this time). Intermittent reinforcement is therefore a mixture of a conditioning process and an extinction process.

Even greater resistance to extinction results from *variable-ratio* and *variable-interval* schedules of reinforcement, in which either the number of unreinforced responses or the time interval between reinforced responses is permitted to vary around some average value. In everyday life, most social reinforcers are dispensed on *variable-combined* schedules, in which both the number of unreinforced responses *and* the time intervals between reinforced responses are allowed to vary. Moreover, social reinforcement is likely to depend on the frequency as well as the nature and magnitude of the response.

If variable reinforcement is administered when the subject is responding at a high rate, the outcome will be a stable *high* rate of response. Variable reinforcement administered only when the subject is responding at a low rate results in stable *low* rates of response. Variable schedules of reinforcement therefore result in behavior sustained at the frequency at which it is maximally reinforced. For example, a compulsive gambling habit may be exceedingly difficult to overcome in spite of continued heavy losses because of the erratic reinforcement schedule. This is only one of the many forms of maladaptive behavior that are learned by trial and error, and perpetuated by the unintentional intermittent reinforcement of undesirable responses having high magnitude and/or frequency. Such behavior is therefore persistent, difficult to extinguish, and baffling for the reinforcing agents (e.g., parents or spouse) who have been responsible for its origin and maintenance.

Imitation

Bandura and Walters emphasized the role of imitation in acquiring deviant, as well as socially con-

forming, behavior. There is considerable evidence that learning may occur through observation of the behavior of others, even when the observer does *not* reproduce the model's responses during acquisition, and therefore receives no *direct* reinforcement. Since eliciting and maintaining imitative behavior are highly dependent on the response consequences *to the model,* an adequate social learning theory should recognize the significance of vicarious reinforcement, by which the behavior of an observer is modified by the reinforcement administered to the model.

Effective social learning requires both adequate generalization and sharp discriminations. Thus, mild physical aggression toward peers is often rewarded as a sign of masculinity in boys, but more intense responses of this kind are often punished. Even mild physical aggression toward parents or siblings is considered undesirable and consequently goes unrewarded or may be punished. On the other hand, specific forms of physical aggression may be permitted, encouraged, and rewarded in certain social contexts. Highly aggressive boys have been found to have parents who strongly disapprove of aggression *in the home,* and who reprimand and punish them for it while encouraging and rewarding aggression *outside the home.* Similarly, prejudices against minority groups, and the scapegoating of out-group members, may result from discrimination learning in which hostile-aggressive attitudes and behavior toward members of these groups have long been observed and rewarded.

Social training is viewed largely as teaching a child to express aggressiveness, dependency, and other social responses only in certain ways. Social learning concepts of personality development consequently emphasize the *continuity of behavioral responses within the individual, and differences between individuals* (which may result from biological, psychological, or sociocultural determinants). In this respect these concepts differ from the stage theories of personality development that emphasize variations within the individual over periods of time, and similarities among individuals at specified ages.

Escape and Avoidance Learning

Escape learning results from negative reinforcement of behavior that leads to termination of aversive stimulation. *Avoidance learning* consists of learning to avoid or prevent aversive stimulation before it occurs. These two forms of learning appear to involve elements of both respondent conditioning and operant conditioning. The learning of avoidance behavior is generally preceded by learning how to escape from the unpleasant situation, as in the following classical experiment:

A dog was placed in a shuttle box divided in two by a low partition over which the dog could easily jump. Each side of the floor consisted of an electric grid through which shock could be administered to the dog. In each training trial, a buzzer was turned on, and after ten seconds the floor on the dog's side of the compartment was electrified. The shock continued until the dog jumped over the partition. Since the jumping response was instrumental in terminating shock, this *escape* behavior was reinforced. Initially there were long intervals between onset of shock and successful escape by jumping the barrier. Then the dog abruptly learned prompt escape behavior, and within a few more trials was consistently *avoiding* any shock by jumping within the ten-second warning period.

In analyzing this learning experiment, there were three recognizable stages. The first involved the classical conditioning of a fear response to the buzzer that was associated with unpleasant shock. Operant conditioning then involved negative reinforcement of escape behavior, and finally avoidance of any further aversive stimulation.

Once such avoidance learning has taken place it is *extremely resistant to extinction*. In some experiments, dogs have been known to jump on signal for thousands of trials after the shock was completely turned off. This is because the avoidance response is reinforced by relief from fear, and it continues to keep the subject away from the primary reinforcement so that there is no opportunity for extinction. However, it may be possible to extinguish the avoidance response experimentally by repeatedly presenting the signal (i.e., the buzzer) in the absence of the aversive stimulation (i.e., shock) while preventing escape or avoidance behavior from taking place.

PUNISHMENT (AVOIDABLE vs. INESCAPABLE)

Punishment may involve either the addition of a negative reinforcer (aversive stimulus) or the removal of a positive one. While punishment may result in escape or avoidance learning, and may produce *suppression* of an existing learned response, it does *not* lead to extinction (which results only from nonreinforcement). In general, punishment reduces or eliminates learned responses only temporarily, and does *not* diminish the total number of responses obtained during a subsequent program of extinction. When a response is strongly motivated and there is no alternative response available, punishment is relatively ineffective in eliminating that response. In the case of child training, frequent or severe punishment by parents has the disadvantage that it tends to drive the child away from the potential source of most positive reinforcement for socially acceptable behavior.

What made punishment effective in the avoidance learning situation described above is the following: failure to make a response, rather than a previously established habit, was punished. The motivation to make any response at all was low, but a response permitting avoidance of the punishment was readily available. There was a definite cue, in this case the stimulus buzzer, that warned of impending punishment. This punishment was consistently administered for failure to make the correct response. Finally, the punishment was a strong one.

By contrast, mild punishment may sometimes serve as a secondary *positive* reinforcer in the learning of new responses, and in maintaining them once they have been learned. If a hungry animal is fed only after a mild electric shock to its leg, it will soon learn to welcome the shock as preliminary to feeding. Human infants have shown pleasurable interpretation of a previously resented needle prick if it was followed repeatedly by feeding. A sexual masochist may first attain orgasm under circumstances of discomfort or pain, and subsequently continue to obtain sexual gratification by submitting himself to whipping or other painful experiences. Punishment may sometimes act as a generalized positive reinforcer since this type of attention may be preferable to being completely ignored. Such findings are compatible with Freud's hypothesis of the repetition compulsion, whereby an individual repeatedly re-enacts certain life situations regardless of seemingly unpleasant emotions and consequences.

Unpredictable and Inescapable Punishment

The dog in the experiment described above had no previous experience with electric shock, and ran frantically around the shuttle box until it accidentally scrambled over the barrier and escaped the shock. Seligman and his associates have shown a strikingly different pattern of behavior in dogs that had previously received inescapable shock. The dog's first reactions to shock in the shuttle box were much the same as those of the naive animal — it ran around frantically for about thirty seconds. But then it stopped moving, lay down, and quietly whined while continuing to experience painful electric shock. On all succeeding trials the dog failed to escape, a finding referred to as *learned helplessness.*

Helplessness with respect to one aversive experience generalizes to another, and reduces motivation to initiate responses of any kind. On the basis of these and further extensive studies, Seligman and his associates elaborated the following theory of helplessness: "The expectation that an outcome is independent of responding (1) reduces the motivation to control the outcome; (2) interferes with learning that responding controls the outcome; and, if the outcome is traumatic, (3) produces *fear* for as long as the subject is uncertain of the uncontrollability of the outcome, and then produces *depression."*

This theory suggests a way to cure induced helplessness, and a way to prevent it from occurring. Cure is accomplished by placing the dog in a situation of escapable punishment and forcing it repeatedly to escape. Prevention may be accom-

plished by *behavioral immunization* — by first exposing the animal to a series of escapable shocks, and only subsequently to inescapable shock (the response to which is then readily reversible).

Imprisonment and Brainwashing, or Thought Reform

These studies on helplessness in animals have a poignant parallel in observations on human prisoners subjected to abuse and/or indoctrination. The past three wars in Southeast Asia have all yielded accounts of debility, dependency, and dread, with prolonged survival based on hope, or death based on helplessness and despair.

Whether in military prisons, or in the civilian communist population, *brainwashing,* or *thought reform,* consists of two basic elements that have been analyzed at length by Lifton. These are *confession,* the exposure and renunciation of past and present "evil"; and *reeducation,* the remaking of a man in the communist image. In a well-known speech delivered to party members in 1942, Mao Tse-tung laid down the basic principles of punishment and cure that were repeatedly elaborated on by later writers. He specified that two principles must be observed. The first is "Punish the past to warn the future," and the second, "Save men by curing their ills."

These two principles appear to involve a combination of external force, or coercion, with an appeal to inner enthusiasm through evangelistic exhortation. Coercion and breakdown rather than exhortation have often been more prominent aspects of prison and military programs, along with various techniques of interrogation and indoctrination. Among the techniques used to extort false confessions of germ warfare from captured American military personnel were periods of solitary confinement (with associated sensory isolation) and sometimes sleep deprivation. Both of the latter processes have been studied in recent years and shown to be capable of precipitating episodes of psychotic reality distortion, with clouding of consciousness, hallucinations, and the possible development of delusional ideation. Both processes may also precipitate or accentuate the symptoms of naturally occurring psychoses such as schizophrenia.

CRITICAL PERIODS IN EARLY EXPERIENCE

There are at least three ways in which early experience differs from experience occurring later in life: (1) Susceptibility to stress is high in young animals and decreases sharply to a level that then remains relatively constant. Mild or moderate developmental stress may improve adaptation, but severe stress is likely to have permanently adverse or fatal consequences. (2) The probability of certain social responses is higher in young animals than in older animals that have passed through the critical period for developing such responses. (3) The consequences of early experience are often more generalized and less specific than those of the same experience at a later age. An adult rat that receives an electric shock while eating from a white dish learns to avoid white dishes, but is otherwise much the same as before. A younger rat shocked in a similar manner shows excessive emotionality in many situations.

At the beginning of the present century, Craig noted that certain animals developed sexual fixations on objects that were not members of their own species. In order to cross two species of wild pigeons, he found that the young of one species had to be reared with foster parents of the other species. On reaching adulthood, the birds that had been reared in this manner were found to prefer mates of the same species as their foster parents. Heinroth reared several species of birds himself and found that social responses became directed toward the human keeper rather than toward members of the same species. Konrad Lorenz extended these experiments using geese, and termed this process *imprinting,* since there appeared to be a rapid and lasting stamping of the impression of the mother object on the young animal. He noted a critical period early in the life of the animal during which the experience must occur in order for it to develop such an attachment. The critical period for imprinting in chicks and ducklings is the first 32 hours after hatching, with maximum effectiveness from 13 to 16 hours after hatching.

Critical periods for the formation of social bonds have also been established in a variety of species of fish, insects, and mammals. John Paul Scott analyzed critical learning periods in the puppy, and found a period of great change in sensitivity to social relationships between the ages of 3 weeks and about 10 weeks. The puppy's experiences during this time were found to determine which animals and human beings would become his closest social relatives. Scott and Fuller therefore defined a critical period as a *special time in life when a small amount of experience will produce a great effect on later behavior.*

They drew the analogy of pulling the trigger on a high-powered rifle, whereby a small amount of effort causes the bullet to travel at high speed and produce a smashing impact at a great distance. However, *the critical period is a relative rather than an absolute concept.* Scott and Fuller stated, "The difference between the amount of effort needed to produce the same effect at different periods determines just how critical the period is. In the case of the puppy it looks as if a small amount of contact shortly after three weeks of age will produce a strong social relation, which can be duplicated only by hours or weeks of patient effort at later periods in life — if, indeed, it can be duplicated at all."

This development of social bonds does not appear to depend on feeding or contact comfort. Whether rewarded, punished, or treated indifferently, the young animal of the proper age proceeds to form an emotional attachment to whatever is present in the environment at that time. However, the presence of a mother or mother substitute appears to greatly diminish the impact, and possible fatal consequences, of stress or aversive stimulation in infancy.

By contrast, Seymour Levine showed that both painful shocks and gentle handling may enhance the development of normal stress responses in infant rats, whereas isolation and understimulation may lead to disturbed physiology and behavior when the animal matures. The original experiment was repeated many times, subjecting infant rats to a variety of stresses and degrees of handling. Invariably, it was the nonmanipulated controls that exhibited deviations of behavior and physiology when they were tested as adults. When placed in unfamiliar surroundings, the animals that had not been manipulated tended to cower in a corner or to creep cautiously about, frequently urinating or defecating. Animals that had been handled and subjected to stress in infancy explored their surroundings freely and showed no evidence of undue emotionality. The impaired behavioral response of nonmanipulated animals in strange situations corresponded with diminished output of steroid hormones by the adrenal cortex.

Even more adverse consequences from *developmental isolation* were reported by Harlow and his associates in a series of well-known experiments on rhesus monkeys. Some infant monkeys were raised and nursed by their mothers, while others were separated from their mothers 6 to 12 hours after birth and suckled on tiny nursing bottles. Among the latter group, some were raised in isolation in a wire cage, while others were permitted to establish physical contact with, and emotional dependence on, a cloth-covered substitute, or mother surrogate. In all cases the surrogate was preferred to a similar plain wire frame without the cloth covering. The inanimate cloth mother surrogate could readily become an object loved with intensity and for a long period of time. Harlow concluded that satisfactory body contact is an extremely strong affectional variable, and may well prove to be the most important affectional variable for primates.

In an attempt to establish experimental neuroses in infant monkeys, various mother surrogates were constructed that subjected the monkeys to unpleasant stimuli or experiences. These all seemed ineffective in destroying the security and satisfaction obtained from clinging to this surrogate, or in producing evidence of subsequent abnormal behavior.

Monkeys living with their own mothers and some of the monkeys reared with cloth surrogates were permitted interaction, in a controlled playpen or playroom, with other young monkeys of the same and of the opposite sex. An outstanding finding in both the playroom and playpen was that male and female infants showed differences in behavior from the second month of life onward. Young males demonstrated a much higher frequency of threatening behavior toward animals of both sexes, whereas young females demonstrated a much higher frequency of withdrawal and immobility. Young males initiated play contact with other animals much more frequently than did young females, while rough-and-tumble play was largely restricted to pairs of young males.

On reaching adult life, male and female monkeys reared in isolation showed many abnormalities of behavior, including fear of and aggression toward other monkeys, an absence of grooming responses, and an inability to participate in normal sexual union with other mature monkeys. After prolonged and patient education by sexually sophisticated male monkeys, some of the isolated females became sexually receptive, but none of the isolated males ever mated with sexually experienced females. Although a number of isolated females became pregnant, they became rejecting and abusive mothers (at least toward the firstborn), from whom the offspring had to be rescued in order to ensure survival. There is a close resemblance between this behavior and the learned transmission of emotional deprivation from human parents to their own offspring.

PARENTAL DEPRIVATION IN HUMANS

Freud remarked that adults with psychopathology often have a chronic scar rather than an acute bleeding wound. There have since been many searches for the original traumas or childhood roots of adult psychopathology. It is generally conceded that traumatic situations operating over long periods of time are more likely to have lasting adverse consequences than are isolated traumatic events. It has still proved difficult to identify and measure the traumatic situations of childhood that are relevant to adult psychopathology.

Permanent loss of a parent during childhood represents one situation that may increase vulnerability to certain forms of psychopathology. George Pollock write as follows: "The death of a parent in childhood is always a traumatic event affecting the development of the survivor's personality. The trauma is not only mediated through the separation, loss, and absence of the deceased parent, but also contact with the surviving parent and family members who may themselves have mourning reactions that may alter their contact with the child."

Along similar lines, Felix Brown stated, "Our hypothesis is that a child can be *sensitized* by situations of loss of love and emotional deprivation, so that he breaks down in various ways in later life when faced with subsequent situations of loss and rejection." However, it is important to recognize that the *impact* (as well as the frequency) of such loss and deprivation may be greatly increased or reduced by membership in a given family or socioeconomic group.

In the well-known monograph *Maternal Care and Mental Health,* John Bowlby reviewed three major classes of evidence concerning the effects of parental deprivation. Many studies involve the direct impact of separation from parents on the physical health and behavior of young children. Another large group of studies concern retrospective reports on childhood parental loss among adolescents or older persons who have developed various forms of psychopathology. Relatively few studies involve long-term anterospective (follow-up) comparisons between the behavior of groups of persons who have or have not been subjected to various forms of earlier parental deprivation.

Direct studies of children separated from their parents do indicate a high probability of a severe grief reaction, with social withdrawal and impaired appetite, that may also be associated with increased mortality. Children surviving in impersonal institutions have also shown a high frequency of subsequent delinquent behavior.

A number of early *retrospective studies* of delinquent adolescents showed that a high proportion came from homes that were broken by the death of a parent or by permanent separation. In one of the best controlled of these studies, Sheldon and Eleanor Glueck compared 500 persistently delinquent boys with 500 nondelinquent boys matched for age, intelligence, ethnic background, and residence in underprivileged neighborhoods. They found that delinquents had experienced all varieties of parental loss during early childhood much more frequently than had the nondelinquent control group. However, one aspect of this study that did not receive sufficient recognition is that permanent loss of the father was much more frequent than permanent loss of the mother among these delinquent boys.

Anterospective studies appear to confirm this association between loss of the father and delinquency in boys, and also to reveal an association between loss of the mother and delinquency in girls. A number of studies also suggested an unduly high frequency of parental death (particularly of the mother) during the childhood of adults who develop schizophrenic psychoses. However, the latter finding may well be attributable to low socioeconomic status, which in turn is correlated with high frequencies both of mortality and of schizophrenia (as well as certain other forms of psychopathology).

A number of studies have indicated an association between death of a parent during childhood and vulnerability to depression during adult life. Beck and his associates reported increased frequencies of childhood bereavement among adult patients with various psychiatric diagnoses who also scored high on an inventory designed to measure depression. These findings were independent not only of clinical diagnosis, but probably also of the age of the patient.

RELATIONSHIPS WITH PARENTS, SIBLINGS, AND PEERS

It is difficult to establish objective evidence on qualitative aspects of childhood relationships and vulnerability to development of psychopathology many years later. Retrospective information based on subjective recall is subject to distortion. The harder we search for adverse childhood experiences, the more we are likely to find, even in those who adapt successfully. However, clinical experience dictates that childhood relationships continue to be accorded a major role in the determination of adult psychopathology. This is true regardless of success or failure with psychotherapy. Learned psychopathology may still be very resistant to change.

Parental behavior may modify childhood personality development in a variety of ways: by various forms and schedules of reinforcement; by the conditions under which behavior is ignored and extinguished; by the nature and consistency of punishment that may be avoidable or inescapable; and through the child's imitation of the attitudes and behavior of parents, siblings, and other models. Actions speak louder than words, and children are sensitive to the nonverbal communications of affect and role expectation that may belie the accompanying words. Parents and peers may reinforce inappropriate affect and maladaptive behavior in a variety of subtle ways.

For normal social development it appears that children require close and enduring relationships with a parent or parent substitute of each sex, and with peers of both sexes outside of the family (which normal parents start to encourage during the preschool years). It has been remarked that discipline without love is revenge, whereas love without discipline is anarchy. An emotionally secure parent is able to accept the emotional lability and periodic anger of a young child, to enforce firm but compassionate controls on the child's behavior, and to encourage gradual appropriate emancipation and independence. Discipline is not based on inconsistent angry feelings of the parent, as is often found in the histories of delinquent children (and antisocial adults). Disapproval or punishment is directed toward the prevention of socially harmful behavior, rather than the provocation of guilt within the child, as is often found in neurotic and depressed patients.

The harsh superego of the typical neurotic tends to be associated with a history of excessive demands for conformity during childhood (reinforced by rewards and punishment), and identification with parents having high ideals and standards of behavior. The defective superego of the delinquent tends to be associated with a history of parental absence or indifference, inconsistent rewards and punishment, and identification with persons having antisocial ideals and standards.

Those reared in an atmosphere of acceptance, reasonable indulgence, and consistent, firm limit-setting, tend to develop confidence, trust, and affection. Those reared in an atmosphere of danger (e.g., inconsistent harsh punishment), indifference (e.g., absence of adequate rewards), rejection, and humiliation are likely to develop prevailing emotions of fear and hostility. These learned emotional responses tend to be generalized from the original person or situation onto others. There may, however, be specificity in the *displacement* of emotion from its original source onto other persons, as from a hostile, punitive parent onto other representatives of authority, or onto other persons of the same sex as that parent. Many wives appear to suffer from the earlier behavior of their husbands' mothers, and many husbands are punished for the earlier behavior of their wives' fathers.

The human family is unique in that it frequently contains two or more dependent offspring of different ages. The different children in a family do not all grow up in an identical environment, but may each have unique relationships with each parent as well as with brothers and sisters. Experiences that appear to affect the entire family, such as moving from one city to another, may have quite a different impact on each individual member of that family.

Sibling rivalry involves feelings of competition and jealousy between siblings, primarily for the attention, approval, and affection of the parents. This is most likely to be accentuated when siblings are close together in age and are of the same sex. Evidence of rivalry is often noted immediately after the birth of a new baby, in the form of aggressive or regressive behavior in the child who was previously the youngest member of the family. Such behavior is apt to be most severe and persistent when excessive attention is showered on the baby (e.g., an only son occurring after the birth of several girls, or vice versa), or when the displaced child is ignored, punished, or invited to display rivalry (by the parents' expectations that there would inevitably be difficulty). Signs of sibling rivalry are likely to be more marked in the first-born (who has never previously competed with other children for his parents' attention) at the time of the second birth than in the case of subsequent additions to the family. Displaced fathers also may regress and manifest hostility toward the firstborn or toward the eldest son, or toward the wife who has redirected some of her affection elsewhere. However, the nature and outcome of such conflicts are quite variable and do not bear a similar relationship to family structure or birth order of the children involved.

Note: Review questions for Chapters 5 and 6 are combined, and appear at the end of Chapter 6.

SELECTED REFERENCES

1. Bandura, A., and Walters, R.H. (1963). *Social Learning and Personality Development.* New York: Holt, Rinehart, and Winston.
2. Bowlby, J. (1952). *Maternal Care and Mental Health.* Geneva: World Health Organization (Monograph Series No. 2).
3. Fuller, J.L., and Waller, M.B. (1962). Is early experience different? In *Roots of Behavior,* edited by E. L. Bliss. New York: Hoeber.
4. Harlow, H.F. (1962). The heterosexual affectional system in monkeys. *American Psychologist,* vol. 17, pages 1–9.
5. Hulse, S.H. (1975). *The Psychology of Learning.* New York: McGraw-Hill.
6. Lifton, R.J. (1961). *Thought Reform and the Psychology of Totalism.* New York: W. W. Norton & Co.
7. Scott, J.P., and Fuller, J.L. (1965). *Genetics and the Social Behavior of the Dog.* Chicago: University of Chicago Press.
8. Seligman, M.E.P. (1975). *Helplessness.* San Francisco: W. H. Freeman and Co.
9. Skinner, B.F. (1953). *Science and Human Behavior.* New York: Macmillan.

6. Psychotherapies

If you will believe well of your fellow man, you may create the good you believe in.
William James

Psychotherapy is any form of treatment for mental, emotional, or behavioral disorders that is based primarily on verbal or nonverbal communication with the patient. Among the most important ways in which psychotherapies differ from one another are in the goals that they seek to achieve.

The goals of therapy may consist of improving adaptation by increasing insight into hitherto unconscious dynamics and disabling conflicts (psychoanalysis); of relieving symptoms and alleviating stress by means of ego support and reassurance (supportive psychotherapy); of fostering maturation and self-actualization (client-centered therapy); or of changing maladaptive behavior by applying learning theory (behavior therapies).

These goals may be accomplished by a variety of techniques, which may foster expression or suppression, verbalization or role-playing, clarification of conscious processes, or interpretation of hitherto unconscious motivation. The *role of the therapist* may be active or passive, directive or nondirective. *Patients in therapy* may be individuals, groups of patients, or two or more members of a single family. Various forms of psychotherapy differ in their conceptual framework and analysis of therapeutic transactions, as well as in their relative emphasis on past origins, present functioning, or future adaptation.

Although psychoanalytic theory and therapy have constituted the prevailing model for American psychiatry, the typical therapist's attitude toward his patient cuts across various theoretical orientations as the most important determinant of prognosis, treatment plan, and diagnosis. As therapists gain experience, they tend to assume a more active role in therapy, to take more initiative, make more interpretations, and behave more as individuals. With the confidence born of experience, trained therapists are not afraid to be themselves or to use their particular style of communication with their patients. There are many common elements in all approaches to psychotherapy as well as considerable differences between therapists of the same theoretical persuasion.

Those interested in technical similarities and differences may wish to refer to Harper's small volume comparing 36 systems of psychoanalysis and psychotherapy. The remainder of the present chapter will focus on the following six major approaches: (1) psychoanalytic therapy; (2) supportive psychotherapy; (3) client-centered therapy; (4) behavior therapies; (5) group and family therapies; and (6) transactional analysis.

PSYCHOANALYTIC THERAPY

Psychoanalysis and analytically oriented psychotherapies are *reconstructive* and *uncovering* forms of therapy. They not only seek to relieve symptoms but to effect changes in maladaptive character or personality. The attainment of more effective adaptation is fostered by the development of conscious awareness and insight into hitherto unconscious conflicts, fears, and inhibitions.

In their early publications on hysteria, Josef Breuer and Sigmund Freud described their technique of *cathartic hypnosis* for the recovery of early memories and feelings about some traumatic event. Hysterical symptoms resulting from the latter were removed by catharsis or *abreaction* of the repressed feelings associated with the forgotten traumatic event. Freud soon found that the results of hypnosis were not lasting, and for a brief period he employed a *concentration* technique in which the conscious subject was encouraged to remember previous events related to the symptoms. This in turn was soon abandoned and replaced by the method of *free association,* in which the patient reported verbally everything that came to mind without conscious reservation. This latter injunction was termed the *fundamental rule* of psychoanalytic treatment, and led to expression of hitherto unconscious feelings, impulses, fantasies, and ideas. *The analysis of dreams* during free association was discovered to be an important means of access to unconscious motivation: Freud referred to the dream as the royal road to the unconscious.

In spite of the patient's conscious attempts to free-associate, obstructions to the associative process become evident. These obstructions to the acquisition of insight into unconscious motivation are called *resistances.* An important part of the therapist's effort involves the recognition of resistances and the utilization of *interpretation* to improve the patient's insight. Interpretation may involve inferences about the patient's emotions or motives, the pointing out of similarities in certain life situations, the increasing awareness of cause-and-effect relationships in the patient's life, or the revelation of hidden or symbolic meanings. The goal of interpretation is not to persuade the patient to believe something about himself, but to enable him to perceive something about himself. There is an analogy between the process of interpretation and the holding up of a mirror so that the person may see his unconscious motives for the first time. What he sees may be frightening, discouraging, or disgusting, and he may even need to deny its existence. If a patient remains blind to reality, it is because he needs his blindness. Resistance to the development of insight may be shown by such reactions as silence, denial, blocking, forgetting, evasion, embarrassment, or strong emotions, including anger toward the analyst. Therapeutic progress is accomplished by cautious and tentative interpretation, as the patient becomes ready to accept and tolerate additional insight.

A major feature that distinguishes psychoanalytic therapy from psychoanalysis involves emphasis on the development, analysis, and resolution of the transference relationship, or transference neurosis. *Transference* has been defined as a special form of displacement, involving the unconscious attachment to the analyst of emotions and attitudes that were originally associated with significant persons in the patient's early life (such as parents and siblings). The patient reacts toward the therapist as if the latter were the person responsible for the original development of these positive, negative, or ambivalent feelings — and expects that the therapist will behave toward him in the same manner as did the significant person in the earlier relationship.

Fenichel described transference as follows: "The patient misunderstands the present in terms of the past; and then, instead of remembering the past, he strives, without recognizing the nature of his action, to relive the past and to relive it more satisfactorily then he did in childhood. He transfers past attitudes to the present."

The aim of psychoanalytic therapy is to replace unconscious acts by conscious acts, or in the words of Freud: "Where there was id, ego shall be." Loewald wrote that the patient who comes to analysis for help is led to self-understanding by the understanding he finds in the analyst. This understanding is fostered by the analyst's recognition that his own attitudes and behavior toward the patient may sometimes reflect displacement of his own unconscious motives through *countertransference.* Hence, an important part of training involves personal analysis for the therapist, and close supervision and control by a training analyst during his early analytic work with patients.

Fenichel classified psychiatric disorders according to their *accessibility to analysis,* in the following sequence: hysteria; compulsion neurosis and pregenital conversion neuroses; neurotic depressions; character disturbances; perversions, addictions, and impulse neuroses; and psychoses, severe manic-depressive episodes, and schizophrenias. In addition to diagnosis, certain other criteria are recognized as influencing the outcome of psychoanalysis and related forms of psychotherapy. These include the age of the patient (preferably 15 to 40 years); his intelligence, education, socioeconomic background, and ability to communicate effectively with the therapist; the duration of symptoms, and the presence or absence of marked secondary gain from them; and the reality situation of the patient, particularly his current relationships with other members of his family and of society.

The following are among the major problems of psychoanalytic therapy: Some object to its high cost and thus its relative inaccessibility. Some analysts and other therapists disagree with the fostering of regression within the transference neurosis, which is generally accompanied by an initial period of worsening symptoms and maladaptive behavior. Classical analytic techniques tend to foster undue dependence on the therapist, with morbid introspection and narcissism, fixation on past events to the exclusion of present and future adaptation, or a tendency toward acting out of sexual and aggressive impulses. However, such criticisms may be based on limited personal knowledge or understanding of psychoanalytic techniques, whose ultimate goal is to improve current and future adaptation to reality.

Psychoanalytic, or dynamic, psychotherapy in the United States has continued to evolve since the time of Freud, and has been profoundly influenced by neo-freudian analysts such as Karen Horney, Erich Fromm, and Harry Stack Sullivan. There has been increased emphasis on the interpersonal and sociocultural context within which personality traits and maladaptive behavior develop. Most analytic therapists today analyze the patient-therapist relationship, the patient's adaptation to his environment, and the development of maladaptive social patterns. They still rely on the interpretation of dreams, transference, and resistance, but are more active in the therapeutic role and tend to employ less frequent interviews, using a face-to-face interview situation rather than having the patient reclining on a couch, unable to see the analyst.

There has also been increased emphasis on the role of the patient's relationship with the therapist in providing a *corrective emotional experience,* since the therapist's response to the patient's behavior and expectations is, it is hoped, different from those responses experienced from parents and others during the developmental years.

SUPPORTIVE PSYCHOTHERAPY

Supportive psychotherapy seeks to reinforce the patient's defenses, and uses those techniques that will make him more secure, reassured, accepted, protected, encouraged, and safe, as well as less anxious and alone. The therapist assumes an authoritarian but usually nondirective role, and attempts to boost the patient's self-esteem. He is warm, friendly, and reassuring, and permits the patient considerable temporary dependence on

him. He attempts to remove external stresses by environmental manipulation or by hospitalizing the patient. He may provide guidance, advice, and a variety of measures for the relief of symptoms, including psychotropic medication.

Supportive psychotherapy may be described as *expressive* when it fosters verbal expression by the patient, emphasizing such techniques as verbalization (ventilation) and clarification. Verbalization, or ventilation, concerns such matters as conscious problems, worries, doubts, fears, impulses, conflicts, and sources of anxiety and guilt. It is an extension of talking things out, getting things off one's chest, or confession (with implied or actual absolution) such as many people employ in everyday relationships with friends and counselors. The therapist may discuss these problems with the patient, and assist in the conscious clarification of their nature, origin, and solution.

Supportive psychotherapy is sometimes *directive,* in the sense that the therapist takes responsibility for making decisions and directing the course of treatment. This approach implies that the physician understands the patient's problems and needs better than the patient himself, and accepts responsibility for seeing that his recommendations are carried out. The latter may include environmental manipulation; voluntary or involuntary admission to hospital; administration of drugs or other somatic therapy; or deliberate efforts to change the patient's attitudes and behavior by conscious persuasion, prestige suggestion, or example.

In *prestige suggestion* the therapist assures the patient directly or indirectly that unpleasant or disabling symptoms are being relieved (e.g., paralysis due to conversion hysteria). The suggestibility of the patient may be increased by means of hypnosis, narcosis, or the administration of other medication (or a placebo), and is greater when the patient has little psychiatric sophistication and the therapist is perceived as having high status, prestige, and power.

Some forms of directive therapy may be described as *suppressive.* These involve such techniques as authoritative firmness and commands, the ignoring of symptoms and complaints, the use of placebos with dogmatic assurance, hypnotic suggestion for the repression of symptoms, the introduction of similar suggestions while the patient is awake, exhortation, and persuasion. In suppressive therapy, the therapist acts as a dictator, or as an omniscient and omnipotent father who expects to be obeyed. Such an approach was more common prior to World War II.

Sometimes direct coercion has involved deliberate attempts to frighten patients out of their symptoms and habits. One such report concerned an 8-year-old boy with nocturnal enuresis who was told by his family physician: "Your little wee-wee will be burnt off with electricity if you don't quit wetting the bed." The boy promptly stopped bedwetting, but developed nightmares and a marked general passivity and dependency that lasted for years. Suppressive therapy of this nature may be not only damaging, but also ineffectual, since other symptoms and maladaptive behavior may replace those that are suppressed.

The preceding example should be contrasted with the desirable application of supportive psychotherapy for patients with an acute situational reaction to a sudden loss or severe stress.

CLIENT-CENTERED PSYCHOTHERAPY

Client-centered psychotherapy was introduced by Carl Rogers, and found widespread acceptance among clinical psychologists. It is a form of *nondirective relationship therapy,* based on a belief in the patient's right to self-determination and his capacity for emotional growth (self-actualization). The therapist is expected to act as a catalyst of growth, and not to impose his own opinions or decisions on the patient. The therapist remains permissive, tolerant, and nonjudgmental, but encourages the patient to verbalize his problems and emotions. The therapist may then rephrase the patient's words, and reflect to the patient the feelings he originally expressed. Clarification of the patient's problems and emotions are believed to lead to an increased self-understanding and capacity for adaptive behavior.

Rogers wrote that success in psychotherapy is effected by the presence of certain attitudes in the therapist that are communicated to and perceived by his client. He believed that if the therapist can provide three specific conditions in his relationship with the client, and if the client can perceive to some degree the presence of these conditions, then therapeutic movement will ensue. These three conditions are (1) the therapist's congruence, or genuineness; (2) unconditional positive regard, a complete acceptance; and (3) a sensitively accurate empathic understanding.

Client-centered therapists have become somewhat more active in the interview than formerly, but most psychiatrists would agree with Bruno Bettelheim that "love is not enough," and consider that a single type of therapeutic relationship is unlikely to have universal effectiveness. Unconditional positive regard may be undesirable in relation to maladaptive aspects of the patient's behavior. The therapist's congruence, or genuineness, may require the expression of negative feelings about such behavior, rather than about the patient as a person. The patient should learn that there is a difference between antisocial wishes and antisocial behavior. The relationship as well as the verbal content of therapy may need to be different for a neurotic patient as opposed to one who is antisocial or psychotic.

BEHAVIOR THERAPIES

Behavior modification therapies, or behavior therapies, attempt to eliminate maladaptive behavior and symptoms of psychiatric disorder by applying the principles of learning theory. The latter principles have been established through laboratory experiments on animals and humans, as outlined in the preceding chapter. Behavior therapies analyze the various types and contingencies of reinforcement that have led to the development or perpetuation of an existing psychopathology, and then develop a detailed schedule for eliminating these maladaptive behaviors and replacing them with socially acceptable or desirable behavior. The various forms of behavior therapy differ according to the major learning processes involved: (1) extinction (nonreinforcement) of deviant behavior; (2) reinforcement and shaping of desired behavior; (3) desensitization and reciprocal inhibition of maladaptive fear (e.g., specific phobias) developed through overlearning of escape and avoidance behavior; (4) aversive conditioning intended to reduce or eliminate undesirable behavior (e.g., drinking) by pairing it with aversive stimulation; (5) remotivation by demonstrating the effectiveness of behavior that has been inhibited because of learned helplessness.

The **extinguishing** of maladaptive behavior involves *nonreinforcement* rather than criticism or punishment. The latter is generally more effective in discouraging the adoption of new patterns of maladaptive behavior than in eliminating those that are already well developed. Moreover, it should be recognized that either undue negative reinforcement or aversive stimulation will tend to drive the patient away from the therapist, who might otherwise be a potent source of behavior modification through positive reinforcement.

In **shaping through successive approximation,** any response that approximates the desired result is reinforced initially. As such behavior becomes more frequent, closer resemblance to the desired end result is required before reinforcement takes place. Many small steps are required to teach increasingly complex social behavior. One form of operant-conditioning program is known as a *token economy,* which may be applied to the residents of a classroom or of a psychiatric ward. Conditioned reinforcers, or tokens, are given to subjects for specified behaviors, and may be accumulated and exchanged for various rewards or privileges.

Systematic desensitization and *reciprocal inhibition* were introduced by Joseph Wolpe in order to overcome neurotic anxiety and overlearned fear responses. In Wolpe's words, "Neurotic behavior consists of persistent habits of learned (conditioned) adaptive behavior acquired in anxiety-generating situations . . . If a response incompatible with anxiety can be made to occur in the presence of anxiety-evoking stimuli so that it is accompanied by a complete or partial suppression of the anxiety responses, the bond between these stimuli and the anxiety responses will be weakened."

The opposite approach to treating phobias or maladaptive anxiety is **implosion therapy,** or **flooding with aversive stimuli**. This may consist of repeated accounts of the dangerous consequences that can be produced by the object or situation feared. Such stimuli are continued until the object or situation is no longer frightening. However, this method has received less widespread acceptance than the better-known techniques of desensitization and reciprocal inhibition.

The use of **aversive conditioning** to treat alcoholism was introduced in many countries prior to World War II. Various techniques were employed, but all involved the concurrent administration of alcohol with emetics (such as emetine and apomorphine) in doses sufficient to produce severe nausea and vomiting. This method involves punishing a well-established behavior and inducing a motivational conflict between the desire for alcohol and a fear of extremely unpleasant consequences. Hence, such aversive therapy is likely to suppress the alcoholism temporarily, but requires repetition at periodic intervals. This form of treatment is only applicable to certain alcoholic patients, namely, those with neurotic rather than antisocial personalities who have good motivation and are in good physical health. It should be contrasted with the preventive administration of drugs that produce vomiting only through interaction with alcohol (in the event that it is later ingested). These drugs, disulfiram (Antabuse) and citrated calcium carbimide (Temposil) were introduced after World War II and largely replaced the earlier aversive therapy of alcoholism.

In recent years aversive conditioning has been employed in the treatment of sexual deviation. Such therapies involve a combination of aversive stimuli paired with deviant behavior, with concurrent positive reinforcement of socially acceptable heterosexual attitudes and behavior. Similar techniques have been applied to coerce delinquents or criminals into the abandonment of antisocial attitudes and behavior, but their use has aroused public indignation over ethical concerns such as the right of the subject to refuse treatment and determine his own destiny. Those who persist with such unpleasant treatment voluntarily are likely to have a strong masochistic component involving guilt and the need for punishment. Even among such patients, the therapist is likely to be perceived as a punitive figure who will ultimately be avoided, and this avoidance may be generalized to other therapists who would otherwise have been in a position to help the patient.

Remotivation is a term that has been applied to techniques employed by therapists of varying persuasions. One of the better-known approaches consists of group treatment undertaken by nursing personnel in mental hospitals, in order to stimulate communication and interest among chronically withdrawn patients (usually schizophrenic). However, the concept is equally applicable to deliberate efforts that are made to force depressed patients to initiate responses previously abandoned because they had been inappropriately extinguished or inhibited (as by aversive contingencies that no longer exist).

There is still considerable controversy over the effectiveness and future role of the behavior therapies. They are based on scientific principles, but hitherto their utility has been limited by the complexity of man's experiences and interpersonal relationships. While all psychotherapists should be familiar with the principles of learning and unlearning, many will not wish to limit themselves to the relatively few simple techniques of behavior therapy that have so far been developed.

GROUP AND FAMILY THERAPIES

Group Therapy

Group therapy involves the application of psychotherapeutic techniques in the simultaneous treatment of a group of patients. Almost every system of psychotherapy has been applied to groups, and the latter have shown a corresponding diversity in size and degree of heterogeneity (e.g., in age, sex, and diagnosis). Group approaches have been applied widely in hospitals and outpatient clinics, and in the treatment of patients with neuroses, psychoses, and behavior disorders. Many therapeutic groups consist of six to eight persons, and sessions are usually scheduled for about 90 minutes

(or roughly twice the length of individual interviews).

The widespread development of group therapy arose out of three major considerations: (1) the desire to bring psychotherapy to a larger number of patients than could be reached on an individual basis; (2) an assumption that greater benefit would be attainable through group interaction than from individual therapies; and (3) an increasing recognition of the sociodynamic nature of human maladjustment.

The shortage of professional personnel is probably the least satisfactory reason for recommending group therapy. It is not a substitute for individual therapy, and many patients are concurrently involved in both individual and group therapies, often with different therapists. However, there are some patients for whom group therapy may be more effective than individual therapy, namely, those who are insecure in social relationships, and delinquents or paranoid patients who may better accept the reality perceived by their peers than that perceived by the therapist.

Frank suggested that all varieties of psychotherapy share three aims: (1) to strengthen the patient's self-respect, (2) to help the patient maintain a level of tension or distress sufficient to keep him working toward better solutions (but not so great as to force him back into his maladaptive patterns), and (3) to supply some guides or models to the patient as he struggles to modify his attitudes. The various approaches to psychotherapy each offer the patient a different kind of emotional relationship and present him with some sort of task. The main advantages of group therapy result from the interactions with a variety of other persons (with each of whom identification may occur, and onto whom there may be unconscious displacement of emotions and expectations related to earlier relationships).

Groups are described as *open* when their membership is continually changing (with some patients leaving and new members being added) or *closed* when membership is restricted to the original group throughout the duration of therapy. Psychoanalytic groups with reconstructive goals tend to be closed, restricted in numbers (from 4 to 12 members), relatively homogeneous in composition (age, sex, and type of problem), and to meet relatively frequently over a long period of time. In such groups three phases of development are usually recognized: a phase of *unification* with development of group identity and cohesiveness; a phase of *interaction* with observation and analysis of dynamic relationships; and a phase of understanding and *resolution* with development of insight and increasingly adaptive behavior.

As with individual therapy, some groups may have limited or superficial goals, particularly that of emotional support during crisis. The latter types of group are usually *open-ended,* with changing membership and infrequent sessions. Another form of group therapy, developed by Jacob Moreno and known as *psychodrama,* involves role-playing, discussion, and interpretation.

A *sensitivity group* is one in which members try to increase self-awareness and their understanding of the group's dynamics. An *encounter group* emphasizes confrontation as a means of developing emotional rather than intellectual insight. A *T-group* is a sensitivity-training group whose members meet to learn about themselves, interpersonal relationships, group processes, and larger social systems. A *marathon group* is a single, very long meeting (from 8 to 72 hours) with the goal of developing intimacy and the open expression of feelings.

Family Therapy

Treatment involving more than one member of the family simultaneously in the same session is known as family therapy. Such treatment is based on the assumption that the family is the unit in which psychiatric problems develop and is therefore the unit toward which psychiatric treatment should be directed. This concept has long been held in the field of child and adolescent psychiatry, where individual therapy with the child has traditionally been accompanied by casework, counseling, or therapy with one or both parents. However, some therapists now consistently involve more than one member of the primary family group in all or

most of their interviews. Such family groups usually consist of husband and wife, or parents and children.

Although family therapy may involve interpretation, support, or direction, it should not be equated with other forms of group therapy. Each family is a kind of subculture, with its own valued role structure and its own unique family mythology. In many families one of the important functions of this mythology is supporting the denial of any conflict among its members. Observing the interaction of such families may be very helpful in learning factors that have contributed to overt psychiatric disorder in one or more of its members. Therapeutic change by one person may affect the dynamic equilibrium of all, and various family members may learn to modify their behavior as a matter of enlightened self-interest.

TRANSACTIONAL ANALYSIS

Transactional analysis is a neo-freudian form of psychoanalytic (dynamic) psychotherapy that may be applied to individual, group, or family therapy. It interprets human interactions in terms of role theory, beginning with current, well-defined, and explicit roles, that are readily recognizable by peers in a therapeutic group. As therapy progresses, patients develop increased awareness and understanding of implicit emotional roles, and of the developmental experiences that are compulsively repeated in maladaptive transactions. In addition to fostering insight into hitherto unconscious processes, the therapist seeks to liberate the patient from the bondage resulting from inappropriate programming by parents and other significant persons during childhood.

Much of the basis of transactional theory was developed by Eric Berne during the period from the mid-1950s until his death in 1970. His early concepts of ego-states, transactions, and games were summarized in his best-selling book *Games People Play* (1965). Berne defined an *ego-state* as a coherent system of feelings and behaviors (i.e., posture, viewpoint, tone of voice, and vocabulary) which represents the person's current psychic attitude. Each individual has a basic repertoire of potential ego-states, the sum total of which constitute his personality, and which may be classified into three broad categories of psychic functioning. To prevent ambiguity, the names of the three categories are always capitalized. (1) The *Parent* consists of ego-states that were mostly learned early in life, largely due to the influences of one's parent figures; it is concerned with morals, values, prejudices, and automatized reactions. (2) *Adult* ego-states are those that are autonomously directed toward an objective appraisal of reality, serving the function of processing of data from three basic sources (the Parent, the Child, and the external world) to produce logical decisions. (3) *Child* ego-states are those aspects of personality that are archaic or fixated relics of early childhood experiences, especially feelings. In the Child reside fantasy, intuition, creativity, spontaneous drive, and enjoyment, as well as various negative responses such as whining or withdrawal. Berne's view was that "All three aspects of personality have a high survival and living value, and it is only when one or another of them disturbs the healthy balance that analysis and reorganization are indicated. Otherwise each of them, Parent, Adult, and Child, is entitled to equal respect and has its legitimate place in a full and productive life."

The unit of social intercourse is termed a *transaction*. When one person by some means acknowledges the presence of another, or otherwise initiates a social exchange, the event is a transactional stimulus. The response it elicits is the transactional response. Transactional analysis is concerned with diagnosing which ego-state initiated the transactional stimulus and which one executed the transactional response (which may in turn be the stimulus for the next transaction). Berne distinguished between *complementary* transactions (e.g., Adult-Adult, Child-Parent) leading to continuing communication, and *crossed* transactions in which a stimulus at one level elicits an inappropriate response from another ego-state. He also distinguished between *simple* transactions involving only one ego-state in each direction, and complex or *ulterior* transactions involving the activity of more than two ego-states simultaneously (in at least one of the participants).

According to Berne, *games* are sets of ulterior transactions that are repetitive in nature and have a well-defined psychological payoff. All games involve a *con*, with the *agent* pretending to do one thing while he is really doing something different. The con can only work because of some weakness, handle, or gimmick in the *respondent* (or mark) such as fear, greed, irritation, or sentimentality. After the respondent, or mark, is hooked, the agent, or player, pulls some kind of a switch in order to get his payoff. This is followed by a moment of confusion or cross-up while the mark tries to understand what has happened to him, after which both players collect their payoffs. The payoff consists of pleasant or unpleasant feelings that the game produces in each of the players. These payoffs are like *trading stamps,* with good feelings spoken of as gold trading stamps, and unpleasant feelings spoken of as brown or blue trading stamps.

Berne and his colleagues subsequently focused on the analysis of *life scripts,* elaborated in a subsequent book, *What Do You Say After You Say Hello?* (1972). The object of script analysis is to turn "frogs" (i.e., losers) into "princes and princesses" (i.e., winners). The patient fights becoming a winner because he is not in treatment for that purpose, but only to be made into a braver loser who can follow his script more comfortably.

From the study of many losing scripts, it appeared that the person's ultimate destiny was determined by childhood decisions rather than by grown-up planning. It seemed that human life plans have been constructed like myths and fairy tales, having a *script apparatus* consisting of at least seven components, as follows:

1. *The script payoff,* or *curse,* in which the parents tell the child how to end his life. The four significant alternatives found in clinical practice are: be a loner, be a bum, go crazy, or drop dead.

2. *The script injunction,* or *stopper,* consists of an unfair negative command from the parents that will keep the child from lifting the curse. This is viewed as the most important part of the script apparatus, implanted at such a tender age that the parents look like magical figures to the child (e.g.,

the fairy godmother, the witch mother, the "jolly green giant," or the ugly troll).

3. *The script provocation,* or *come-on,* which consists of parental encouragement of behavior that will lead to the payoff. This is accomplished by the Child ego-state of the parent, particularly the parent of the opposite sex.

4. *The antiscript slogan* consists of a parental prescription from a nurturing Parent ego-state. This is in the form of a moral precept towards socially acceptable behavior that will fill in time while waiting for outbursts of maladaptive script behavior.

5. *The patter,* or *program,* represents a form of parental instruction, usually by the Adult ego-state of the parent of the same sex. Thus, the example of the father's behavior may show his son how to carry out the script injunction, or stopper, received from his mother's Child or Parent ego-state.

6. *The demon* consists of intrinsic "scripty impulses" and urges to fight against the whole script apparatus laid on the child by the parents.

7. *The antiscript,* or *internal release,* consists of a spell-breaker, or a way to lift the curse of the losing script payoff.

The preceding analysis of the script apparatus implies a rigid determinism based on early childhood conditioning or programming. This is illustrated by Berne's concept of the subject sitting at the player piano, from which the music pours forth in a pattern that he cannot change. However, he still works hard at pumping the pedals to provide the air and the mechanical unwinding of the roll of paper punched out long ago by his ancestors. He and his friends and relatives may believe that he is playing his own tune (and applaud or boo accordingly).

The *script matrix* is a diagram, first used by Claude Steiner, to illustrate and analyze the directives handed down from parents and grandparents to the offspring (patient). As indicated previously, the most decisive controls appear to come from the Child ego-state of the parent of the opposite sex (injunctions and come-ons such as "Don't think; drink."). The Adult ego-state of the parent of the same sex then gives the person the example

of a pattern to follow that determines his life course while he is carrying out his script (e.g., "Here's how. Work and drink."). Meanwhile, both parents, through their Parent ego-states, transmit socially acceptable messages in the form of prescriptions or slogans that determine the counterscript (e.g., "Work hard."). These concepts are illustrated in the following script matrix that shows these messages in the case of one male alcoholic patient (Fig. 6-1).

Berne wrote of psychiatric treatment as consisting of three main ingredients: "being there"; "handy household hints"; and "flipping in." The latter refers to getting the patient out of his script and into the real world, ideally by one single intervention, which would be the most effective *script antithesis.* This requires the therapist to be *potent* enough to prevail over the pathogenic parental injunction; he must give the patient *permission* to disobey the script control, and he must *protect* him from the consequences of disobedience.

Script matrices have been widely used in group therapy to foster clarity in communication and promote shortcuts in the attainment of dynamic insight. However, the approach is neither as stereotyped nor as superficial as some critics have maintained. The language of transactional analysis (and of dreams) has been referred to by Berne as Martian, but many of the basic concepts are easily recognizable by others who are familiar with psychoanalytic therapy. Whether this approach continues its growth and popularity may well be determined by how much therapeutic change is accomplished, and how enduring such change remains following termination of therapy.

As Steiner remarked, an inexperienced therapist is often trapped into responding to the patient as though the latter were a powerless Victim of circumstances beyond his control. If the patient behaves as a good little Victim, the therapist is likely to react by assuming the role of Rescuer. If the patient acts like a bad little Victim, the therapist may respond more as Persecutor (with the hostile behavior rationalized as beneficial for the patient). In either event, the therapist is now cast in a role of power and superiority, and the patient

Father 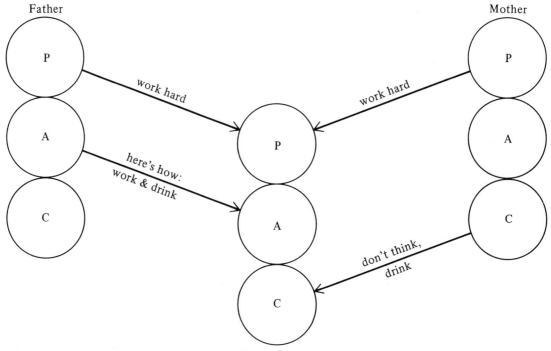 Mother

Figure 6-1. Script matrix in the case of one male alcoholic patient.

has ceased to accept any responsibility for helping himself.

There has therefore been an increasing tendency for transactional analysts (and other therapists) to base therapy on an explicit *contract* between patient and therapist. This is regarded as the indispensable first step in therapy, and certain legal aspects of the patient-physician contract will be considered further in Chapter 10.

REVIEW QUESTIONS FOR CHAPTERS 5 AND 6

56. A neurotic patient insists on using an entire therapy hour to describe a recent dream in great detail. A psychoanalytically oriented therapist would probably view this behavior as:
    (A) positive transference
    (B) regression
    (C) countertransference
    (D) resistance
    (E) ventilation

57. A 30-year-old unmarried male patient is

referred to a psychiatrist by his family physician because of depression related to continued active homosexual behavior. The patient says that he very much wants to be rid of his homosexual feelings. The best course of treatment would be:
    (A) therapy directed primarily at relieving the depression
    (B) supportive therapy aimed at encouraging the patient to actively seek heterosexual experiences
    (C) aversive conditioning to remove the homosexual tendencies
    (D) an authoritarian, directive approach to help him suppress his homosexual feelings
    (E) use of hypnosis or other methods to remove the symptoms by suggestion

58. Psychoanalytic therapy is more likely to be effective than other treatments for:
    (A) antisocial personality
    (B) acute situational reaction
    (C) involutional melancholia

(D) hysterical neurosis

(E) alcoholism

59. The most useful treatment for chronic ambulatory schizophrenia is a combination of chemotherapy and:
    (A) behavior therapy
    (B) supportive psychotherapy
    (C) psychoanalytic psychotherapy
    (D) family therapy
    (E) brief psychotherapy

60. Systematic desensitization is a psychotherapeutic technique based on:
    (A) learning theory
    (B) psychoanalytic theory
    (C) positive reinforcement
    (D) conditioned avoidance
    (E) the pleasure-pain principle

61. The extinction of a learned response
    (A) occurs if the response repeatedly goes unreinforced
    (B) may be accomplished by means of a mild punishment
    (C) results in a state the same as if the response had never been learned
    (D) all of the above
    (E) none of the above

62. Punishment of a child is most likely to produce adaptive forms of behavior if it has *each* of the following characteristics *except*:
    (A) it is applied to new behaviors
    (B) it is severe
    (C) it is consistently applied
    (D) it is accompanied by a reward
    (E) an alternative unpunished response is available

63. Which of the following is *not* a behavior modification technique?
    (A) shaping by successive approximations
    (B) implosion therapy
    (C) unconditional positive regard
    (D) aversive conditioning
    (E) reciprocal inhibition

64. Corrective emotional experiences are emphasized as important in:
    (A) supportive psychotherapy
    (B) client-centered therapy

(C) behavior modification therapy

(D) psychoanalytic psychotherapy

(E) all of the above

65. Negative reinforcement of a behavior refers to the situation in which the occurrence of the behavior
    (A) results in termination of noxious stimulation
    (B) results in noxious stimulation
    (C) results in termination of desirable stimulation
    (D) fails to receive reinforcement it previously received
    (E) either B or C

Summary of Directions

A	B	C	D	E
1, 2, 3 only	1, 3 only	2, 4 only	4 only	All are correct

66. In contrast to classical psychoanalysis as developed by Freud, in modern psychoanalytic psychotherapy there is:
    (1) little or no use of free association
    (2) a focus on current conflicts and dynamics rather than on early life experiences
    (3) less tendency to encourage regression and dependency
    (4) little or no attempt to interpret and overcome resistance

67. An experienced psychoanalytically oriented therapist who is selecting patients to be included in a new therapy group would be likely to agree that:
    (1) patients who have problems with authority figures are often helped by group therapy
    (2) group therapy initially increases anxiety in patients whose problems involve relationships with peers
    (3) for children and adolescents it is preferable that all group members be approximately the same age
    (4) group therapy is contraindicated for patients who tend to project their feelings onto others

68. The relationship between patient and therapist is considered to be an important component of:
    (1) supportive psychotherapy
    (2) client-centered therapy
    (3) psychoanalytic psychotherapy
    (4) behavior modification

SELECTED REFERENCES

1. Ackerman, N.W. (1958). *The Psychodynamics of Family Life.* New York: Basic Books.
2. Berne, E. (1965). *Games People Play.* New York: Grove Press.
3. Berne, E. (1972). *What Do You Say After You Say Hello?* New York: Grove Press.
4. Colby, K.M. (1951). *A Primer for Psychotherapists.* New York: The Ronald Press Co.
5. Fenichel, O. (1945). *The Psychoanalytic Theory of Neurosis.* New York: W.W. Norton & Co.
6. Frank, J.D. (1973). *Persuasion and Healing.* New York: Schocken Books.
7. Harper, R.A. (1959). *Psychoanalysis and Psychotherapy: 36 Systems.* Englewood Cliffs, New Jersey: Prentice-Hall.
8. Shapiro, A.K. (1976). The behavior therapies: Therapeutic breakthrough or the latest fad? *American Journal of Psychiatry,* vol. 133, pages 154–159.
9. Steiner, C. (1974). *Scripts People Live.* New York: Grove Press.
10. Ullman, L.P., and Krasner, L. [Eds.]. (1965). *Case Studies in Behavior Modification.* New York: Holt, Rinehart, and Winston.
11. Wolpe, J. (1958). *Psychotherapy by Reciprocal Inhibition.* Stanford, California: Stanford University Press.

7. Biological Determinants of Personality and Psychopathology

Cruelty and compassion come with the chromosomes; all men are merciful and all are murderers.
Aldous Huxley, Ape and Essence

HEREDITARY DIFFERENCES

The biographies of eminent people contain many examples of childhood adversity, apparently similar to that reported in the childhood of patients with psychiatric disorders. One possible explanation for the difference in outcome lies in their different genetic potential and vulnerability. This concept is implied in the old truism, "The same fire that hardens steel melts butter." A similar concept is expressed in the statement that life is like a grindstone, which either wears us down or polishes us up, depending on the stuff we are made of. However, the "stuff we are made of" depends on interaction between inherited potential (or vulnerability) and subsequent experiences that affect both body and behavior.

Various data may provide information relevant to the inheritance of behavioral tendencies and psychopathology, such as the following: (1) pedigrees; (2) family correlations and expectancies; (3) twin correlations and concordances; (4) foster child correlations and expectancies; and (5) cytogenetics.

The Study of Pedigrees

A given gene *A* is described as completely *dominant* to an allele *a* when it is impossible by any known test of the trait in question to distinguish between *AA* and *Aa* individuals. A gene *a* is described as completely *recessive* to an allele *A* when there is no detectable effect of *a* in *Aa* individuals.

Characteristics transmitted by a single, rare, completely dominant autosomal (not sex-linked) gene are clearly evident in a simple pedigree study, as in the case of Huntington's chorea. Affected individuals are nearly all heterozygous *Aa* individuals, and (barring new mutations) result from a mating of one heterozygous *Aa* (affected) individual with one homozygous *aa* (unaffected) individual. The criteria for identification of this form of inheritance are therefore as follows: (1) The trait is transmitted directly from affected parent to affected child without skipping of generations; (2) the two sexes are affected with equal frequency; (3) approximately half the children and half the siblings of an affected individual also show the trait.

Transmission by a dominant gene usually is followed by some phenotypic variation among individuals carrying the allele in question. Among the factors to which such variations may be attributed are: (1) the amount of *penetrance* of the gene in each case (i.e., the capacity for the gene to express itself); (2) the *expressivity* of the gene (i.e., the exact nature of the phenotypic traits it tends to produce); (3) the influences of other genes on the phenotypic traits under consideration; and (4) the extent to which environmental events are also able to influence these traits. Huntington's chorea tends to be relatively little affected by these factors. Other disorders of interest to psychiatrists that are believed to be transmitted by single rare dominant genes and that tend to show greater phenotypic variability include the following: (1) Pick's presenile dementia; (2) the acute intermittent form of porphyria; (3) neurofibromatosis, or von Recklinghausen's disease; and (4) tuberous sclerosis, or Bourneville's disease. The first two result in organic brain syndromes and will be discussed in Chapter 11; the latter two are primarily associated with mental retardation and will be described in Chapter 20.

Family Correlations and Expectancy Rates

Characteristics transmitted by a single pair of rare *recessive* autosomal genes include phenylketonuria (PKU) and many other inborn errors of metabolism that may lead to brain damage and mental retardation, various cerebral lipidoses, galactosemia, glycogenosis (von Gierke's disease), and hypoglycemosis. Affected persons are all homozygous *aa* individuals, and are usually the offspring of two heterozygous *Aa* (unaffected) individuals. The criteria for recognition of simple recessive inheritance are: (1) Father, mother, and more remote ancestors of an affected individual are usually normal; (2) about one-quarter of the siblings of the affected individuals will be similarly affected; (3) the two sexes are affected with equal frequency; and (4) there tends to be a higher frequency of consanguinity among the parents of affected individuals than in the general population (including marriages between first cousins).

Such characteristics are not likely to be established by simple pedigree studies, but require statistical comparison between *lifetime expectancies* (estimated lifetime incidence or risk) for various classes of relatives versus the corresponding expected frequencies computed according to the hypothesized mechanism of genetic transmission. Precise frequencies predicted among various classes of relatives will depend on the frequency of the gene (and hence of affected individuals) in the population.

The two preceding types of autosomal transmission may be described as simple mendelian inheritance. This may also be termed *monogenic inheritance,* since differences between individuals are attributable to the presence or absence of a single major gene or pair of genes at a given genetic locus. However, some differences between individuals are due to the cumulative effects of multiple minor genes, which is termed *multifactorial,* or *polygenic, inheritance.* The following criteria are considered suggestive of polygenic, or multiple-gene, inheritance: (1) continuous quantitative variation or gradation of measurements (e.g., height, weight, and intelligence); (2) suggestion of a strong hereditary component resulting from twin and foster-child studies, as outlined below; (3) correlations between the values for different classes of relatives, decreasing according to the degree of their blood relationship, i.e., decreasing in the following sequence; between uniovular twins, between midparental values (the average for *both* parents) and their children, between binovular twins or other full siblings (brothers and sisters),

between *one* of the parents and his or her children, between grandparents and grandchildren, between uncles or aunts and nephews or nieces, and between first cousins (Table 7-1).

It may be noted in Table 7-1 that correlations for intelligence between siblings, and between children and *each* parent, approximate + 0.50. Even higher correlations (up to + 0.75) have been reported between the intelligence of children and *midparental* intelligence (averages for *both* parents combined). However, there is a *regression toward the mean,* so that the average intelligence of offspring in a family tends to be somewhat closer to the population mean of 100 than to the average IQ of their parents.

Twin Correlations and Concordance Rates

Uniovular twins, arising from a single fertilized egg, are always of the same sex, and are known as monozygous, monozygotic (MZ), or identical twins. Binovular twins, arising from two fertilized eggs, may be alike or unlike in sex, and are known as dizygous, dizygotic (DZ), or fraternal twins.

A rough index of the proportion of population variance in a trait that may be attributed to *heredity* (H) may be obtained by comparing pairs of MZ with pairs of DZ twins, and applying a simple formula that depends on the nature of the characteristic to be compared. If this characteristic is distributed along a *continuous* range of values (e.g., height, weight, or intelligence), the contribution of *heredity* may be estimated by means of the statistic:

$$H = \frac{r_{MZ} - r_{DZ}}{1 - r_{DZ}}$$

where r_{MZ} is the (intraclass) correlation coefficient between pairs of monozygotic twins and r_{DZ} is the correlation coefficient between pairs of DZ twins (Table 7-2).

Table 7-2 shows an index of heritability for intelligence amounting to 0.68, or 68 percent. This means that roughly two-thirds of the sample variation in IQ should be attributed to heredity, and one-third to other factors. Some personality vari-

Table 7-1. Correlations for Height and Intelligence, According to Degree of Relationship

Degree of Relationship	Correlation for Height	Correlation for Intelligence
Siblings	0.54	0.51
Parents and children	0.51	0.49
Grandparents and grandchildren	0.32	0.34
Uncles or aunts and nephews or nieces	0.29	0.35
First cousins	0.24	0.29

Adapted from data from Burt, C., and Howard, M. (1956). The multifactorial theory of inheritance and its application to intelligence. *Br. J. Statist. Psychol.,* 9:59.

ables have also been found to have a significant heritable component. Among these are several scales of the MMPI, particularly scale 2 (depression), scale 4 (psychopathic deviate or antisocial traits), and scale 0 (social introversion). It may seem paradoxical at first, but the greater the similarities in environmental opportunities, the greater will be the extent to which remaining differences result from heredity.

If the characteristic under consideration is discrete (i.e., present or absent, as in the case of schizophrenia or manic-depressive psychosis), data for assessing heritability consist of samples of twins in which at least one member of each twin pair has the trait. Each pair in this sample is assessed as either *concordant* (if both twins develop the trait) or *discordant* (if only one of the two develops it). The contribution of heredity in determining the development of the characteristic in the population may then be estimated by the statistic

$$H = \frac{CMZ - CDZ}{100 - CDZ}$$

where H represents heritability, while CMZ and CDZ are the percentages of concordant MZ and DZ twins respectively. Twin studies do suggest a substantial contribution by heredity to the development of some forms of schizophrenia and manic-depressive psychosis, as will be discussed in later chapters.

Foster-child Correlations and Expectancy Rates
Foster-child studies involve comparisons of similarities observed between: (1) children and their biological parents from whom they were separated at birth; and (2) children and their adoptive or foster parents with whom they have lived all their lives. Such data are increasingly hard to obtain in a mobile population that has grown extremely sensitive to the rights and privacy of human subjects. However, some well-controlled foster-child studies of intelligence were undertaken many years ago and are summarized in Table 7-3.

The correlations for intelligence between children and their two biological parents are of the same order as previously noted in Table 7-1, and

Table 7-2. Correlations Between Pairs of Monozygotic and of Dizygotic Twins

Characteristic	Intraclass Correlations		Index of Heritability
	MZ Twins r_{MZ}	DZ Twins r_{DZ}	H
Height	0.93	0.65	0.81
Weight	0.92	0.63	0.78
IQ	0.88	0.63	0.68

Data from Newman, Freeman, and Holzinger (1937).

Table 7-3. Correlations for Intelligence of Children Adopted at Birth Compared with Their Foster Parents and with Their Biological Parents

Characteristic	Correlations	
	Children and Foster Parents r	Children and Biological Parents r
Data from Burks (1928)		
M.A. (father vs. child)	0.07	0.45
M.A. (mother vs. child)	0.19	0.46
Data from Leahy (1935)		
Otis score of father vs. child	0.15	0.51
Otis score of mother vs. child	0.20	0.51

much higher than those with the foster parents with whom they had lived all their lives. These findings support those from twin studies and indicate that heredity is of considerable importance in determining parent-child similarities in intelligence. In recent years attempts have also been made to estimate (1) the frequency of schizophrenia among the adopted offspring of schizophrenic parents, and (2) the frequency of schizophrenia among the biological relatives of adopted children developing schizophrenia. Both the latter types of study support data from twin and family statistical studies, indicating some type of genetic predisposition for at least certain forms of schizophrenia.

Cytogenetic Studies

About a dozen gross chromosomal anomalies have been reported among patients with psychiatric disorders, the most frequent of which involve *mental retardation*. *Down's syndrome* (mongolism) has an incidence of about one in 600 live births, and is usually associated with severe mental retardation and is due to *trisomy 21*. This involves the presence of an extra autosome in group G, resulting in a total of 47 (in place of the usual 46) chromosomes. However, Down's syndrome may also be due to *translocation* of chromosomal material between two chromosomes, in which case the total number remains 46 chromosomes, or to *mosaicism*, in which some cells have 46 chromosomes and some have 47.

In *Turner's syndrome* one of the two female sex chromosomes is missing, so that the total count is only 45 chromosomes. This anomaly appears in about one out of 4,500 liveborn females, and some patients show mental retardation, but it is usually mild. As in Down's syndrome, there is a variant of Turner's syndrome due to mosaicism.

Klinefelter's syndrome is an anomaly of the male sex in which there is an extra X chromosome, making a total of 47. It occurs in about one out of 800 male live births, and among 1 percent of all mentally retarded male patients in institutions.

The *superfemale* is a female with three X and a total of 47 chromosomes. Such persons often are sexually infantile and amenorrheal, and usually infertile, but show no consistent psychiatric disorders. The incidence is about one in 800 liveborn females.

The *supermale* is a male with an extra Y chromosome (and a total of 47). The incidence is about once in every 500 liveborn males. Supermales have been reported to be tall and mentally retarded, to have acne, and to show aggressive behavior. One of these was Richard Speck, who murdered eight nurses in Chicago in 1966, and who based his unsuccessful insanity defense on this chromosomal anomaly.

CONSTITUTION, TEMPERAMENT, AND PREDISPOSITION

Constitution may be defined as a person's intrinsic physical and psychological endowment. The term *intrinsic* should imply relative constancy or stability of bodily structure, physiology, and behavior over relatively long periods of time. Sometimes, however, the term *constitution* is used in a much narrower sense as synonymous with either *genetic endowment* (from the time of conception), or *congenital predisposition* (present from the time of birth).

Various aspects of constitution may be distinguished, the most important of which are as follows: (1) *body structure,* morphology, physique, or somatotype; (2) *body physiology,* endocrinology, and chemistry, particularly functions mediated through the nervous system; (3) *temperament* or *character,* consisting of relatively fixed and enduring personality traits and habitual emotional and behavioral responses; and (4) *predisposition,* susceptibility or vulnerability to various forms of bodily illness or psychiatric disorder.

Many typologies or systems of classifying constitutional types have been proposed. The ancient Hindus classified men into types designated the hare, the bull, and the horse; and women into types referred to as the mare, the elephant, and the deer. In the second century A.D. Galen gave detailed descriptions of nine temperamental types that he considered to be based on various mixtures of the four humors (blood, lymph, black bile, and yellow bile). This is the origin of subsequent classification of temperaments into the sanguine, phlegmatic, choleric, and melancholic types.

Most recent typologies recognize three or four extremes, based on relative development of one of the major embryonic layers of tissues. One well-known system is that of Ernst Kretschmer, who distinguished between (1) the *asthenic,* or leptosomatic, type (slender persons with long bones and poor muscle development), associated with schizoid personality traits and vulnerability to schizophrenia; (2) the *athletic* type (sturdy and strong with wide shoulders and well-developed muscles), associated with aggressiveness and sometimes antisocial behavior; (3) the *pyknic* (stocky, plump, rounded persons), associated with cyclothymic personality traits and vulnerability to manic-depressive psychosis; and (4) the *dysplastic* type, with disproportionate development and endocrine disturbances.

The best-known typology in this country was developed by William Sheldon, who rated individuals on a seven-point scale in each of three dimensions of *somatotype.* High correlations were obtained (in the order of + 0.8) between the following physical and temperamental characteristics: (1) The *endomorphic* body build tended to be associated with *viscerotonic* characteristics such as relaxation, love of physical comfort, and sociability; (2) the *mesomorphic* body build corresponded with *somatotonic* characteristics such as assertiveness, energy, and competitiveness; and (3) the *ectomorphic* body build tended to be found with *cerebrotonic* personality characteristics such as restraint, love of privacy, and sensitivity. These associations are epitomized in the following anonymous verses that appeared many years ago:

Oh, I'm a little *endomorph,* asittin' in the sun.
I dote on beer and skittles; and I like my bit of fun.
I'm just a trifle lardy, just a trifle fat,
I may be somewhat tardy, but I like to be like that.

Oh, I'm a busy *mesomorph,* encased in gorgeous
  muscle,
My thinking is a trifle short, I'm long on vim and
  hustle.
I'm a certified go-getter; I'm the boy who will
succeed.
(Minus reason even better) perspiration is my creed.

Oh, I'm a spectral *ectomorph,* full of ratiocination.
The mind's my happy hunting ground, and I loathe
  participation.
Lonelier than any cloud, I'm always quite superior
To the mouthings of the motley crowd and grunts
  of the inferior.

Some of the earlier studies were poorly controlled for factors such as age. Some slim or athletic young people tend to overeat and become more endomorphic with the passage of time. Some reported associations with psychiatric diagnosis may therefore have been partly attributable to such factors (since delinquency and schizophrenia are more prevalent among the young, whereas manic-depressive psychosis becomes more prevalent with advancing age). However, controlled studies still indicate some statistical associations between: (1) predominant endomorphy and manic-depressive psychoses; (2) predominant meso-morphy and delinquency; and (3) ectomorphy and schizophrenias.

SLEEPING AND DREAMING

Sleep involves recurring episodes of readily reversible relative disengagement from sensory and motor interaction with one's environment, usually associated with recumbency and decreased motility. There are two major types of sleep, characterized by the presence or absence of *rapid eye movements* (REM). This discovery by Aserinsky and Kleitman (1953) was followed by further analysis of sleep and its disorders by means of all-night polygraph recordings, usually including electroencephalogram (EEG), electromyogram (EMG), and electro-oculo-graph (EOG).

Non–rapid-eye-movement (non-REM) sleep, also known as *orthodox* or *synchronized* sleep, is present throughout most of the night. EEG tracings show four different stages of non-REM sleep: Stage 1 starts immediately after the onset of sleep, with low-voltage, relatively fast waves. Stage 2 is characterized by the presence of *K-complexes* and *sleep spindles* on the EEG, and the absence of sufficient high amplitude slow waves to define stage 3 or 4. The appearance of relatively high-voltage waves of two cycles per second or slower accompanies the deepest levels of sleep, and is labeled as stage 3 or 4, depending on the relative frequency of such waveforms.

During non-REM sleep there is an overall low level of activity. Eyeball movements are present only in stage 1, where they are slow and pendulous, from side to side. Progression through all four stages of non-REM sleep is usually accomplished in about ninety minutes.

Rapid-eye-movement (REM) sleep is also termed *paradoxical* or *desynchronized* sleep. Studies of physiological changes in animals and humans have found striking differences between REM and non-REM sleep. In addition to the bursts of conjugate rapid eye movements from which the phenomenon gets its name, REM sleep in healthy individuals is accompanied by changes in both the rate and the variability of many functions.

During REM, temperature, oxygen utilization, and many metabolic processes in the brain are increased. Pulse, blood pressure, and respiration show an increase in average rate and dramatically more variability. Gastric acid secretion has been reported as slightly increased in most persons and greatly increased in peptic-ulcer patients. In males of all ages (including infants) there are spontaneous penile erections. The EEG shows a low-voltage, relatively fast, mixed-frequency pattern similar to stage 1, but including *sawtooth waves,* which are unique to REM. There are episodic twitching movements of limbs and facial muscles and also a marked increase in spontaneous neuronal discharge. All of these changes are similar to those that would characterize *hyperarousal* in the waking state.

Another important feature of REM sleep is a generalized tonic inhibition of motor output. With the exception of a few special muscle groups (e.g., sphincters and extraocular muscles), the organism is completely flaccid during REM sleep. There is also a complete suppression of many reflex discharges.

In a healthy young adult, the first episode of REM occurs after about 70 to 100 minutes of non-REM sleep has elapsed. Episodes last about twenty minutes and occur cyclically at about ninety-minute intervals, for a total of four to six per night. About 20 to 25 percent of the total sleep time of a healthy adult will be REM sleep. The figure is greater for infants (up to 50 percent) and is slightly decreased in old age.

When awakened during REM sleep, most persons report complex dream experiences, and the length of the dream corresponds roughly to the length of the REM sleep period. Some dreaming or mentation may also occur in non-REM sleep (particularly during stage 1), but these dreams are not nearly as vivid, emotional, and bizarre as those that occur during REM sleep. However, the original conception of REM sleep as dreaming sleep must be recognized as inaccurate.

In earlier studies, **total sleep deprivation** appeared to precipitate an acute brain syndrome or aggravate a preexisting functional psychosis. During studies involving selective deprivation of

REM sleep over a period of several nights, Fisher and Dement noted the occurrence of psychological changes in their subjects. Combining this observation with the results of long-term REM deprivation in animals (which resulted in increasingly disturbed behavior and eventually in death), they hypothesized that the effects of sleep deprivation might be attributable to REM deprivation alone. However, subsequent research has failed to confirm this theory.

The effects of drugs on sleep may be significantly modified by a differential impact on REM sleep. The amount of REM sleep is *increased* by relatively few drugs — most notably LSD. REM sleep is selectively *blocked* by drugs that affect monoamine activity, including amphetamines, MAO inhibitors such as tranylcypromine (Parnate), tricyclic antidepressants such as imipramine, and reserpine. REM sleep is also inhibited by most hypnotic drugs, including all barbiturates and alcohol, but *not* moderate dosages of benzodiazepines. After REM-suppressing drugs have been used repeatedly and are then discontinued, there is a *REM rebound,* in which REM time increases to unusually high levels and may remain increased for more than a month. Nightmares and insomnia often accompany REM rebound, and may lead the individual to resume the use of the drug.

Primary Sleep Disorders

Primary sleep disorders are those in which disordered sleep is the only sign or symptom of abnormality. Evalution is facilitated by a careful history and all-night polysomnograph recordings in a well-staffed sleep laboratory. The best recognized of these disorders are as follows:

INSOMNIA. Insomnia may be defined as difficulty in initiating or maintaining sleep. It rarely occurs as a primary sleep disorder, but is quite commonly associated with psychiatric illness (especially depression), with physical illness or pain, and with a variety of environmental stresses (e.g., change of working shifts, jet lag, and emotionally charged events) to which people respond differentially. Sleep laboratory studies of insomniacs have generally found an increased level of physiological arousal throughout sleep. Hypnotic drugs are occasionally helpful, but their usefulness is limited by rapid development of tolerance, and it should be remembered that the primary insomniac may have a reduced baseline requirement for sleep.

NIGHTMARES. Nightmares are episodes of anxiety and fear associated with dreaming. Especially in children, they are usually transient and situational; if persistent at any age, they are then usually indicative of neurosis or other psychopathology, which will benefit from psychotherapy and possibly adjuvant medication. Nightmares are also frequent during the REM rebound phenomenon following withdrawal from REM-suppressing drugs. In contrast with night terrors (discussed below), nightmares usually occur during REM sleep and are recalled easily and in vivid detail. They are accompanied by little or no autonomic reaction.

NIGHT TERRORS. Night terrors (also called *pavor nocturnus* in children and *incubus* in adults) are much less frequent than nightmares. In children this is usually a primary sleep disorder that disappears during the normal course of maturation and that requires no treatment except education and reassurance. In adults this condition usually is an indicator of a more basic psychopathology requiring diagnosis and treatment. In contrast with nightmares, night terrors occur during stage 3 or 4 of non-REM sleep, and dream content is recalled poorly or not at all. Often there is amnesia for the entire experience, even though the associated autonomic arousal is intense. The episodes are also accompanied by severe autonomic discharge and by motility and vocalization. Treatment, when indicated, is usually by a stage 4—suppressing drug such as diazepam or flurazepam.

ENURESIS. Enuresis (bedwetting) and somnambulism (sleepwalking) both occur primarily in children and will therefore be discussed in Chapter 19.

NARCOLEPSY. Narcolepsy is characterized by repeated, uncontrolled, irresistible sleep attacks of brief duration. Some combination of three auxiliary symptoms may also be found: (1) episodes of *cataplexy* (sudden, usually generalized loss of muscle tonus during the waking state, often initiated by emotional or other stimulation); (2) *hypnagogic hallucinations* (false perceptions, usually visual or auditory, during the period immediately preceding sleep); and (3) *sleep paralysis,* which occurs during the transition between wakefulness and sleep. In patients who experience cataplexy as well as the sleep attacks, the latter usually consist of REM sleep, and nocturnal sleep is usually found to begin with REM. Narcoleptics who do not also have cataplexy are often found to have a more normal sleep pattern, with the first occurrence of REM about 90 minutes after falling asleep. Treatment is usually a psychomotor stimulant medication such as amphetamine for prevention of the sleep attacks. Imipramine is effective against the auxiliary symptoms but may not be effective against the sleep attacks. However, the combination of amphetamine or other stimulant with imipramine is considered dangerous by some authorities. A recent report suggests that protriptyline, a more stimulating tricyclic antidepressant than imipramine, may be the ideal drug for treating narcolepsy.

HYPERSOMNIA. Hypersomnia refers to a number of syndromes, characterized by excessive sleepiness (day or night), that are often followed by post-dormital confusion (extreme difficulty in achieving full wakefulness, sometimes referred to as sleep drunkenness), but not by known EEG sleep-stage abnormalities. Hypersomnia is theoretically distinguished from narcolepsy by the absence of the auxiliary symptoms of the latter, by the normal sleep EEG, and by the nature of the excessive sleep. The latter is not irresistible (as in narcolepsy) and tends to be of much longer duration. Chronic hypersomnia may be symptomatic of various other functional disorders (e.g., depression) or organic disturbances (e.g., brain injury or intracranial tumor).

KLEINE-LEVIN SYNDROME. The Kleine-Levin syndrome consists of periodic episodes of hypersomnia occurring at intervals of about six months. The disorder usually occurs in adolescent boys, is associated with overeating (bulimia), and tends to disappear spontaneously after a time. The **Pickwickian syndrome** consists of chronic hypersomnia accompanied by respiratory insufficiency (sleep apnea) and sometimes by obesity.

SLEEP APNEA. Sleep apnea has been found in hypersomniacs, narcoleptics, and even in insomniacs. In this syndrome, sleep is punctuated by episodes of apnea (cessation of breathing) which may be fatal. It has recently been linked to the sudden infant death syndrome (Steinschneider, 1972).

NEUROCHEMISTRY AND PHARMACOLOGY

Attempts to find some kind of anatomical or humoral basis for psychiatric disorders date back more than 2,000 years. In his *Anatomy of Melancholy* (1621) Burton wrote of Hippocrates finding Democritus dissecting various animals in the hope of finding the black bile that he assumed responsible for his own melancholic temperament. Many psychiatric disorders are known to result from *organic brain syndromes* (see Chap. 11) and from brain damage associated with some forms of mental retardation (see Chap. 20). Technological advances in the past few decades have provided new impetus in the search for biological causes or correlates of the major functional psychoses.

Many positive findings have been reported, and the history of the Akerfeldt test for schizophrenia illustrates the type of problem encountered. Around 1956 Akerfeldt reported a simple colorimetric test that gave a positive reaction with the serum of most schizophrenics tested. It soon became evident that the test was positive in chronic, institutionalized schizophrenics, but rarely in acute and recently admitted patients. The result was also positive in some general-hospital patients without schizophrenia, and was in fact due to changes in the ceruloplasmin content of the serum due to ascorbic acid deficiency. Similarly, a number of other positive results were often found to result from dietary, drug, or other non-disease variables that had been inadequately controlled.

Modern chemical and pharmacological studies of schizophrenias and depressions involve one or more of the following three approaches: (1) the search for abnormal metabolites or metabolic pathways in persons with the specified psychiatric disorder; (2) investigation of the mode of action of drugs that counteract the disorder; and (3) examination of the mode of action of drugs that precipitate, aggravate, or mimic the disorder. These approaches have all contributed to current hypotheses on possible biochemical bases for schizophrenias.

Transmethylation Hypothesis

In 1952 Harley-Mason speculated that schizophrenia might result from faulty transmethylation of catecholamines, leading to accumulation in the body of hallucinogenic methylated metabolites chemically related to mescaline. He singled out one substance as being of special interest, since it had been reported to produce catatonic behavior in animals. This was 3, 4-dimethoxyphenylethylamine (DMPEA) which was identified 10 years later as the substance in the urine of schizophrenic patients that had been found to produce a pink spot on paper chromatography. The same pink spot was, however, reported in the urine of some nonschizophrenics, and the matter was complicated by the fact that phenothiazines produced metabolites that also produce a pink spot in a similar position. Other techniques have been used to demonstrate DMPEA in the urine of both normals and schizophrenics, but the significance of the finding remains in doubt.

Dopamine Hypothesis

Soon after the introduction of phenothiazines in the treatment of schizophrenia, it was noted that they produced extrapyramidal side effects similar to those of Parkinson's disease. The discovery that dopamine was deficient in the caudate nucleus of patients suffering from Parkinson's disease led to the suggestion that antipsychotic drugs acted by blocking dopamine receptors. It has since been established that this blockade of dopamine receptors does in fact occur. In addition, several drugs are known to exacerbate schizophrenia among schizophrenic patients in remission. These include amphetamine, methylphenidate, and L-dopa. The psychosis due to amphetamine appears to be mediated by release and potentiation of dopamine at its brain receptors, and is aborted by dopamine receptor blockers such as the phenothiazines.

An imbalance between dopamine and norepinephrine activity was suggested by Seymour Kety (1976) to explain certain aspects of the findings to date. Whereas overactivity of dopaminergic synapses might explain some features of schizophrenia (stereotyped behavior, paranoid delusions, and auditory hallucinations), other manifestations are more likely related to decrease in norepinephrine activity (e.g., anhedonia, withdrawal, and autism or flatness of affect). He therefore proposed a single mechanism that could produce both increased dopamine activity and decreased norepinephrine activity. This hypothesis involves deficiency, or "throttling," of the enzyme dopamine-beta-hydroxylase, which converts dopamine to norepinephrine at the noradrenergic nerve endings in the brain.

Another provocative finding concerns a significant decrease in the level of MAO in the platelets of schizophrenic patients, which was also reported for the nonschizophrenic monozygotic twins among pairs of twins who were discordant for schizophrenia. Unfortunately, the results of studies attempting to measure MAO in the brains of schizophrenics have hitherto proved inconsistent.

Research concerning the synaptic functions of the biogenic amines and their relationships to behavior continues to appear promising. Such research is relevant both to etiology and to treatment by means of pharmacological agents that will be discussed in the next chapter.

REVIEW QUESTIONS

69. Onset of REM during the first ten minutes of sleep is a frequent finding in the sleep records of:
    (A) healthy adults

(B) narcoleptics
(C) patients currently taking barbiturates
(D) enuretic adults
(E) chronic insomniacs

70. Pavor nocturnus (night terror) occurs during:
    (A) REM sleep exclusively
    (B) Stage 1 of non-REM sleep
    (C) Stage 2 of non-REM sleep
    (D) Stages 3 and 4 of non-REM sleep
    (E) atypical periods of sleep which cannot consistently be assigned to one of the usual categories

71. A subject in a sleep laboratory is most likely to report that he was dreaming if awakened when the polygraph records show:
    (A) K-complexes on the EEG
    (B) "sleep spindles" on the EEG
    (C) high voltage slow waves on the EEG
    (D) rapid eye movements on the electro-oculograph (EOG)
    (E) slow eye movements on the EOG

72. An etiologic theory for schizophrenia that led to trials of nicotinic acid therapy was:
    (A) the transmethylation hypothesis
    (B) the drift hypothesis
    (C) the dopamine hypothesis
    (D) the catecholamine hypothesis
    (E) none of the above

73. A healthy young adult who has a regular sleeping pattern and is not taking medication spends most of his sleeping time in:
    (A) REM sleep
    (B) Stage 1 of non-REM sleep
    (C) Stage 2 of non-REM sleep
    (D) Stage 3 of non-REM sleep
    (E) Stage 4 of non-REM sleep

74. Each of the following drugs is a complete or partial suppressor of REM sleep *except*:
    (A) barbiturates
    (B) imipramine
    (C) tranylcypromine
    (D) reserpine
    (E) LSD

Directions: Following are five genotypic descriptions, prefixed with the letters A through E. For items 75 to 81, select the correct genotypic description from the list. Each of the lettered choices may be used once, more than once, or not at all.

(A) gross autosomal anomaly
(B) sex chromosomes XXY
(C) sex chromosomes XYY
(D) simple mendelian transmission by a dominant gene
(E) none of the above

75. Klinefelter's syndrome
76. Turner's syndrome
77. Huntington's chorea
78. Phenylketonuria
79. Supermale
80. Down's syndrome
81. Tuberous sclerosis

Summary of Directions

A	B	C	D	E
1, 2, 3 only	1, 3 only	2, 4 only	4 only	All are correct

---

82. Fruitful studies of hereditary transmission of schizophrenia *that control for the effects of environment* include:
    (1) twin studies
    (2) family expectancy studies
    (3) foster child studies
    (4) pedigree studies

83. In comparison with non-REM sleep, during REM sleep there is a higher degree of:
    (1) variability in respiratory rate
    (2) spontaneous penile erections in males
    (3) variability in heart rate
    (4) muscular tension

84. *Polygenic* transmission is believed to make a significant contribution to the incidence of:
    (1) cerebral lipidoses
    (2) borderline mental retardation
    (3) acute intermittent porphyria
    (4) schizophrenia

SELECTED REFERENCES
1. Hartmann, E. (1970). *Sleep and Dreaming.*

International Psychiatry Clinics, vol. 7, no. 2. Boston: Little, Brown and Co.

2. Kety, S. (1976). Recent Genetic and Biochemical Approaches to Schizophrenia. *Drug Treatment of Mental Disorders,* edited by L. L. Simpson. New York: Raven Press. (Chapter 1.)

3. Matthyse, S., and Kety, S. [Eds.] (1975). *Symposium on Catecholamines and Their Enzymes in the Neuropathology of Schizophrenia.* Oxford: Pergamon Press.

4. Newman, H.H., Freeman, S.N., and Holzinger, K. (1937). *Twins: A Study of Heredity and Environment.* Chicago: University of Chicago Press.

5. Rosenthal, D., and Kety, S. [Eds.] (1968). *The Transmission of Schizophrenia.* Oxford: Pergamon Press, Inc.

6. Sheldon, W.H. (1964). Constitutional Factors in Personality. *Personality and The Behavior Disorders,* vol. 1, edited by J. McV. Hunt. New York: The Ronald Press Co.

7. Shields, J. (1962). *Monozygotic Twins Brought Up Apart and Brought Up Together.* New York: Oxford University Press.

8. Steinschneider, A. (1972). Prolonged apnea and the sudden infant death syndrome: Clinical and laboratory observations. *Pediatrics,* vol. 50, page 646.

9. Vandenberg, S.G. (1962). The hereditary abilities study: Hereditary components in a psychological test battery. *American Journal of Human Genetics,* vol. 14, pages 220–237.

8. Psychotherapeutic Drugs and Electrotherapy

The competent physician, before he attempts to give medicine to his patient, makes himself acquainted not only with the disease which he wishes to cure, but also with the habits and constitution of the sick man . . . .
Marcus Tullius Cicero

Prior to the present century, physical interventions in the treatment of severe mental illnesses included such methods as isolation, physical restraint or immobilization, enforced dieting or starvation, heating, chilling, burning, bleeding, abdominal and cranial surgery, beating, water immersion, and the administration of various medicinals (e.g., purgatives, emetics, opioids, sedatives, and stimulants). The effectiveness of these approaches was poor, and there were occasional public outcries against excesses. However, a belief that such severe disorders must have a biological basis persisted, as did attempts at innovative therapies.

The first success was reported in 1917. *Julius Wagner von Jauregg*, a psychiatrist in Vienna, had deliberately transfused blood from a patient with malaria into several patients with general paresis, and noted a marked improvement in the psychosis following recovery from the malarial fevers. Like many discoveries, his was based on a chance observation — that a patient with general paresis improved following an attack of fever. Malarial treatment had demonstrable therapeutic efficacy, and produced partial remission in many patients with paresis, but attempts to treat other forms of psychosis with fevers were unsuccessful. Nevertheless, interest and hope for somatic treatments of other disorders were greatly increased.

The following 20 years were marked by many advances, including Jacob Klaesi's introduction of *prolonged sleep therapy* (Switzerland, 1922), Manfred Sakel's development of *insulin coma treatments* (Austria, 1933), Laszlo von Meduna's redis-covery of *pharmacological convulsive therapy* (Hungary, 1933), and Egas Moniz's surgical technique known as *prefrontal lobotomy* (Portugal, 1936). In 1937 *electroconvulsive therapy* (ECT) was introduced by Ugo Cerletti and Lucino Bini in Italy. With the notable exception of ECT, each of these innovations later became obsolete or nearly so. Malaria fever therapy was displaced by penicillin and other antibiotics. Sleep therapy and insulin coma therapy involved substantial risk and great expense. Ethical objections were raised against lobotomy, which also proved less effective than was originally hoped. However, the principal reason for the decline of these methods has been the discovery of *specific pharmacological agents,* which have proved more successful, less dangerous, and more readily accepted by patients and society.

Early History of Psychopharmacology

The use of drugs having depressant or stimulant effects on the central nervous system can be traced far back in history, for human beings always seem to have had a need to mask the realities of life. For example, hashish was used by the Assyrians as early as the eighth century B.C. Other drugs that have been used for centuries include opium, caffeine (in beverages), and cocaine (in coca leaves). Alcohol has found application in a particularly wide variety of circumstances.

The first report of a systematic scientific investigation of the effects of different psychoactive drugs in healthy subjects was by *Emil Kraepelin*. In 1892 he published a book describing experimental investigations with morphine, tea, alcohol, ether, chloral, and paraldehyde. He remarked, "We will sometimes be able, from the particular effect a quite well-known substance exerts on a given psychic process, to better understand the workings of the latter . . ." A few examples of Kraepelin's prophetic observation are mentioned below and elsewhere in the present volume.

PSYCHOTROPIC DRUGS. These may be loosely defined as those chemical agents that have an effect on the mind. *Psychotherapeutic drugs* comprise the relatively small subset that have established indications in the treatment of mental disorders. It is usual to place in a separate category those drugs whose only mental effects involve a reduction in the level of consciousness (sedatives, hypnotics, and anesthetics), and to exclude entirely the vast majority of medicinals that have psychic effects only indirectly, as in the treatment of organic brain syndromes resulting from generalized systemic or localized intracranial pathology (e.g., antibiotics or thyroid extract).

The widespread application of modern psychotherapeutic drugs and ECT during the past few decades has dramatically improved the prognosis for major mental disorders. *There has not been decreased emphasis on psychotherapies;* on the contrary, these may now be employed more selectively and effectively than ever before. Judicious use of medication or ECT can alleviate overt and covert symptoms. These treatments can bring a severely ill patient within the reach of psychotherapy, and they enable some patients to be treated by methods less sophisticated and expensive than would otherwise be required. They *cannot* change poor life situations nor alter adverse environmental circumstances; they *can* change both the impact of these factors on the patient's functioning and the impact of the patient's functioning on the environment.

CLINICAL MANAGEMENT OF PSYCHO-THERAPEUTIC DRUGS

Although these agents are still far from ideal, treatment "failures" and "disasters" can often be attributed to one of four basic errors: (1) selection of the *wrong basic type of drug;* (2) the prescription of the correct type of drug, but at *inadequate dosage;* (3) the prescription of the correct drug and dosage, but for an *inadequate period of time;* or (4) *the failure by the physician to obtain the patient's reliable cooperation* with the treatment regimen, even when he makes no technical errors.

In many respects the clinical management of psychopharmaceuticals is identical with other specialties of medical pharmacology. The following discussion will summarize the differences that do exist, and suggest how to avoid these four basic mistakes.

CLASSIFICATION. Psychotherapeutic drug classification is controversial, but for clinical purposes it is useful to think of groups of similar drugs that alleviate specific types of *target symptoms*. There are three types of major psychopharmaceuticals: *antipsychotics, antidepressants,* and *antimanics.*

These drugs appear to have *specific effects on the pathophysiology of their target symptoms*. It is well documented that these effects are neither restricted to, nor dependent on, a simple alteration in the level of arousal (i.e., sedation or stimulation). Moreover, if taken in nontoxic doses by "normal" persons (i.e., in good physical and mental health), *the only discernible psychotropic effect is usually a reduction in alertness* (i.e., sedation). Antidepressants do not usually produce euphoria, antimanics do not produce depression, and antipsychotics do not interfere with normal cognitive processes (except by sedating). The same side effects occur in patients and in "normals," but generally with greater severity and at lower dosages in the latter. *Psychotic patients appear to have a greater biological tolerance* to the sedation and other side effects than do nonpatients.

Less specific psychotherapeutic drugs can be grouped into *antianxiety drugs (anxiolytics), psychomotor stimulants,* and *sedative-hypnotics.* Unlike the preceding groups, these drugs are of little value in the treatment of functional psychoses and mood disorders. They produce similar psychic effects in most persons who use them, regardless of diagnosis. They are therefore frequently abused, and hence subject to stricter legal control than the major psychopharmaceuticals.

The term *tranquilizer* is applied in some contexts to any sedating drug. A more correct usage would restrict it to the antipsychotics and anxiolytics (sometimes referred to as "major tranquilizers" and "minor tranquilizers," respectively).

Drug Selection
Selection of drug should be deferred until the *type of drug* needed has been determined. It is a serious

and potentially dangerous error to prescribe any drug before all of the following information is available:

1. *A tentative diagnosis based on adequate clinical evaluation.* The physician must remember that patients with psychiatric disorders may not be reliable informants. A patient who appears to be an anxious neurotic may actually have frightening delusions that he will conceal, or a floridly psychotic patient may fail to admit having taken illicit drugs.

2. *Adequate knowledge of the expected course of the illness.* Treatment should usually be conservative and supportive if the condition is sharply time-limited or has a good prognosis. If the diagnosis is unclear and there is no dramatic urgency, a drug-free period of observation is recommended.

3. Assessment of *the risks of the illness if left untreated* and the *differential risks associated with alternative forms of treatment available.* Dramatically beneficial drugs involve risks, and trivial illnesses should not be treated with dangerous drugs, but neither should dangerous illnesses be treated with trivial drugs.

Within broad groupings, the individual drugs differ little in specificity for various constellations of their target symptoms. Therefore, choice of a drug within the group is usually based on other factors, such as: (1) *The previous history of the patient.* It is very likely that a drug that has been satisfactory in past episodes will be successful again. (2) *The psychopharmacological history of close relatives.* Both therapeutic response and side effects are greatly determined by genetic factors. (3) *The side effects profile.* The patient's current physical status and past history of drug side effects may suggest specific drugs to select or avoid. (4) *The physician's familiarity with the drug.* Nonspecialists are advised to select a few drugs of each type and to restrict most of their prescribing to these drugs. They will thereby become confident in the use of these agents, and will acquire a good practical knowledge of both main effects and side effects. (5) *Financial cost* may be quite important to some patients and lead to comparison shopping. (6) Once a drug has been adequately

tried and determined to be a failure, the items outlined above should be reconsidered. If trial of another drug of the same basic type is indicated, *the next drug selected should be as different as possible* from the one found to be unsuccessful. (A more complete discussion of therapeutic failures will be given below.)

Dosage

There is a high correlation between the severity of target symptoms and the minimum drug dosage that produces optimal response. However, there is also an amazing variability of response across patients. It is not unusual for clinically "identical" patients (e.g., same age and body weight, same physical status, and similar type and intensity of target symptoms) to differ by a factor of 20 or more in optimal dosage requirements for a specific agent. It therefore makes little clinical sense to adhere rigidly to printed dosage guidelines — such data should be recognized as averages that apply to many patients but for which exceptions will occur. *The important considerations are safety and quality of therapeutic response.*

Some drugs (e.g., antidepressants) have a "therapeutic window" outside of which response will be unsatisfactory, and the established dosage limits should rarely be exceeded. However, for some other drugs (e.g., certain antipsychotics), the limits printed in the package insert or in the *Physicians' Desk Reference* (PDR) are quite conservative, and experienced clinicians recognize that dosages in excess of these limits are both safe and helpful for some patients. Careful monitoring, the absence of side effects, and a demonstrated therapeutic advantage should be the important *clinical* considerations. However, the package insert has great, though probably unwarranted, *legal* significance.

A few patients, notably the elderly and the very young, respond best to quite small dosages of certain drugs, and may manifest toxic signs in the "normal" therapeutic dosage range. However, as Klein and Davis have remarked, *most psychotherapeutic drug treatment suffers from being too conservative rather than too radical.* The same idea was expressed many centuries earlier by Hippocrates: "Extreme remedies are very appropriate for extreme diseases." Certain psychiatric disorders are acutely life-threatening, and others may involve years of suffering or lifetime incapacitation. Undue timidity about ordering adequate dosages of medication known to be safe and effective can be as disastrous as careless overdosage.

Stages and Duration of Treatment

Following mental and physical evaluation and diagnostic formulation, the drug treatment of a schizophrenic or affective psychosis proceeds through four distinct stages:

The *first stage* begins with initiation of medication, and its goals are the *interruption* of psychotic symptoms, the *reduction* of any acute danger, and the *determination of optimal dosage.* The starting dosage should be as low as the clinical situation will permit, especially if the patient's vulnerability to side effects is great or unknown. Small portions should be administered three or four times daily, or even at intervals of one to six hours around the clock if necessary. Careful initiation is followed by escalation of dosage and titration to determine the optimal level. Tolerance is acquired for many side effects, and therefore the speed of dosage increase should be regulated as carefully as the absolute dosage level.

The *second stage* of treatment begins when the optimal dosage has been determined, and is directed at *resolution,* or *normalization,* of the psychosis. This period ranges from a few days to many months, during which the total daily dosage of medication remains relatively constant. However, with antipsychotics and antidepressants there may be a gradual consolidation of the small frequent doses into a single daily dose (usually taken at bedtime). The advantages and disadvantages of a once-daily schedule were summarized by Frank Ayd (1972).

The *third stage* of treatment is entered after complete normalization has been achieved. At this time there may be increased concern about side effects, and some side effects may become more intense. The dosage may therefore be reduced somewhat, but *patients often suffer serious relapses if beneficial medication is discontinued prematurely.* Even if recovery has been excellent, the usual practice is to continue adequate dosage of medication for at least several months. Unless psychotherapy of a specialized type is continuing, many patients may be returned to the care of their primary physician or to a nearby community mental health center or clinic for this stage of their treatment. *A most dangerous error is to reduce or discontinue medication at the time of discharge from the hospital* – the very time when the patient will return to a stressful situation, often with the stigma of a "nervous breakdown" as an additional pressure.

The value of a *fourth stage* of *long-term maintenance treatment* is now well established, and two excellent review articles by Davis have been included in the reference list at the end of this chapter.

Clinical monitoring of mental and physical status is an important aspect of both acute and long-term care. Such monitoring, even if brief, should be done on a regular and frequent basis; the responsible physician should be available for telephone consultation or an unscheduled office visit if necessary; and monitoring should *increase* in frequency for a period after reducing or terminating medication.

Route of Administration

Dosages administered by injection will be two to four times as potent as the identical dose taken by mouth, since the drug reaches circulation without being partially metabolized by the liver. There will be a more rapid rise and a higher level of plasma concentration, with consequent enhancement of therapeutic effects, sedation, and peripheral side effects. The latter may be dangerous if there is overwhelming hypotension or cardiac arrhythmias, especially if the patient is agitated.

Intravenous injections of antipsychotics and antidepressants are not recommended. However, intramuscular injections of antipsychotics may be ordered for any of three reasons: (1) the need for rapid relief of dangerous symptoms; (2) the inability or unwillingness of the patient to take medication by mouth; and (3) possible poor absorption of medication taken by mouth. The latter two reasons apply to tricyclic antidepressants as well, but *there is no increase in speed of onset of antidepressant effects associated with injections.* In addition to the danger of overwhelming side effects, two other disadvantages of injections should be mentioned: (1) Psychotic patients may interpret an injection as an assault; and (2) a few drugs, most notably *chlorpromazine,* are quite painful when injected and may produce local tenderness, irritation, or even abscess formation.

Intravenous injections of sedatives are relatively safer than those involving antipsychotics, and occasionally may be life-saving, as in the treatment of status epilepticus. Such injections must be given *very slowly,* and intramuscular injections are safer if instantaneous response is not needed. However, unlike most drugs, *the benzodiazepines are poorly absorbed from muscle tissue,* and such injections will act more slowly and less predictably than the same dose taken orally.

Detection and Management of Side Effects

The effectiveness of treatment with psychotherapeutic drugs depends in large measure on the patient's acceptance and cooperation. A patient may unilaterally discontinue prescribed medication because of the belief that it is not helpful, the belief that it once was helpful but is no longer needed, or the presence of distressing side effects *(or symptoms incorrectly assumed to be side effects)* that outweigh any advantages he may perceive. In this regard his confidence in the therapist is crucial, and the effectiveness of the latter depends on attitude and nonverbal communication as well as technical skill. He must be concerned about his patient's day-to-day comfort as well as long-range recovery from a major illness. This is achieved through both *systematic monitoring* for dangerous side effects and *appropriate responsiveness* to the patient's complaints, even if only concerned with medically trivial problems.

The first step in the management of side effects is *detection.* This is often not as simple as it sounds, for the following reasons: (1) Psychoses are accompanied by physical as well as mental changes; (2) because of apathy, diminished responsiveness to pain, inability to communicate, or delusional beliefs, psychotic patients may fail to report problems that are painful or even life-threatening (e.g., urinary retention); (3) delusional or extremely anxious patients may report nonexistent problems (and the therapist or nurse may thereafter treat all complaints as unworthy of evaluation); and (4) symptoms of concurrent physical illness may be hidden or greatly modified by the psychosis, the medication, or both. These possibilities may cause some side effects to remain undetected, and may also make it quite difficult to decide whether any observed physical change represents: (a) a true side effect of the medication; (b) a somatic complication or manifestation of the psychosis; (c) a normalization of a previously disordered physical function due to improvement in the psychosis; (d) a manifestation of a physical illness unrelated to the mental illness and the medication; or (e) some combination of these factors.

If high doses or injections of medication are ordered, or if the patient is in poor physical health, *routine measurement of vital signs* is advisable. The somatic status of psychotic patients should be carefully observed by trained nursing personnel, with special attention to bladder and bowel functions. Even though some patients are very suggestible, a structured interview covering all organ systems should occasionally be done; after therapy is well underway, this may be shortened to evaluation of any problems previously detected (whether drug-related or not) and to any special vulnerabilities of the patient. Spontaneous complaints by the patient should always receive attention.

The important approaches to minimization and elimination of side effects of psychotherapeutic drugs may be summarized as follows: (1) regular monitoring for insidious problems; (2) prompt and concerned attention to all complaints; (3) prescribing the smallest dosage that produces the desired effect; (4) practical advice and realistic reassurance; (5) symptomatic treatments and in some cases adjunctive medication; (6) if necessary, reduction of dosage, perhaps followed by increases at a slower rate as tolerance develops; (7) for major problems, discontinuation or change of drug; (8) regular reevaluation, and drug holidays if appropriate; and (9) avoidance of polypharmacy.

It may be impossible to find an effective therapeutic regimen that is devoid of side effects. However, any particular side effect can usually be minimized or avoided. Most patients are willing to accept the first fact if the therapist makes an effort to apply the second; the patient may then be able to accept reassurance about those trivial problems that cannot be avoided.

Combinations of Psychotherapeutic Drugs

Combinations of two or more drugs of the same basic type are almost never desirable. This was once common practice, based on the rationale that combining drugs with differing side effects would permit increased dosage of therapeutic medication without any single side effect becoming excessive. There was also a mistaken impression that the drugs differed in specificity for various target symptoms. However, efforts to justify this practice by well-controlled studies have disproved these intuitively appealing arguments. The current consensus is that a combination of two or more drugs of the same basic type involves increased risk, and in the vast majority of cases offers no advantage over an appropriate dosage of some single drug (not necessarily one of those in the combination). Rather than minimizing side effects, such combinations seem to potentiate them. Therefore, they are only justified in the exceptional case of a truly idiosyncratic drug response, and should only be attempted after careful trials of several different individual drugs.

Combinations of different types of drugs are sometimes correct, but should be ordered because of, and not instead of, a careful diagnostic evaluation. It is usually advisable to start the drugs at different times, and the continuing need for each should be periodically reassessed; a combination that is beneficial early in therapy may have no long-term advantage.

Teratogenicity

Teratogenicity is a major consideration whenever a drug is considered for a pregnant or fertile woman. This risk must always be weighed against the risks of the illness, and it is never correct to assume that any drug is completely safe. There is special concern with psychotherapeutic drugs, since they easily cross membrane barriers and are therefore readily transported across the placenta. The data known about those drugs approved for use in the United States, and current clinical practice based on these data, are summarized below.

Antipsychotics and antidepressants have never been convincingly associated with birth defects. These drugs, especially the older ones, have been taken by millions of women, certainly including many in every stage of pregnancy, and even anecdotal reports of fetal malformations have been extremely rare (and have usually involved other factors such as additional medications or a family history of similar defects). Since the principal indications for these drugs are major illnesses, and since the statistics are so impressively favorable, many therapists have found the risk justifiable for many patients. If the patient or spouse needs reassurance, involvement of a trusted obstetrician or family doctor may be helpful.

Lithium has been widely used only in recent years, and some animal studies suggested a possibility of increased risk. However, animal data are of limited value, and the human data available so far (which *overestimate* the risk) have been more favorable. The current norm is to prescribe lithium for pregnant or fertile women *only when it is clearly indicated* (e.g., for acute mania, or for prophylaxis in a highly vulnerable patient) *and only if it clearly offers greater benefit than any alternatives* (e.g., convulsive therapy or antipsychotic medication).

The data for *anxiolytics and sedatives* are more controversial. The Food and Drug Administration has recently required package inserts to carry warnings that some studies have found increased incidence of birth defects associated with the use of these drugs during the first trimester of pregnancy. The drugs most frequently implicated are *meprobamate* and *benzodiazepines.* The indications for these drugs are generally far less urgent than those for antipsychotics, antidepressants, and lithium, so it is likely that most therapists will avoid prescribing them for most pregnant patients.

Many psychotropic drugs are excreted in breast milk, and therefore many therapists advise mothers against nursing their infants while taking such drugs.

Advice to the Patient

Advising the patient is an important aspect of prescribing psychotherapeutic drugs. If the patient is unreliable, confused, mentally retarded, or seriously ill, it is usually desirable to include a responsible family member in these discussions. In the case of a child, the parents should of course receive this information, but the child patient should also receive such information as he is capable of understanding. The physician should devote an adequate amount of time to such discussions, encourage the patient to ask questions, and mention that telephone consultations or even unscheduled office visits will be available in case of problems. Many physicians find it helpful to give the patient a standardized written summary of important information, but this should not take the place of direct verbal discussion.

Topics to be discussed with the patient include: (1) *Anticipated benefits,* and how these will be assessed. It is important to mention that relief from symptoms may be a gradual process over many weeks; patients may understand this more readily if it is pointed out that acquisition of symptoms was also gradual. (2) *Side effects,* including (a) potential signs of rare but dangerous problems (jaundice, blood dyscrasias), (b) individual vulnerabilities of the patient (e.g., difficulty with urination), (c) extrapyramidal reactions, if an antipsychotic is prescribed, and (d) common but relatively benign side effects for which practical advice may be given (e.g., frequent sips of water for dryness of mouth). (3) Possible *increased vulnerability* to accidents or toxic reactions to other drugs, especially alcohol.

Therapeutic Failures

Therapeutic failures can often be attributed to one of the four basic errors mentioned previously, but even error-free treatment and cooperation does not always lead to immediate satisfactory results.

Failure to benefit from one treatment should never be interpreted as inability to benefit from any treatment. Indeed, if the proper technique is followed, an unsatisfactory response to one drug may provide valuable information that increases the probability of success on the next attempt.

A logical approach to evaluation of therapeutic failures must be based on data. First, one should review and if necessary reverify all of the information on which the original treatment choice was based: (1) the nature of target symptoms and the possibility of the patient's concealing important data; (2) the previous psychiatric history of the patient, including the possibility of unrecognized or misdiagnosed episodes (e.g., brief hypomania); (3) the exact nature of all previous psychiatric treatment and the response to these treatments; (4) a family history of mental illness, types of treatment, and the response to treatments; and (5) the physical status of the patient.

Second, this information should be updated on the basis of the patient's response to the treatment just attempted. It is important to obtain data from as many different observers as possible. The patient himself should be questioned, as well as relatives with whom he is living or who have visited him in the hospital. For inpatients, the most valuable data often come from the nursing staff, who have more frequent and extensive contacts with the patient than the physician does, who have observed him at all times of day and night, and who can best report his attitude toward the medication and the frequency and nature of his complaints. Data of special importance include: (1) any changes observed in the target symptoms; (2) the emergence of any new psychopathological symptoms; (3) the nature and severity of any side effects or other physical changes noted, or the absence of all side effects (suggesting malabsorption or surreptitious noncompliance); (4) the patient's attitude toward the medication; and (5) the temporal relationship of all these factors to (a) changes in medication (dosage, route of administration, time of day medication was given), and (b) any potentially stressful experiences (e.g., visitors, hospital leaves, interpersonal relationships with hospital staff or with other patients).

Only after all of this information is available can the therapist judge the extent to which each of the following factors may be involved: (1) incorrect diagnosis; (2) incorrect dosage of medication (too low or too high); (3) surreptitious avoidance of some or all of the medication; (4) side effects that have been incorrectly diagnosed (e.g., akathisia) or that are unreported but distressing to the patient (e.g., disturbance of sexual function); (5) a psychiatric side effect of the medication prescribed (e.g., depression caused by an antipsychotic); (6) a synergistic effect of several medications being taken concurrently; (7) the covert use of illicit drugs; (8) pharmacodynamic factors such as poor absorption or unusually rapid metabolism; (9) a natural change in the course of the psychiatric illness; (10) concurrent physical illness; and (11) idiosyncrasy of drug response.

Possible responses may be summarized as follows: environmental changes (admission to hospital, exclusion of visitors, or removal of hospital privileges); (2) continuing the same medication, but with alterations in dosage, frequency, or route of administration; (3) discontinuing certain medications; (4) addition of another psychotherapeutic drug to the regimen; (5) changing the main psychotherapeutic drug to a different agent of the same basic type; or (6) changing to a different type of treatment.

Idiosyncratic Response

Idiosyncratic response to treatment is relatively more common in psychiatry than in some other medical specialties. An occasional patient may not respond to one medication and then show excellent response to a different but similar drug. There are also many anecdotal reports of patients who derive no benefit from any standard treatment but unexpectedly improve when some highly unusual approach is employed. While this psychopharmacological idiosyncrasy of some patients can be a vexing problem, the clinician who is a good observer and maintains an open-minded approach will often be able to use this individuality to his patient's advantage. It is not recommended that nonspecialists attempt bizarre or highly unusual

treatments — or even that specialists do so until the situation warrants novelty — but every physician should be aware of the possibility and be ready to seek help from an experienced colleague before giving up.

ANTIPSYCHOTIC DRUGS (NEUROLEPTICS)

The molecular configuration of *promethazine* (Phenergan) includes a central tricyclic nucleus consisting of two benzene rings joined by a nitrogen and a sulfur atom (the *phenothiazine* nucleus). In the mid-1930s this drug was reported to have antihistaminic, antiemetic, and sedative properties, and thereafter it found application in anesthesiology. It was later tried as a treatment for psychotic agitation, but with poor results.

In 1950 a number of new phenothiazine compounds were synthesized from promethazine in an attempt to find drugs having greater central nervous system (CNS) action. An anesthesiologist made use of one of these drugs (later known as *chlorpromazine*) in combination with pethidine (meperidine) and promethazine. He administered this "lytic cocktail" to surgical patients to produce *artificial hibernation* — not unconsciousness, but indifference to the environment, reduced concern about pain, decreased fear, and relaxation. Somewhat later the French psychiatrists Jean Delay and Pierre Deniker decided to try chlorpromazine as a treatment for psychotic agitation, at doses of 75 to 150 mg per day. They became convinced that its benefits went much further than symptomatic relief of agitation, and hypothesized that it would have an ameliorative effect on diverse psychotic symptoms. Their enthusiasm was "supported by the sudden, great interest of the nursing personnel, who had always been reserved about innovations."

In 1953 chlorpromazine was made available for clinical use in the United States. The approved applications were as an antiemetic, a potentiator, a sedative, and a hypothermic, but the great interest was in its novel application in psychiatry.

The antipsychotic effects of another new drug, *reserpine*, were also attracting attention following a favorable report by Nathan Kline (1954). Delay and Deniker subsequently proposed the name *neuroleptic* to be applied to drugs that, like reserpine and chlorpromazine, produced a characteristic triad of (1) decreased psychomotor activity, (2) emotional apathy, and (3) affective indifference. Such drugs have also been called *major tranquilizers, neuroplegics, antipsychotics, psychostatics,* and *ataraxics;* the latter term, however, is also sometimes applied to the minor tranquilizers (antianxiety agents).

Classes of Antipsychotic Drugs

In 1956, for the first time in 175 years, the total number of patients residing in mental hospitals in the United States decreased from that of the preceding year. This was attributed to the widespread use of new antipsychotic drugs, thereby stimulating a vigorous search for others. Based on extensive animal studies, a battery of screening tests was devised that determines whether a given drug has a potential for effects similar to those of chlorpromazine. Although this methodology has produced a great many new neuroleptics, its implicit limitation is that only drugs with properties similar to those of existing drugs can be thus identified.

There are currently six different chemical classes of neuroleptic drugs available in the United States: (1) *Rauwolfia alkaloids;* (2) *phenothiazines* (subdivided into *aliphatics, piperidines,* and *piperazines*); (3) *thioxanthenes* (similarly subdivided); (4) *butyrophenones;* (5) *dihydroindolones;* and (6) *dibenzoxazepines.* Not every drug in each group is a neuroleptic, nor do these groups exhaust the known possibilities; there are already at least four additional groups in use abroad. The most numerous group by far is the phenothiazines, and each of the last three groups named contains only a single antipsychotic drug currently available.

All known neuroleptic drugs are synthetic except for the Rauwolfia alkaloids. Table 8-1 lists many of those available for clinical use in the United States. Certain other drugs also have neuroleptic properties but are unsuitable for use as antipsychotics because of their very short duration of action (e.g., droperidol) or because they are significantly less effective (e.g., promazine and mepazine) than those listed. *All of the drugs listed should be considered equally effective as antipsychotics, though the dosage ranges vary approximately a hundredfold.*

The second column of the table lists the approximate oral dosage or range (in milligrams) that will have the same antipsychotic action as a standard 100 mg oral dose of chlorpromazine. The drugs that are roughly one to four times as potent as chlorpromazine on a milligram basis (e.g., thioridazine or triflupromazine) are often referred to as *low-potency (or high-dosage) neuroleptics,* while those at the other extreme (i.e., those that are about 20 or more times as potent as chlorpromazine, such as trifluoperazine or haloperidol) are called *high-potency (or low-dosage) neuroleptics.* This terminology is widely used, since it provides an extremely handy way of predicting the relative frequency of most side effects. However, the word *potency* should not be confused with *efficacy,* since the drugs are equally efficacious as antipsychotics. Also, the terms *low-dosage neuroleptic* and *high-dosage neuroleptic* should never be interpreted as guidelines for maximum safe dosage. In fact, *megadose neuroleptic therapy is done only with the "low-dosage" neuroleptics.*

Rauwolfia Alkaloids

Various extracts from plants of the genus *Rauwolfia* have been used as medicinals since ancient times, most notably to sedate the mentally deranged or to reduce anxiety. In 1952 *reserpine* was isolated from the root of *Rauwolfia serpentina* and identified as one of its pharmacologically active constituents. Following Kline's report of its antipsychotic effects, this drug enjoyed a brief period of popularity. However, it fell into disuse only a few years later, for two basic reasons: (1) It became apparent that reserpine is slower-acting, less effective, and less often effective than other antipsychotics; and (2) the adverse effects of antipsychotic doses of reserpine are relatively greater than those of other neuroleptics. The most serious of these side effects is psychotic depression, which is insidious in onset and is often accompanied by suicidal ideation. Other disadvantages include pronounced hypotension, gastric hypersecretion

Table 8-1. Selected Antipsychotic Drugs Currently Available in the United States, with Approximate Oral Dosages Equal in Antipsychotic Potency to a Standard 100 mg Dose of Chlorpromazine

Chemical class, generic name, and trade names	Milligram oral dosage range approximately equal in antipsychotic potency to 100 mg of chlorpromazine
Phenothiazines	
Aliphatics	
Chlorpromazine (Thorazine and many others)	100
Triflupromazine (Vesprin)	25—35
Piperidines	
Thioridazine (Mellaril)	100
Mesoridazine (Serentil)	50—60
Piperacetazine (Quide)	10—20
Piperazines	
Carphenazine (Proketazine)	25—30
Acetophenazine (Tindal)	20—25
Prochlorperazine (Compazine)	12—15
Thiopropazate (Dartal)	10—12
Butaperazine (Repoise)	8—12
Perphenazine (Trilafon)	9—10
Trifluoperazine (Stelazine)	2—5
Fluphenazine hydrochloride (Prolixin, Permitil)	1—4
Thioxanthenes	
Aliphatics	
Chlorprothixene (Taractan)	40—100
Piperazines	
Thiothixene (Navane)	2—5
Butyrophenones	
Haloperidol (Haldol)	1—4
Dibenzoxazepines	
Loxapine (Loxitane, Daxolin)	10—20
Dihydroindolones	
Molindone (Moban)	6—15

(which exacerbates peptic and other ulcers), and relative lack of safety in combination with other treatments (ECT or insulin therapy).

The use of reserpine and two related antipsychotics (deserpidine and rescinnamine) is today virtually limited to the treatment of hypertension. Their only remaining psychiatric application is for psychotic patients who are refractory to all other treatments or unable to take standard neuroleptics because of allergy or some other problem.

Indications for Antipsychotic Drugs

The target symptoms best alleviated by these drugs are: (1) *thought disorders* (delusions, autistic thinking, association defects); (2) *hallucinations;*

and (3) *psychomotor disturbances* (agitation and retardation). Antipsychotics reduce these target symptoms in all types of functional psychoses and in many psychotic brain syndromes, but their preeminent application is in the treatment of *functional cognitive psychoses* (i.e., schizophrenias and paranoid states). They are superior to all other treatments for schizophrenias, and are therefore sometimes referred to as *antischizophrenic* drugs. However, they are more effective against the acute psychotic manifestations than the underlying schizophrenic process; they arrest or alter the course of schizophrenia, and may greatly improve the prognosis, but they do not cure the disease.

In the absence of the target symptoms, neuroleptics are *not* very effective against such other manifestations of schizophrenia as maladaptive social behavior, withdrawal, defective insight, or affective disturbance (e.g., apathy, depression, elation, anxiety). Therefore, the "process" schizophrenias such as the simple and hebephrenic subtypes tend to respond less favorably than those in which the target symptoms constitute the primary disturbance. However, it should not be overlooked that such symptoms may be *secondary to the target symptoms* (e.g., maladaptive social behavior motivated by delusional beliefs) and in these cases will respond well to neuroleptic therapy.

Secondary indications for neuroleptics include: mania and hypomania; agitated or anxious depression; hyperkinetic and aggressive behavior disorders in children and adolescents; panic disorders; and certain psychotic brain syndromes. These indications are considered "secondary" because there are other treatments that are either more effective than neuroleptics or equally effective but safer. However, neuroleptics may be helpful when the standard treatments are ineffective or cannot be used, or for short-term control of dangerous symptoms (e.g., agitation or suicidal behavior).

CNS Effects of Neuroleptic Drugs

The CNS pharmacology of neuroleptics has been extensively studied; Byck (1975) and Longo (1973) summarized much of this knowledge. A comprehensive presentation is beyond the scope of this text, but selected highlights deserve consideration.

The antipsychotic action of neuroleptic drugs is not associated with a comparable level of CNS depression and is not due to sedation. Far from being general depressants, these are among the most selective of CNS drugs. In fact, some of their actions are exactly opposite to those of depressants. For example, neuroleptics *lower the threshold for epileptic seizures.* The frequency of seizures in epileptic patients may be increased, or a latent convulsive disorder may be unmasked. This epileptogenic effect may be counteracted by increased dosage of anticonvulsant medication, but neuroleptics must be used cautiously in patients with seizure disorders (for whom the preferred drug is haloperidol).

The central effects most consistently related to the antipsychotic action have involved catecholaminergic functions, particularly those of *dopamine.* All known neuroleptics *inhibit dopaminergic function* in the CNS, and conversely every drug known to have this effect also has antipsychotic properties (not necessarily clinically useful). Rauwolfia alkaloids achieve this by depletion of intracellular stores of dopamine, norepinephrine, serotonin, and possibly other monoamines. None of the drugs listed in Table 8-1 is a dopamine-depleter, but most are known and all are hypothesized to cause *postsynaptic blockade* of dopamine-sensitive receptor sites. In recent years the most widely held theory about the antipsychotic mechanism of neuroleptics has involved dopaminergic inhibition at three neuroanatomical sites: the *reticular formation,* the *hypothalamus,* and the *limbic system.*

One of the clinically important effects of neuroleptics on the hypothalamus involves *temperature regulation.* Animals treated with these drugs are unable to adjust their body temperature properly when exposed to a hot or cold environment. Human patients taking an antipsychotic typically manifest mild hypothermia. However, in extreme environmental temperatures hypothermia or hyperthermia may become severe. *Hyperpyretic crises* may occur either in combination with other drugs (e.g., severe lithium toxicity) or as a result of *anticholinergic toxicity* (possibly due to the neuroleptic itself) which prevents sweating by an overheated person.

Decreased dopaminergic activity in the *basal ganglia* is now known to be the pathological basis of Parkinson's disease. A major factor in this discovery was the observation that neuroleptics can produce *extrapyramidal side effects (EPS),* including a *pseudoparkinson syndrome* that is clinically indistinguishable from the natural disease but fully reversible when the drug is discontinued. It was once thought that basal ganglia effects of neuroleptics might be essential for their antipsychotic action, but proponents of this theory are now a minority.

With the notable exception of thioridazine (Mellaril), even low doses of neuroleptics have powerful *antiemetic effects* due to depression of the chemoreceptor trigger zone. Prochlorperazine (Compazine) is advertised primarily for its antiemetic effects. This is based solely on the marketing policy of the manufacturer, for this drug is neither a better antiemetic nor a poorer antipsychotic than others, and it has the same spectrum of side effects. It is *not* true that all centrally acting antiemetics have neuroleptic properties (e.g., promethazine does not).

Neuroleptics *depress vasomotor reflexes,* producing a centrally mediated fall in blood pressure, a reflexive increase in heart rate, and orthostatic hypotension. These effects are marked for low-potency drugs such as chlorpromazine, and are minimal for high-potency drugs such as haloperidol. Long-term or high-dosage neuroleptic therapy may *suppress the cough reflex,* and this has resulted in deaths following aspiration of food or vomitus.

Peripheral Effects of Neuroleptic Drugs

Chlorpromazine was first marketed under the trade name Largactil, which drew attention to a diversity of peripheral effects already noted (long before the CNS effects had been adequately investigated). Although there are important differences in intensity, every neuroleptic drug manifests some combination of: (1) anticholinergic effects; (2) antihistaminic effects; (3) alpha-adrenergic blocking effects; (4) adrenergic agonist effects (due to interference with re-uptake processes); (5) antitryptaminergic effects; (6) complex effects on hormones; (7) direct depressant effects on the heart; (8) direct vasodilating effects on blood vessels; (9) reduction of gastrointestinal secretions and motility; and (10) local anesthetic properties (following topical application or injection). Many different types of adverse effects result from interaction of these properties with each other, with biological idiosyncrasies of individual patients, and with the many neurovegetative changes that accompany psychoses. However, a detailed enumeration will not be attempted until after discussion of the *tricyclic antidepressants,* since the latter share many of these same properties and therefore have a similar spectrum of side effects.

Interactions of Neuroleptics with Other Drugs

Neuroleptics interact with many other drugs. A useful generalization is that *a neuroleptic will interact in at least an additive fashion, and possibly by true potentiation, with any other drug having any similar effect* (e.g., antihypertensives, anticholinergics, antihistamines). A few special cases and a few exceptions deserve additional comment.

CNS DRUGS. The antiparkinson effects of *levodopa* are antagonized, as are most CNS effects of stimulants such as amphetamine and other sympathomimetics, caffeine, and nicotine, but not strychnine. *Anticonvulsant effects are antagonized, but other effects of CNS depressants are potentiated.* Ataxic, sedating, and hypnotic effects are prolonged and intensified, which may contraindicate neuroleptics for persons acutely intoxicated from ethanol, barbiturates, and similar drugs. The *analgesic effects* of opiates (including synthetics) are potentiated strongly, leading to a valuable nonpsychiatric application.

PERIPHERAL DRUGS. Chlorpromazine and perhaps other neuroleptics antagonize the antihypertensive effects of *guanethidine* (Ismelin) by blocking the receptors at which it acts. *The pressor effects of epinephrine may be reversed,* depending on the amount of alpha-receptor blockade. There is a possibility of a decreased effect of oral anticoagulants, and an increased effect of oral hypoglycemics.

Conversely, other drugs may affect the pharmacokinetics of neuroleptics. *Anticholinergic antiparkinson drugs* may cause reduction in plasma and tissue concentrations, thereby diminishing the antipsychotic effect. *Barbiturates* and other stimulators of hepatic microsomal enzymes may dramatically increase the speed of metabolic deactivation, and *antacids* may reduce the efficiency of gastrointestinal absorption.

CLINICAL TESTS. Clinical tests known to be occasionally altered by neuroleptics include: alkaline phosphatase; urine and serum bilirubin; CSF proteins; cholesterol; diacetic acid in urine; estrogens in urine; fasting glucose; certain pregnancy tests from urine; catecholamines and 17-hydroxy-steroids in urine; phenylketonuria tests; protein-bound iodine; porphyrins; transaminase; uric acid; and urobilinogen.

Differences Among Neuroleptics

All of the neuroleptics listed in Table 8-1 are considered equally efficacious as antipsychotics (i.e., for the target symptoms listed previously), and all have the same spectrum of potential side effects. Important differences among these drugs include: (1) relative frequencies and intensities of various side effects; (2) possible antidepressant or antimanic properties of a few specific drugs; (3) relative safety of high doses (especially injections); and (4) idiosyncratic side effects of thioridazine. Many attempts to show that certain neuroleptics have differential effects against particular constellations of target symptoms (e.g., paranoid ideation or catatonia) have been conspicuously unconvincing.

In retrospect it appears that most differences reported (which were modest at best, and usually not replicated in other studies) were artifacts of dosage.

The important differences in frequency and severity of various side effects can be estimated on the basis of the *relative antipsychotic potencies* of the drugs. Chlorpromazine and haloperidol are at the extremes of the potency scale implied in Table 8-1, and are also at or near the extremes for many types of side effects. They may therefore be taken as prototypes of low- and high-potency neuroleptics respectively, and Table 8-2 contrasts their profiles of side effects.

The antipsychotic potency scale for neuroleptics correlates highly with each of the scales implied by the contrasts in Table 8-2; drugs that are similar to chlorpromazine or haloperidol in antipsychotic potency may be expected to be similar in these other characteristics as well. These are empirical generalizations, based on data derived from animal experiments, human experi-

Table 8-2. Some Important Empirical Differences Between Chlorpromazine and Haloperidol, which may be Generalized to Other Neuroleptics of Low and High Antipsychotic Potency

Clinical property	Chlorpromazine (and low-potency neuroleptics)	Haloperidol (and high-potency neuroleptics)
Antipsychotic efficacy	Equal	Equal
Amount of sedation	Great	Relatively small
Acute EPS (pseudoparkinsonism, acute dystonias, akathisia)	Less frequent, less severe	More frequent, more severe
Chronic EPS (tardive dyskinesias)	Possibly more	Possibly less
Anticholinergic effects	Relatively strong	Relatively weak
Peripheral adrenergic blocking	Relatively strong	Relatively weak
Allergic reactions (blood dyscrasias, rashes)	More frequent	Less frequent
Jaundice	More frequent	Less frequent
Cardiovascular problems (hypotension, orthostatic hypotension, arrhythmias)	More frequent and severe	Less frequent and severe
Endocrine changes	More frequent	Less frequent
Weight gain	Greater	Less
Activation of seizures	Greater	Less
Safety of high oral dosage	Increased risk	Relatively safer
Safety of high-dosage IM injections	Increased risk	Little or no increased risk

ments, and clinical experience with the drugs. Some pharmacologists assert that the higher potency neuroleptics are more selective for the central nervous system, thereby requiring lower dosages and having fewer peripheral side effects of all types. However, the data may be incomplete for the high-potency neuroleptics, which are newer and have been taken by fewer patients to date.

Most neuroleptics have poor antidepressant effects and may even cause depression as a side effect. However, some studies have found thioridazine (Mellaril), chlorprothixene (Taractan), and especially thiothixene (Navane) equal in efficacy to tricyclic antidepressants for some types of depressed patients (notably those with prominent anxiety, hostility, or agitation). At least one well-controlled study has found haloperidol superior to chlorpromazine and comparable to lithium during the first few weeks of treatment of *mania,* but the same study found lithium superior to both antipsychotics after several weeks of therapy.

Thioridazine (Mellaril) has the significant advantage of being the *least likely to produce EPS,* and is often prescribed for patients having high empirical risk, especially adolescents and children. However, it also has several important disadvantages to remember: (1) *The upper dosage limit must never exceed 800 mg per day.* This is the only drug listed in Table 8-1 that has any appreciable risk of causing *retinitis pigmentosa,* which may lead to blindness, and nearly all reported cases involved dosages in excess of 800 mg per day. (2) This drug frequently causes characteristic *electrocardiographic changes,* possibly by a direct toxic effect on the heart. Although these changes are usually asymptomatic, are believed to be benign, and reverse when thioridazine is discontinued, many clinicians prefer to avoid the drug for this reason. (3) Male patients are frequently disturbed by *ejaculatory disorders* that are relatively frequent with this drug, and may refuse all further therapy for this reason.

Depot Injections of Fluphenazine
Fluphenazine is available in three different forms. The hydrochloride form is similar to other high-

potency neuroleptics, and may be injected or taken orally in tablets or liquid concentrate. *Fluphenazine enanthate* and *fluphenazine decanoate* are esterified forms for injection only, and have the significant advantage of *extremely long duration of action* (one to three weeks). Patients who are unreliable about managing their own medication and might otherwise require long-term custodial care may be managed as outpatients if arrangements can be made for periodic injections (e.g., by the family doctor or an outpatient clinic). The dosage and interval between injections must be determined empirically for each patient, and it is recommended that the mental status be stabilized and response to fluphenazine be determined by administration of the hydrochloride form before switching to one of the esters.

Nonpsychiatric Uses of Neuroleptic Drugs
Many of the CNS and peripheral effects of neuroleptics described above can be applied therapeutically in certain nonpsychiatric situations. Although these applications are not officially approved for many individual drugs, it is likely that most or all neuroleptics would be equally effective, and rational selection of the drug should involve consideration of the possible side effects. These applications include: (1) control of nausea and vomiting in a wide range of disorders, such as radiation sickness, uremia, gastroenteritis, carcinomatosis, and side effects of certain other drugs (but *not* levodopa); (2) reduction of hyperpyrexia due to certain infectious diseases, brain syndromes, etc.; (3) reduction of need for narcotics by potentiating opiates; (4) control of hyperkinetic extrapyramidal symptoms in certain neurological disorders (e.g., Huntington's chorea, Gilles de la Tourette's syndrome); (5) in lytic cocktails, producing relaxation and reducing autonomic reactivity associated with surgery or childbirth; (6) prolongation of the action of barbiturates or other hypnotics, thus producing increased duration of sleep; (7) termination of intractable hiccough; and (8) treatment of hypertensive crises with chlorpromazine (not yet an "approved" application).

ANTIDEPRESSANT DRUGS

Two major groups of antidepressant drugs are currently available: the *tricyclic antidepressants (TCAs)*, of which the prototype is imipramine, and the *monoamine oxidase inhibitors (MAOIs)*, of which the prototype is iproniazid. TCAs are chemically classified as dibenzazepines, dibenzo-cycloheptadienes, and dibenzoxepins, but all have very similar properties and all have a tricyclic molecular structure. MAOIs are chemically classified as hydrazines and nonhydrazines; however, this entire group of antidepressants is now virtually obsolete, for reasons mentioned below.

Imipramine

Imipramine was one of more than 40 derivatives of iminodibenzyl synthesized in 1948 by the Geigy Company for possible trials as antihistamines, sedatives, analgesics, and antiparkinsonian agents. Following discovery of the antipsychotic properties of chlorpromazine, several of these drugs (which have chemical and pharmacological properties closely resembling phenothiazines) were investigated for possible use as antipsychotics. Imipramine was selected for clinical trials on the basis of its structural resemblance to chlorpromazine, but was found ineffective as a neuroleptic. However, Roland Kuhn in Switzerland noted improvement in the depressed patients in his sample, and suggested the possible application of imipramine as an antidepressant. Following his report at the Second World Congress of Psychiatry (1957), which he read "to an audience of barely a dozen people," other investigators became interested and confirmed his results. (Exactly four months earlier, others had reported the antidepressant effects of *iproniazid*, a drug originally developed for use in the treatment of tuberculosis.)

Mechanism of Action of Antidepressant Drugs

The discovery during the 1950s of reserpine, a drug that causes depression, and of imipramine and iproniazid, which alleviate it, has facilitated 20 years of fruitful study of the pathophysiology of depression. The biochemical and pharmacological differences between imipramine and iproniazid

were found to be greater than their similarities, and the search for a common link implicated monoaminergic functions in the CNS. Successive refinements of technique focused attention on the catecholamines, especially *norepinephrine (NE)*, leading to Joseph Schildkraut's formulation of the catecholamine hypothesis of affective disorders, which is discussed in Chapter 14.

The original concepts describing the mechanism of action of antidepressant drugs involved *potentiation of CNS noradrenergic function.* Monoamine oxidase is the enzyme that deactivates NE and certain other amines while free in intraneuronal cytoplasm. Inhibition of this enzyme permits accumulation of increased amounts of these neurotransmitters. Imipramine has not been shown to interfere with enzyme activity, but in animal experiments appears to inhibit the re-uptake pump which returns NE to the cytoplasm of the effector cell following release into the synaptic cleft. This delay of inactivation permits the neurotransmitter to stimulate receptor sites for an increased duration of time, presumably potentiating its effect.

Such simple concepts are intuitively appealing, but no longer account for all data. Further refinements of technique, originally expected to close the few remaining loopholes in this elegant theory, have raised more problems than they have solved. Studies of biochemical indicators of CNS amine activity in depressed and nondepressed persons have produced grossly inconsistent results. Also, certain TCAs appear to affect other neurotransmitters besides NE, in some cases to a much greater extent. For example, amitriptyline potentiates the indolamine *serotonin* much more strongly than NE, and potentiates NE much less than does imipramine, but is equivalent to imipramine in antidepressant effect.

In recent years, much research has attempted to identify homogeneous subgroups of depressed patients on the basis of biochemical and other clinical findings, in the hope of shortening the time required to find optimal treatment. Although a reliable method may eventually be found to take the guesswork out of treating depression, more traditional methods are currently in use. The recommended approach is based on a combination of careful history taking, systematic clinical observation, evaluation of risks and benefits of different treatments, and clinical judgments based in part on empirical data presented here and in Chapter 14.

Monoamine Oxidase Inhibitors

Many observers have reported qualitative differences in the types of target symptoms that respond to treatment with TCAs and MAOIs. Such distinctions may be valid, and are still recommended by some experts, but are often difficult to apply in specific cases. Moreover, current psychiatric practice has de-emphasized the use of MAOIs, which have several significant disadvantages that for most patients override any possible advantage. Specifically:

MAOIs are less effective and less often effective than TCAs. The hydrazine compounds (isocarboxazid and phenelzine) are also slower acting.

MAOIs are considerably more toxic than TCAs. A detailed presentation of their many side effects will not be attempted, but one very dangerous problem may be mentioned: hydrazines may cause *irreversible hepatocellular jaundice.* The exact mechanism is unknown, but this disorder has a 25 percent mortality, and several MAOIs (including the prototype iproniazid) were withdrawn from the market because of an intolerably high incidence of jaundice. Those still available are safer, but have also been reported to cause this side effect.

All MAOIs cause pronounced hypotension during therapy. Therefore, the occurrence of *hypertensive crises* in some patients was puzzling until Blackwell succeeded in recognizing the mechanism. MAO in the liver serves the very important function of deactivating exogenous pressor amines that occur in many foods. Since these drugs inhibit the enzyme in the liver as well as the CNS, subsequent ingestion of any food containing such substances leads to abnormal levels in the circulation, resulting in marked increases in blood pressure, headaches, and possibly intracranial bleeding and even death. This is commonly known as the *cheese reaction,* since certain cheeses contain high concentrations of *tyramine.* However, the list of foods that must be avoided during MAOI therapy is now quite extensive, and the risks and disadvantages of such stringent dietary restrictions for depressed patients are obvious. This problem is especially severe with tranylcypromine (a nonhydrazine).

MAOIs interact with a great many other drugs, often dangerously and in unexpected ways. Even some nonprescription medications are contraindicated for patients taking an MAOI, and the physician must cross-check very carefully before attempting any other treatment. The potential for such interactions persists for several weeks after MAOI therapy is discontinued, since return to normal enzyme levels is a slow process.

For reasons such as these, MAOIs have been largely relegated to research laboratories; even many psychiatrists prefer to use them only as a last resort. *Their use by nonspecialists is not recommended.*

Tricyclic Antidepressants

Like many illnesses characterized by a multiplicity of causes and manifestations, depressions do not respond uniformly well to any single treatment approach. Some comparisons of the modalities currently available will be presented in the section on electroconvulsive therapy, which is the treatment having the highest empirical rate of success for severe depression.

The extensive research on TCAs permits only two firm conclusions. First, they are the most effective medications available for the treatment of some types of depression. Second, a minority of severely depressed patients obtain little or no relief from these drugs, and a large number of others will respond equally well or better to some different type of medication.

Endogenous, or *endogenomorphic, depressions* are the clearest indications for TCAs. These are potentially severe illnesses, usually with prominent melancholia (feelings of sadness), but obvious precipitating factors such as loss, conflict, or frustration may or may not be present. Clinical signs and complaints suggestive of this syndrome include early morning awakening with inability to fall asleep again; diurnal variation in mood, with greatest discomfort in the morning; loss of appetite and weight; loss of sexual desire; constipation; inability to obtain even temporary pleasure from previously enjoyed activities; preoccupation with feelings of guilt, sometimes of delusional intensity; excessive inhibitions which may severely impair normal functioning; and bizarre delusions of somatic disease or nihilism. The number and severity of such signs correlate with the likelihood of therapeutic benefit from TCAs, especially if therapy is begun relatively soon after the onset of symptoms. However, acute danger or serious physical illness (e.g., dehydration, exhaustion, malnutrition, cardiovascular disease) may be an indication for immediate use of ECT, or for antipsychotic medication on either a temporary or a long-term basis.

Such depressions are called *retarded* if there are signs of psychomotor slowing, such as decreased speed of movements, speech, and thoughts, diminished volume of speech, and poverty of ideation. Retarded depressions generally have the highest rate of favorable response to TCAs, and also are the group in which these drugs are the most clearly superior to others. *Agitated,* or anxious, depressions are those in which there is excessive purposeless or undirected activity, such as pacing, handwringing, increased volume and speed of speech, difficulty in concentration, and other manifestations of tension. These respond well to TCAs, although not as well as the retarded depressions, and are more likely to respond equally well to other types of medication (usually antipsychotics). Antianxiety drugs are sometimes helpful either in addition to or instead of antidepressants, but if there are obvious signs of hostility and anger the antianxiety drug may exacerbate these symptoms.

Depressions labeled as *neurotic* or *characterological* typically differ from endogenomorphic depressions by being closely related and more appropriate in duration and severity to loss, conflict, or frustration (either acute or chronic). Feelings of melancholia are less prominent and increase or diminish in temporal relationship to life changes or pleasurable activities. Guilt feelings are often absent or minimal; sleep disturbance is likely to consist of difficulty initiating or maintaining

sleep rather than early awakening; and if there is diurnal variation in mood, the evening is usually the time of greatest discomfort. The most important aspect of treatment for such disorders is psychosocial therapy and environmental manipulation. TCAs are usually no better than a placebo, although there are exceptions to this statistical generalization.

The six tricyclic antidepressants currently available in the United States are listed in Table 8-3. The only well-established clinical differences among these drugs concern side effects, and even these are only differences of intensity. The table also shows the usual dosage "windows." At dosages below those listed, the drugs are often ineffective; at dosages above the upper limit, toxicity is markedly increased. Since the drugs have weak postsynaptic blocking effects (similar to those of neuroleptics), excessive dosage may actually antagonize the antidepressant effect.

Imipramine and *amitriptyline* are the two oldest TCAs. Because of the recent expiration of patents on these drugs, they are now available from many manufacturers at competitive prices. They are the most thoroughly studied and probably the most frequently prescribed TCAs, and compare favorably with the others in efficacy and side effects. Amitriptyline is the most strongly sedating of these six drugs, and is frequently the drug chosen for patients with severe insomnia, anxiety, or agitation. It is also the most strongly anticholinergic, which is a disadvantage for many patients, but occasionally may be an advantage (e.g., if a neuroleptic is also prescribed).

Desipramine and *nortriptyline* are the demethylated metabolites of imipramine and amitriptyline respectively. They were initially tested as antidepressants in the hope that they would prove faster acting than other TCAs, but experiments attempting to verify this have not been convincing: at best the differences are clinically insignificant. However, they are effective antidepressants in their own right, and desipramine has the weakest anticholinergic effects among these six drugs.

Protriptyline differs from the other TCAs by having relatively weak and short-lived sedative effects. It is often described as the "most stimu-

Table 8-3. Tricyclic Antidepressants Currently Available in the United States, with Dosage Ranges for Acutely Depressed Patients and Comments about Noteworthy Properties

Generic and trade names	Acute daily dosage range in milligrams	Special properties and comments
Dibenzazepines		
Imipramine (Tofranil and many others)	75–300	The prototype and most extensively studied TCA; patent has recently expired, permitting competitive pricing
Desipramine (Norpramin and Pertofrane)	75–300	The demethylated metabolite of imipramine; least anticholinergic effects of all TCAs
Dibenzocycloheptadienes		
Amitriptyline (Elavil and many others)	75–300	The most sedating TCA; strongest anticholinergic effects; patent has expired
Nortriptyline (Aventyl)	40–100	The demethylated metabolite of amitriptyline
Protriptyline (Vivactil)	15– 60	The most stimulating, or least sedating, TCA; may have special applications in sleep disorders
Dibenzoxepins		
Doxepin (Sinequan and Adapin)	75–300	Highly sedating; least cardiovascular toxicity of all TCAs; not well tested in hospitalized psychotic depressives

lating" of the TCAs, but this is misleading, since only the diminished sedative effect is well documented. Many physicians have avoided protriptyline because the stronger sedative effects of the other drugs are beneficial to insomniac patients; some may also incorrectly consider it in the same class as true stimulants, which are poor antidepressants. Recent reports suggest that this drug may have previously unrecognized applications in the treatment of certain sleep disorders.

Doxepin is the newest of the TCAs available. Advertisements have emphasized its use in treating anxiety-depression syndromes in outpatients, and controlled studies have demonstrated its efficacy for such patients. However, it has not been well studied in populations of hospitalized patients with severe depression. The manufacturer's claim that it may be considered as an antianxiety agent should be disregarded; antidepressants should not be prescribed for the same indications as antianxiety drugs, and the "anxiolytic" properties

may simply be due to the relatively strong sedation (comparable to amitriptyline). Doxepin has weaker anticholinergic effects than several other TCAs, but its greatest merit is that it has the *least cardiovascular toxicity* among these six drugs. For a time it was described as the only TCA that does not block the antihypertensive action of guanethidine. However, this is true only at low dosage (under 150 mg per day), and doxepin is less potent on a milligram basis than imipramine and amitriptyline.

All drugs in Table 8-3 should be considered equally effective in statistical terms, but individual patients often respond better to one drug than others. Good guidelines for selection of the optimal drug are not yet available, beyond the generalizations suggested previously (history, side effects, etc.).

Clinical Considerations with TCAs

It is widely stated that "tricyclic antidepressants have delayed onset of action." This is only partly true. *Proper clinical evaluation requires three to four weeks of therapy at adequate dosage.* If good improvement is not noted after this period, the drug should be considered a failure and discontinued. It may be discontinued sooner if side effects that will obviously limit dosage to less than adequate levels are observed.

However, it is not unusual to note amelioration of some symptoms within the first few days of therapy. The many symptoms of severe depression are usually acquired gradually, and respond to treatment gradually as well. Unfortunately, the mood disturbance itself is usually the last symptom to improve, lagging behind normalization of psychomotor disturbance and vegetative changes. A seriously depressed patient who is responding to treatment will often look improved to persons in his immediate environment long before he is aware of feeling better. The observers note that he is eating and sleeping better and resuming a more normal pattern of activities; the patient notes only that the painful feelings have not decreased.

Suicidal risk is increased during the first few weeks of treatment. This paradoxical phenomenon is well known but not well understood. Several intuitively appealing explanations are the following: (1) Despair increases because the patient feels no better after beginning treatment. (2) His anger and hostility increase when he is told that he is getting better, although he *knows* that he is not. (3) Removal of the crippling inhibitions that prevented routine functioning may also remove the final deterrent to suicidal behavior. (4) Recovery does not follow a smooth uphill course, and minor setbacks may be perceived as signs of a return to intolerable suffering.

Regardless of the reason, the increased risk of suicide is a consideration of major importance. Inpatients should *not* be permitted to leave the hospital for weekend visits during the early stages of recovery. Outpatients should be seen frequently by the physician, and only very small prescriptions should be written. *The lethal dose of an antidepressant is approximately 5 to 30 times the usual daily therapeutic dose.* All depressed patients should be monitored carefully, and the

fact that recovery will be gradual must be explained to them.

SIDE EFFECTS OF ANTIPSYCHOTICS AND TRICYCLIC ANTIDEPRESSANTS

Acute Extrapyramidal Side Effects (EPS)

All drugs which alter dopamine-mediated functioning in the basal ganglia have the possibility of producing extrapyramidal side effects. TCAs have relatively weak effects on dopamine and relatively strong anticholinergic properties; EPS, though possible, are very rare with these drugs.

Antipsychotic drugs have strong antidopaminergic effects, and EPS are a major problem. For any particular drug, the incidence and severity of EPS are directly related to *dosage.* However, at equivalent antipsychotic dosages (which are presumably equivalent antidopaminergic dosages) there are important differences between drugs. These differences are empirically correlated with *antipsychotic potency* (see Table 8-2), and are attributed by some authorities to differences in affinity for specific dopaminergic tracts. A more important factor appears to be the *anticholinergic* (muscarinic blocking) property which is common to all but relatively stronger for the low-potency neuroleptics (Snyder et al., 1974). This also explains why the correlation of EPS with dosage is *curvilinear* (at least for high potency neuroleptics). As dosage increases, both antidopaminergic and antimuscarinic effectiveness increase; EPS increase until the muscarinic blockade becomes significant, and then decrease.

There are three basic types of acute EPS: akathisia, pseudoparkinsonism, and muscular dystonias and dyskinesias. All are fully reversible by discontinuing the medication, but for psychotic patients this is usually unwarranted, as there are other effective means of reducing or removing these side effects.

AKATHISIA. Akathisia is a syndrome of motor restlessness. The term is derived from a Greek word meaning "unable to sit down," which aptly describes the typical patient's driving desire to remain in motion. Attempts to sit down or otherwise remain still are accompanied by intense subjective discomfort, and the combination of undirected hypermotility and psychic distress may be misdiagnosed as an exacerbation of the psychosis and lead to erroneous increase in dosage of the antipsychotic drug. Akathisia should be suspected whenever the patient manifests or complains of poorly described discomfort, especially if he uses words like jittery, uptight, nervous, etc.

PSEUDOPARKINSONISM. Pseudoparkinsonism is clinically indistinguishable from idiopathic or postencephalitic Parkinson's disease, except for its full reversibility. Symptoms may include any of the following: muscular weakness, reduced motility, rigidity, festinant gait, mask-like facies, coarse tremor, "pill-rolling" movements, excessive salivation, and seborrhea. *Akinesia* is a form of drug-induced behavioral toxicity believed to be a variant of the parkinsonian syndrome. Obvious neurological signs are usually absent, but the patient manifests diminished activity level, reduced spontaneity of speech, gestures, and social interactions, inability to participate or disinterest in recreation, apathy, and complaints of feeling excessively drowsy or anergic. Such symptoms may be indicative of depression, chronic schizophrenia, demoralization, or excessive sedation, but may also be a form of EPS and respond well to antiparkinson medication or reduction in dosage of the antipsychotic.

Acute dystonias and dyskinesias are the least frequent but most dramatic form of EPS. Symptoms arise very suddenly and may be quite frightening to the patient and observers who do not understand their etiology. If an outpatient seeks treatment in a hospital emergency room, the use of a neuroleptic may not be reported (especially if prescribed for a nonpsychiatric indication such as vomiting) since uninformed patients typically do not associate these reactions with the medication. Most physicians now routinely inquire about recent drug use whenever examining any bizarre neurological syndrome, but in the past these EPS were sometimes misdiagnosed as hysteria, tetanus, malingering, or catatonia, and treated with surgery

or other completely unnecessary methods. Any voluntary muscle or muscle group may be involved, but those of the neck and the head are most frequently affected. Typical syndromes include torticollis, retrocollis, trismus, laryngospasm, opisthotonos, swollen tongue, and oculogyric crisis (spasm of the external ocular muscles causing painful upward gaze). If breathing or swallowing are impaired the symptoms may be acutely life-threatening.

EPIDEMIOLOGY. Epidemiology of EPS is well known if not understood. In a sample of 3,775 patients treated with phenothiazines, Ayd (1961) reported an overall incidence of 38.9 percent of these patients manifesting EPS. Although females only slightly outnumbered males in this sample, they were disproportionately represented among those showing EPS (63 percent). The most frequent type was akathisia (21.2 percent of the sample); parkinsonism was also relatively frequent (15.4 percent); and acute dystonias and dyskinesias were uncommon (2.3 percent). The approximate 2:1 ratio of females to males held true for akathisia (65 percent female) and parkinsonism (65.5 percent female), but was reversed for dystonias (65 percent male). The type of EPS was strongly related to age, with young patients showing most of the dystonias, middle-aged having akathisia, and the elderly having the highest incidence of parkinsonism. Ninety percent of the dystonias occurred during the first four and a half days of treatment, while akathisia tended to have later onset, and parkinsonism still later (90 percent within the first 72 days). More recent studies involving newer drugs and higher doses have confirmed these statistical trends.

TREATMENT. Treatment of EPS may involve: (1) reduction of neuroleptic dosage; (2) discontinuation of medication; (3) change to a lower potency neuroleptic; or (4) adjunctive medication. In the latter case, the most frequently used drugs are *anticholinergic antiparkinsonian agents* such as benztropine (Cogentin), biperiden (Akineton), cycrimine (Pagitane), procyclidine (Kemadrin), or trihexyphenidyl (Artane). *Anticholinergic anti-histamines* such as diphenhydramine (Benadryl) and orphenadrine (Disipal) may also be used. Depending on the exact circumstances, these may be administered orally or by intramuscular injection; a few are even suitable for intravenous injection in emergencies.

Parkinsonian symptoms are usually relieved by an anticholinergic drug, and unless unusually severe the neuroleptic dosage need not be reduced. However, it must be remembered that *anticholinergic antiparkinsonian drugs reduce the therapeutic effects of antipsychotics,* that they have their own side effects, and that they may potentiate or increase other side effects of the neuroleptic. Therefore, reduction in neuroleptic dosage or change of drug may be a better alternative. *Levodopa and other dopaminergic agonists cannot be used,* since these drugs will either be ineffective or will exacerbate the psychosis. Akathisia may respond to an anticholinergic, but often does not; sedating agents such as a benzodiazepine or barbiturate may then be helpful, but if not it will be necessary to reduce dosage or change the antipsychotic drug. Acute dystonias usually respond well to anticholinergic medication, to benzodiazepines such as diazepam, or to caffeine sodium benzoate. These symptoms are time-limited but frequently recur unless preventive measures are instituted.

PREVENTION. Prevention of EPS is a matter of some controversy, with respected authorities taking directly opposing positions. The majority currently advise against prescribing anticholinergic medication prophylactically, noting that many patients never develop EPS, and that prophylactic medication increases cost, side effects, and risks. A few others are in favor of prophylaxis when high dosages or high-potency antipsychotics are prescribed or when the patient is considered especially vulnerable. However, prophylactic antiparkinson medication seems unwarranted for inpatients, since a routine order can be specified "prn." *Experienced psychiatric nurses are quite skilled at recognizing EPS.*

For outpatients, it is absolutely essential that the possibility of EPS be carefully explained. Depending on the therapist's judgment, there are four alternative approaches: (1) give immediate prophylactic medication; (2) write a prescription to be filled immediately, but instruct the patient to take the medication only if EPS occur; (3) write a prescription and instruct the patient to have it filled only if EPS occur; or (4) instruct the patient to phone for a prescription or other advice if EPS occur. The latter is advisable only if EPS are considered extremely unlikely (e.g., if thioridazine is prescribed).

Maintenance antiparkinson medication is advised whenever an EPS has required treatment (unless the neuroleptic therapy is modified so as to reduce EPS). However, tolerance is acquired to EPS over time, and placebo-controlled studies have found that over 90 percent of patients who initially need antiparkinson medication no longer need it after three months of continuous therapy. It is therefore recommended that this medication be gradually withdrawn after three months, with careful observation for return of EPS. Some patients may need additional reassurance because of psychological dependence on the antiparkinson drug (e.g., if the original EPS was severe or frightening). Some authorities advise against removal of the anticholinergic if the patient is receiving one of the long-acting esterified neuroleptics, because the latter are absorbed irregularly and fluctuations in absorption may lead to episodic EPS.

If the neuroleptic itself is removed, the anticholinergic should also be stopped, but a few days later than the neuroleptic (which is eliminated slowly from tissues). If a tricyclic antidepressant is added to the neuroleptic regimen, a trial off the antiparkinson drug is warranted, since TCAs themselves have strong anticholinergic properties.

Chronic Extrapyramidal Disorders (Tardive Dyskinesias)

The occurrence of acute reversible extrapyramidal disorders in patients treated with antipsychotic drugs had been well studied for nearly a decade before reports of chronic and potentially irreversible EPS appeared in the literature. Such disorders are known collectively as *tardive dyskinesias,* or *persistent dyskinesias,* or sometimes as *terminal extrapyramidal insufficiency,* and are characterized as follows: (1) The syndrome consists of continuous involuntary abnormal movements unaccompanied by other neurological abnormalities: therefore, diagnosis is by sight only. The movements may affect any voluntary muscle or muscle group, but most frequently involve the buccal-lingual-masticatory region. They may be so slight as to be undetectable or grossly obvious to the casual observer. They become more severe when performing a task using different muscles, but often disappear when using or focusing attention on the affected ones, or during sleep. (2) Nearly all cases occur after many years of treatment with antipsychotic drugs, although some may occur after only a few months of drug therapy, and cases have been reported in persons who have never been treated with neuroleptics. (3) The symptoms are usually masked by the continuing neuroleptic therapy, and may only become apparent when the dosage is reduced or the drug therapy discontinued. (4) The course is variable, but in most cases the symptoms are worsened by discontinuation of the antipsychotic medication and persist for many months or years after all medication has been stopped. (5) Conversely, the symptoms are reduced by increasing the dose or changing to a neuroleptic of higher potency. (6) Anticholinergic medication is not helpful, and may exacerbate the disorder. (7) Even severe cases may abate or disappear entirely after several months free of neuroleptic medication, but *there is no universally effective treatment.*

For a time there was debate about whether tardive dyskinesias are indeed drug-related, but accumulated evidence is now convincing. These disorders are rarely seen in acute schizophrenics, but studies have estimated the incidence at around 20 percent among chronic schizophrenics who have received neuroleptic drugs for many years. Although such patients often manifest little concern about the abnormal movements, some cases are so severe as to cause considerable social disability, impairment of gait or other purposive

movements (e.g., dressing or brushing teeth), or even gross inability to speak, swallow, or breathe. Predisposing factors include: sex (females are affected twice as frequently as males); age (over 50 years); duration of therapy with antipsychotic drugs; total lifetime dosage of neuroleptic medication; brain damage or trauma, including ECT; and idiosyncratic vulnerability. There is also evidence that long-term use of antiparkinson medication increases the risk.

Other CNS and Behavioral Side Effects

In addition to acute and chronic EPS, antipsychotics and TCAs may cause a variety of other side effects known or presumed to be mediated centrally. These include: seizures (by lowering the seizure threshold); hypothermia or hyperthermia, sometimes severe; sedation that is dose-related and to which tolerance is usually (but not always) acquired; increased sleep; sleep stage changes (including increased dreams or nightmares); EEG changes; and interactions with other centrally acting drugs, especially depressants.

The most frequent psychiatric side effect of antipsychotics is depression, and of TCAs, precipitation or exacerbation of schizophrenia or mania. With either type of drug, an occasional patient experiences paradoxical insomnia, which will usually be insignificant if the medication is taken early in the day. Rarer but also possible is *paradoxical exacerbation of target symptoms,* usually quite specific to one drug or chemical group of drugs.

Surprisingly, both antipsychotics and TCAs can cause a *toxic psychosis.* This resembles the syndrome due to *atropine poisoning* and is due to excessive anticholinergic medication. Most cases occur when several strongly anticholinergic drugs are combined (e.g., chlorpromazine, amitriptyline, and benztropine). A few patients may become toxic on therapeutic doses of a single drug (a TCA or low potency neuroleptic), but most cases involving only one drug are due to intentional overdosage. *Physostigmine salicylate (Antilirium),* a cholinesterase inhibitor which easily crosses the blood-brain barrier, is a specific and usually dramatic antidote for anticholinergic toxicity (see Chap. 12).

Allergic and Hypersensitivity Reactions

Several *blood dyscrasias* have been reported in connection with antipsychotic or antidepressant drug therapy, including leukocytosis, leukopenia, thrombocytopenia, and *agranulocytosis*. The latter is by far the most dangerous, with an estimated mortality of 30 percent of treated patients. The onset is very abrupt, and usually (but not always) occurs during the first eight weeks of therapy. Typical early signs are those of upper respiratory infection (fever, cough, sore throat); destructive ulcerative lesions may be noted during visual inspection of mucous membranes of mouth, gums, and throat. A complete blood count should be ordered immediately, and a diagnosis of agranulocytosis is confirmed by a drastically lowered white blood count (WBC) and reduction in neutrophils to below one-third the normal level. All medications should be discontinued at once, and aggressive hematological treatment initiated.

The incidence of agranulocytosis has been studied for many years. All authorities agree that it is very rare, and that patients with existing bone marrow depression are more vulnerable than others. Several investigators have noted that *asymptomatic leukopenia* (i.e., reduced WBC) is much more frequent than agranulocytosis and does not justify discontinuation of effective medication. This fact, combined with the abruptness of onset of true agranulocytosis, has led to general agreement that routine blood counts for screening purposes are not justified and in fact may be counterproductive. The objections include: (1) increased cost and discomfort to the patient; (2) the likelihood that any abnormality detected will be relatively benign, but may lead to an unwarranted decision to interrupt effective treatment; and (3) the false sense of security provided by routine testing may decrease interest in investigating real symptoms when they are reported.

Jaundice is another rare hypersensitivity reaction, with onset usually during the first few weeks of therapy. The usual prodrome consists of flu-like malaise, abdominal pain, anorexia, fever, vomiting, and diarrhea. There is bile in the urine and abnormally high levels of alkaline phosphatase associated with elevated bilirubin. Other enzymes are also elevated. Pruritus and other skin reactions may be present but are not usual. Biopsy and autopsy studies have confirmed that this is an obstructive type of jaundice, which usually remits without complication if the offending drug is promptly discontinued and the patient is kept in bed and given a diet high in proteins and carbohydrates. Cross-sensitivity is rare, so that a different drug of the same basic type may be started if necessary. As in the case of blood dyscrasias, there is general agreement that routine laboratory tests are of little value unless the patient is highly vulnerable or has a history of previous reaction (in which case the laboratory tests should be made daily).

Simple allergic skin disorders include maculopapular rashes, erythema multiforme, and localized or generalized urticaria. These are usually mild and transient, and respond well to treatment with a systemic antihistamine. However, if the patient shows severe distress there may be danger of secondary infections or later noncompliance with treatment, so it may be advisable to change medications. Unlike the case of penicillin, appearance of these rashes does not signify an impending anaphylactoid reaction. On very rare occasions angioneurotic edema or exfoliative dermatitis have been reported; these are more dangerous reactions, requiring change of medication and more aggressive treatment (e.g., corticosteroids).

Phototoxicity reactions are not uncommon, especially in young female patients. Caution is highly advisable until this possibility has been ruled out, since some patients have suffered severe burns following minimal exposure to sunlight. Treatment and prevention are the same as for any sunburn.

Cardiovascular Side Effects

Hypotension and *orthostatic (postural) hypotension* are among the most common side effects of antipsychotics and TCAs. The high-potency neuroleptics are notably safer than the other drugs in this regard, and are therefore increasingly preferred, especially for injections. The degree of hypotension depends also on drug dosage, the presence of other drugs, the patient's physical condition and degree of agitation, and idiosyncratic increased vulnerability. *Vasomotor collapse* followed by cardiorespiratory arrest may occur with little or no warning, usually during high-dose therapy but sometimes following a single small injection. In such cases, *epinephrine is contraindicated as a pressor agent.* Alpha-receptor blockade must be assumed, and any drug having beta-stimulating effects will therefore further lower blood pressure. Recommended pressor agents include norepinephrine (Levophed) and phenylephrine (Neo-Synephrine).

Other cardiovascular side effects of these drugs include various arrhythmias and ECG changes of characteristic types (especially with thioridazine). Tricyclic antidepressants and low-potency neuroleptics are relatively dangerous during the acute recovery stage following myocardial infarction. Hypertension associated with these drugs is relatively rare in adults, but one recent study of imipramine reported statistically significant increases in both systolic and diastolic blood pressure in a sample of children with hyperactive behavior disorders.

Endocrine and Endocrinelike Side Effects

It should be noted that many of the phenomena described here are vegetative changes associated with severe psychosis, and therefore are not always drug-related when observed. These include: amenorrhea, dysmenorrhea, and other menstrual changes; inappropriate lactation in females and galactorrhea in males; alterations in glucose metabolism; weight gain (very common with low-potency antipsychotics and TCAs); peripheral edema (excess fluid retention); gynecomastia or feminization in males; and false-positive pregnancy tests (based on urine specimens).

Other Peripheral Autonomic Side Effects

Anticholinergic, antiadrenergic, and other peripheral autonomic effects of these drugs lead to a wide variety of undesirable results. Many of these are included among the most common complaints spontaneously made by patients: blurriness of near vision, dryness of mouth and mucous membranes, nasal congestion, increased or decreased sweating, flushed skin, diarrhea or constipation, disturbance of speech or swallowing, and difficulty with urination. Extremes of some of these are potentially dangerous (e.g., urinary retention, fecal impaction, and paralytic ileus) and may not be promptly detected if the patient is withdrawn or uncommunicative. Patients vulnerable to the latter three problems are usually identifiable before therapy is begun (e.g., by age, history, or physical condition) so that an appropriate drug may be selected and adequate observation arranged. Bethanechol chloride (Urecholine) may be helpful for urinary retention. *Aggravation of narrow-angle glaucoma* is another dangerous possibility, and this condition is considered a relative contraindication for TCAs and low-potency neuroleptics.

Disturbances of sexual function are also quite disconcerting to some patients, and may lead to noncompliance with therapy if not alleviated. These include decreased libido (or, rarely, increased libido), impotence (inability to obtain an erection), and various ejaculatory disorders, especially with thioridazine.

For most of these problems there is no specific treatment other than changing medication, reducing the dosage, or waiting to see if tolerance develops. Nonspecific (symptomatic) treatments may be quite helpful. It should be noted that *additional anticholinergic medication increases the severity* of many of these problems.

Skin and Eye Changes

Skin and eye changes are quite rare, and some may be specific to only one or two drugs. *Pigmentary retinopathy,* similar to the hereditary disease, is associated only with *thioridazine,* and is the reason for a relatively low but strict limit on dosage. Regular eye examinations are recommended, but often the first sign is a complaint by the patient of a brownish tinge in vision. Night vision is impaired first, and prompt discontinuation of thioridazine may enable the patient to overcome the visual impairment, but the pigment deposits are permanent. Other eye changes associated with low-potency phenothiazines include lenticular and corneal opacities.

Skin pigmentation changes have also been reported, and are attributed to either or both of the following mechanisms: (1) increased melanocyte-stimulating hormone levels; and (2) direct deposition of dyes which are phenothiazine metabolites. Typically light-exposed skin is more strongly affected, and various unusual colorations have been described as slate-gray or purple.

Habituation, Tolerance, and Withdrawal

Tolerance is acquired by the majority of patients to most side effects described. This has two important clinical implications: (1) most side effects may be minimized or entirely avoided by increasing the dosage slowly; and (2) dosages that would cause severe, even life-threatening, side effects initially may be well tolerated if approached gradually. However, *there is no evidence that tolerance is ever acquired for the therapeutic (antipsychotic or antidepressant) effects.* A patient whose condition deteriorates after initial stabilization at a constant dosage should be investigated for (1) surreptitious discontinuation of medication; (2) an unrecognized side effect (e.g., akathisia); (3) covert use of nonprescribed medication; or (4) an incorrect diagnosis (e.g., mania misdiagnosed as schizophrenia). If none of these possibilities account for the deterioration, then an alteration in the natural course of the pyschosis is probably responsible.

These drugs are nonaddicting. However, some patients may develop psychological dependence if they "learn" that they cannot function without their medication. Following prolonged usage, abrupt discontinuation may produce a *physical abstinence syndrome,* usually mild in degree; typical symptoms include muscular discomfort, nausea or other gastrointestinal distress, and difficulty sleeping. *Seizures do not occur.* Therefore, abrupt withdrawal is not contraindicated, but should not be done unless necessary because of possible temporary discomfort. *The most serious danger following abrupt withdrawal is relapse of the mental illness* (rapid or delayed).

ANTIMANIC DRUGS (LITHIUM SALTS)

The first report of the antimanic properties of lithium was published in 1949 by the Australian psychiatrist John Cade, but a combination of unfortunate circumstances caused it to be virtually ignored for fifteen years. Clinical trials of lithium were then reinitiated, and in 1970 the carbonate salt was approved for clinical use in the United States as an antimanic agent. A task force was appointed by the American Psychiatric Association to make periodic reports on the subsequent clinical and research experience with this drug.

In its most recent official report (1975), the APA task force concluded as follows: "Lithium is the treatment of first choice in mania if the patient can be managed successfully without additional drug therapy. If hyperactivity demands immediate control, lithium plus a neuroleptic is the best approach." Regarding maintenance therapy, the task force's opinion was, "Lithium carbonate is effective in preventing or diminishing the intensity of recurrences of bipolar affective illness."

Pharmacology of Lithium

Lithium has major endocrinologic, renal, gastrointestinal, and CNS effects which have been summarized by Singer and Rotenberg (1973). Its physical, chemical, and biological properties are quite similar to those of sodium, but it crosses cell membranes relatively slowly, so that plasma steady states and therapeutic response are not reached until after five or ten days of therapy. It is excreted unchanged by the kidneys, although about 80 percent of filtered lithium is reabsorbed. Lithium clearance is highly correlated with creatinine clearance (at about 20 percent the rate of the latter).

The mechanism or even the site at which the antimanic action of lithium takes place is unknown Among the current hypotheses are the following: (1) alteration of plasma cortisol levels; (2) increasing speed of reuptake deactivation of norepinephrine or other neurotransmitters, or inhibiting their release; (3) alteration of physiological processes depending on ion transport or distribution in the CNS; (4) inhibition of hormone-activated adenyl cyclase in the CNS, resulting in decreased production of cyclic AMP; and (5) interference with neuronal carbohydrate metabolism.

Selection of Patients for Lithium Therapy

The criteria for the diagnosis of acute mania are described in Chapter 14. However, not all manic patients can be safely treated with lithium. The only absolute contraindication to lithium therapy is *inability to excrete lithium* (i.e., impaired renal functioning). A major relative contraindication is any *significant cardiovascular disease.* Most authorities list *organic brain damage* as another relative contraindication, but there are sporadic reports of dramatic improvement in aggressive behavior by severely mentally retarded persons treated with lithium. Conditions that greatly increase the risk of lithium toxicity include hyponatremia, diuretic drug therapy, and severe debilitation or dehydration; these are not contraindications but rather *indications for especially close monitoring.*

Before initiating lithium therapy, physical and laboratory examinations ordinarily recommended are the following: (1) renal evaluation (urinalysis, blood urea nitrogen [BUN], creatinine clearance, etc.); (2) cardiovascular evaluation including ECG; (3) blood chemistry studies (at least CBC with differential, and electrolyte evaluation if indicated); (4) thyroid (history, palpation, hormone levels); (5) liver function tests; and (6) EEG if indicated.

Laboratory facilities must be available for evaluation of serum lithium concentrations. Most importantly, the patient (and family when appropriate) should receive adequate information to enable him to cooperate with lithium therapy. This includes: (1) explanation of manic-depressive disease, and description of the signs of hypomania; (2) information about normal side effects of lithium and signs of toxicity; and (3) instructions about maintaining normal fluid and sodium intake, and avoiding overheating, excessive sweating, and dehydration.

Monitoring of Serum Lithium Levels

Monitoring of serum lithium levels is an important aspect of all stages of lithium therapy. A blood specimen should be obtained for laboratory analysis *8 to 12 hours after the last dose of lithium* (ordinarily before the first dose in the morning), since the guidelines for serum lithium levels are based on this assumption and the laboratory result cannot be interpreted if lithium has been ingested more recently. During the acute manic episode, the therapeutic lithium level desired is somewhere between 0.8 and 1.5 mEq/L. The prophylactic level (when the patient is not manic) is between 0.7 and 1.2 mEq/L. Levels below 0.7 mEq/L are considered homeopathic for most patients. Between 1.5 and 2.0 mEq/L many persons will show mild but definite signs of toxicity; from 2.0 to 4.0 mEq/L there will be serious toxic signs; and levels above 4.0 mEq/L have sometimes been lethal. It must be emphasized that these are approximate ranges, and that *serum monitoring must be associated with clinical monitoring of therapeutic response and side effects.* Acutely manic patients are ordinarily started on 600 to 900 mg of lithium carbonate the first day, with dosage increased to 1,200 to 1,800 mg on the second day, and thereafter adjusted somewhere in the range of 1,500 to 3,000 mg per day. *Lithium is always given in divided doses* (two or three times a day). Manic patients require high doses to reach adequate serum levels. When the mania subsides, the dose should be adjusted downward, for otherwise the serum level may continue to rise even though the dose is constant.

Serum levels should be monitored frequently (at two or three day intervals) while the patient is manic and dosage is being adjusted. Thereafter the frequency of monitoring may be *gradually* decreased, but should never be less often than monthly. A stat check of serum lithium should be made: (1) whenever dosage is adjusted; (2) if signs of hypomania appear; (3) if signs of toxicity appear; (4) whenever any but the most trivial illness develops (especially if there is vomiting, alteration of fluid intake, diarrhea, etc.).

Side Effects

During the first few weeks of lithium therapy most patients experience transient side effects which are rarely severe and almost never necessitate discontinuation of the treatment. These include: (1) *gastrointestinal symptoms* such as anorexia, nausea, vomiting, loose stools, and abdominal pain; (2) *neuromuscular distress* such as fatigue, muscular weakness, and fine tremor of the hands; (3) *CNS effects* such as sleepiness, light-headedness, and a dazed feeling; (4) *renal symptoms,* usually polyuria and increased thirst; and (5) *altered taste,* usually metallic. These are all dose-related, so intensity will be greatest at the time of peak plasma levels and subside between doses. Most patients adapt to all these side effects within a few weeks.

LEUKOCYTOSIS. Leukocytosis is a regular phenomenon throughout lithium therapy, with many patients having WBC above 14,000 per cubic millimeter. The mechanism is unknown, and the phenomenon rapidly reverses when lithium is discontinued. Only mature cells are involved, so this leukocytosis can be differentiated from infection by the absence of a left shift.

RARE SIDE EFFECTS. Rare side effects unrelated to dosage include: (1) nephrogenic diabetes insipidus; (2) quinidine-like ECG changes; (3) hypothyroidism, usually mild (and occasionally producing a nontoxic goiter), which is treated with supplementary thyroid hormone; (4) mild skin rashes; (5) EEG changes of a characteristic type; (6) seizures or other signs of neurotoxicity unaccompanied by a full toxic syndrome.

Toxic Signs

Toxic signs usually begin with gastrointestinal distress (nausea, vomiting, diarrhea) and progress with increasing serum lithium levels to neurological manifestations (tremors, weakness, sedation, confusion, ataxia, hyperactive deep tendon reflexes, fasciculations, twitching, clonic movements, etc.). At even higher serum levels other organ systems will be involved (cardiovascular, renal, hepatic, etc.).

TREATMENT. Treatment of lithium poisoning involves: (1) supportive measures as indicated (cardiovascular, respiratory, anticonvulsant, etc.); (2) stabilization of electrolytes; (3) forcing lithium diuresis with urea or mannitol; (4) increasing lithium clearance with aminophylline; (5) alkalinization of urine; (6) dialysis in extreme cases.

Other Uses of Lithium

The clearest indications for lithium therapy are acute mania and prevention of future manic episodes. There is increasing evidence that lithium maintenance also prevents or diminishes the intensity of depressive episodes in bipolar patients. Davis (1976) concluded that the same is true of recurrent unipolar depressions, but some other authorities disagree. There is greater controversy over the question of *acute antidepressant effects* of lithium; the APA task force's conclusion was, "At this time experimental results are not sufficiently conclusive . . . . It should not be considered standard treatment but in selected cases may be considered if the usual methods fail." Some authorities recommend starting with lithium if a patient with a prior manic episode presents with an acute depression; the rationale is that this patient should be taking lithium anyway (to prevent manic episodes) and one should see whether the lithium ameliorates the depression before beginning other therapy.

Lithium has been found inferior to neuroleptics for schizo-affective psychosis, although it may be tried on the grounds of diagnostic uncertainty when the usual treatments are unsatisfactory. Some patients with other forms of cyclical mental disturbance respond to lithium, but such cases are rare. Recent journal articles suggest the possible application of lithium in a wide variety of disorders, even in childhood, if the patient has a close blood relative who has responded well to lithium.

ELECTROCONVULSIVE THERAPY

Although descriptions of similar treatments had appeared in medical journals as early as 1785, the use of convulsive therapy in psychiatry today is generally dated from a report by Laszlo von Meduna of Hungary (1933). Based on a rationale later shown to be incorrect, he had hypothesized that schizophrenia and epilepsy were mutually antagonistic diseases. His treatment consisted of provocation of grand mal seizures, first by intramuscular injections of camphor in oil, and later by intravenous injections of pentylenetetrazol (Metrazol or Cardiazol).

Although Meduna's method was effective in treating some schizophrenic patients, trials by other clinicians soon led to the discovery that its most important application was in mood disorders, particularly psychotic depressions. Ugo Cerletti and Lucino Bini were the first to suggest and use electric current as a convulsive agent in humans (1937–1938). This approach removed several major disadvantages of pharmacological convulsive therapy, and today nearly all convulsive treatments are induced by electrical shock.

Hexafluorodiethyl Ether

Hexafluorodiethyl ether (Indoklon) produces convulsions when the vapors are inhaled, and was an alternative favored by some clinicians until its recent removal from sale by the manufacturer. Indoklon must be handled cautiously to prevent vapor from escaping into the air supply of the treatment team. Nausea is often severe following each treatment, and the acute brain syndrome may be more severe than that following ECT. However, one possible advantage of Indoklon convulsive therapy is avoidance of the negative connotations associated with electric shock.

ECT Machines

ECT machines of several different types are available and usually may be plugged into the standard electrical outlet. The simplest consists of a variable transformer, a voltmeter, and an automatic timer. The seizure threshold varies as a function of age, amount of sedative premedication, and other factors, but a convulsive stimulus typically consists of 70 to 110 volts applied for 0.1 to 0.5 second, with amperage ranging from 200 to 1,600 ma. Ordinarily it is desirable to use the smallest amount of current that produces a *grand mal seizure.* Many versions of *subconvulsive electrical stimulation*

have been studied, but these may be painful and their therapeutic value is questioned by most psychiatrists.

If the patient is not anesthetized, an adequate convulsive stimulus produces instantaneous loss of consciousness without pain. The tonic phase of the seizure begins immediately and lasts for about ten seconds, followed by the clonic phase for about thirty seconds. Vital signs should be monitored and respiration supported until the patient's condition has stabilized, following which he may be moved to an observation area for the remainder of the postconvulsive coma. As with any grand mal seizure, there will be an acute (reversible) organic brain syndrome of variable duration and consisting of amnesia, confusion, and other intellectual impairment.

Indications for Electroconvulsive Therapy (ECT)

ECT is statistically superior to all other known treatments for *psychotic depressions,* especially involutional melancholia. It is also effective for several other types of functional psychosis, although it is usually not the preferred treatment. These include *acute mania* and *schizophrenias* (especially catatonic stupor and schizo-affective depression). However, ECT may be safer if not more effective than drugs in any functional psychosis involving severe agitation or stupor accompanied by deteriorating physical health or persistent refusal of food and fluids.

ECT is less likely to be effective, and may make matters worse, in *neurotic depressions* and other disorders in which it may intensify anxiety, and in which there is exogenous stress that is unaffected by treatment and leads to early relapse. However, if disability is severe and other treatments have failed, a trial of ECT may be justified.

Preparation for ECT

A course of ECT is ordinarily preceded by a careful medical workup and psychological preparation of the patient, which includes obtaining *informed consent* (required by law for any type of treatment involving loss of consciousness). To intelligently give such consent, the patient or his guardian needs to know: (1) the anticipated benefits of the treatment; (2) reasons for selection of this type of treatment; (3) the anticipated adverse effects (e.g., reversible posttreatment amnesia); and (4) the potential risks.

For some patients having serious physical illnesses, ECT may be considerably safer than antipsychotic, antidepressant, or antimanic medication. The risks associated with drugs are relatively constant at all times of day and night. By contrast, the risks from ECT are sharply time-limited to the treatment period. This permits precautionary measures, such as ready availability of emergency equipment, medications, and personnel.

The pre-ECT medical workup should devote special attention to organ systems likely to be involved in an emergency during treatment. Usually included are: cardiovascular evaluation, including ECG; neurological examination and EEG; chest and spine x-rays; and evaluation of any special problems of or risks to the individual patient (e.g., dental problems, recent surgery, etc.). Additional studies and consultations may be indicated by the results of these investigations.

The physician who will actually administer the treatments should be consulted before beginning the workup in case he has additional instructions. Some experts have made ECT almost a subspecialty within psychiatry, and can successfully treat high-risk patients if adequate preparations are made.

If possible, all medications should be discontinued during a course of ECT. If this cannot be done each individual drug should be carefully checked, and dosage adjusted to the minimum possible. The drugs that produce the greatest risks during ECT are those affecting the cardiovascular system (e.g., antihypertensives, antipsychotics, and antidepressants). All drugs given concurrently with ECT should be scheduled so that a maximum drug-free interval precedes each treatment. Patients should take *nothing* by mouth for eight hours prior to each treatment to minimize the possibility of vomiting and aspiration; drugs that are required during this interval may be injected.

The only absolute contraindication to ECT recognized by most authorities is *CNS neoplasm producing increased intracranial pressure.* ECT may stimulate the growth of some neoplasms, but the greater danger is the marked increase in intracranial pressure that occurs during the seizure, which may produce structural damage or herniation of the brain.

All other contraindications to ECT are only relative. For example, serious cardiovascular disease increases the risk, but such patients may be in greater danger from severe agitation. Continued or recent therapy with *reserpine* or other catecholamine-depleting drugs is considered a contraindication; some patients suffer cardiac arrest during ECT and do not respond to resuscitation if peripheral catecholamines have been extensively depleted. Most other possible contraindications may be minimized by alterations to the treatment procedure described below.

Modified vs. Unmodified ECT

ECT was originally given to conscious patients who were not premedicated in any way. Although it produced immediate unconsciousness and was completely painless, this procedure (unmodified ECT) was sometimes complicated by fractures or dislocations, and many patients become quite fearful while awaiting electrode placement and the subsequent stimulus.

Most ECT today is modified by up to three types of pretreatment medications. An injection of *atropine* (0.4 to 2.0 mg) is usually given prior to treatment to reduce secretions, to lessen the possibility of vomiting, and to block vagal stimulation caused by ECT (supposedly the principal cause of cardiac arrest). *General anesthesia* by intravenous infusion of an ultra-short-acting barbiturate (e.g., methohexital sodium) helps to reduce patient discomfort. Following loss of consciousness, a *depolarizing muscle relaxant* such as succinylcholine (Anectine) is administered through the same venipuncture. Adequate dosage of the latter virtually eliminates the possibility of complications due to severe convulsions.

Any of these drugs may be contraindicated or increase the risk for certain patients. If the anesthesia is omitted, *the muscle relaxant should never be administered to a conscious patient.* The muscular fasciculations are quite painful, and loss of voluntary control of respiration is terrifying. Unconsciousness may be produced by a subconvulsive stimulus from the ECT machine, following which the muscle relaxant may then be administered in preparation for the full grand mal convulsive stimulus.

Risks Eliminated by Muscle Relaxation

Many of the risks of ECT are related to the mechanical effects of the convulsion, while the therapeutic benefit is believed to result solely from the CNS seizure activity. Fractures and dislocations are the only mechanical risks significantly frequent, although others have been reported on rare occasions (e.g., ruptures of internal organs or blood vessels). Certain complications are related to preexisting physical disease: perforation of ulcers or diverticuli, aggravation of hernias, retinal detachment, alteration of thrombophlebitis, aggravation of existing musculoskeletal defects, etc.

ECT does not induce labor, but advanced pregnancy is another indication for extra care in obtaining adequate muscle relaxation.

Side Effects

Side effects encountered during a normal course of ECT include: apnea following treatments (respiratory support should be routinely provided); headaches after treatments (responsive to aspirin); EEG changes of a characteristic type and persisting for several months; weight gain; amenorrhea or other menstrual changes, possibly of several months' duration; centrally mediated cardiac arrhythmias and blood-pressure changes during the seizure and for a few minutes afterwards; and transient alterations of certain biochemical parameters. The permeability of the blood-brain barrier is temporarily increased, which may significantly alter the effects of certain medications.

Fractures of poorly supported or weakened teeth and tongue-biting may occur if adequate preventive measures are not undertaken; use of a mouth guard is routine. Minor hemorrhages of

nose, ear, or incompletely healed abrasions are rare. Extremely rare are such side effects as activation of tuberculosis, pulmonary abscess from aspiration, embolisms, and cardiac arrest.

The Acute Brain Syndrome

Acute brain syndrome is the most notable side effect in the vast majority of cases. This consists of a confused state following treatment, variable intellectual impairment, and *amnesia* that may persist for several months following completion of a normal course of ECT. The extent and duration of amnesia are known to be affected by a number of factors, including: (1) Patient idiosyncrasy and predisposition (e.g., preexisting dementia). (2) Electrode placement—*bilateral* stimulation causes greater amnesia than *unilateral* stimulation on the *nondominant* side. The peripheral convulsions caused by unilateral stimulation are bilateral and appear identical to those from bilateral stimulation. The CNS differences are unknown, but there is general agreement that *unilateral ECT may be less effective than bilateral ECT* (i.e., poorer therapeutic response, or more treatments required). (3) Frequency and number of treatments: Ordinarily bilateral ECT is given three times weekly, and unilateral treatment five times weekly, for two to four weeks (but sometimes longer).

The reversibility of amnesia after ECT has long been a subject of controversy. Although the number of anecdotal reports indicates that occasional patients may have long-lasting memory impairment (especially if many closely spaced treatments were given), *controlled studies have repeatedly failed to detect significant impairment persisting beyond a few months* in the majority of patients receiving a *normal* course of ECT. In a recent study by Squire and Chace (1975), six sensitive tests of memory function were administered to three groups of patients who had been hospitalized and treated for depression six to nine months previously. They were unable to find any differences on any of the six tests in comparisons of persons treated with bilateral ECT (5 to 17 treatments), unilateral ECT (5 to 15 right-sided treatments), or no ECT. No patients in any of the three groups appeared to be impaired, but a control group of patients currently receiving bilateral ECT (tested after the sixth treatment) showed considerable impairment on all six tests. Interestingly, a significantly higher proportion (62 percent) of the patients previously treated with bilateral ECT *rated themselves as still impaired,* although no evidence of such impairment could be found. The authors concluded, "These results suggest that memory functions are markedly impaired by bilateral ECT, but recovered to normal levels within six to nine months after treatment." They suggested several explanations for differences in self-estimates of impairment, including the possibility that high levels of initial impairment lead to a persistent belief that impairment exists, even after full recovery.

ECT and Mortality

Even though patients with "calculated risks" are sometimes treated with ECT, the rate of treatment-related deaths is exceedingly small. Somewhat higher rates have been reported in the past, but two changes in practice have been important: curare is no longer used as a muscle relaxant, and precautions against unexpected emergencies are routinely employed (e.g., support of respiration and availability of cardioverter). A 1947 study reported no deaths in a series of 20,645 treatments; a 1956 study reported five deaths in approximately 70,000 treatments; and a 1968 report noted one death in 10,000 treatments. It may be correctly observed that statistics are difficult to interpret without knowing more about methods of patient selection (i.e., which types of risks led to refusal of ECT). However, such data compare quite favorably with those for any minor surgical procedure involving general anesthesia.

It is also relevant to compare death rates due to ECT with the long-term outcome of involutional melancholia. Huston and Locher (1948) reported a follow-up of 93 patients admitted to a mental hospital during the years 1930 to 1939 with this diagnosis. None of these patients had ever received convulsive therapy (which was not in use at that hospital until after 1940). Instead, they were treated with psychotherapy, hydro-

therapy, work therapy, and all other available methods. At follow-up, which averaged 78 months from the date of hospital admission, only 46 percent of these patients were considered recovered, and the mean duration of illness among the recovered group was 49 months. An additional 18 percent were still hospitalized and still considered mentally ill, with an average duration of illness of 115 months thus far. Thirteen percent of the sample had committed suicide, and an additional 23 percent had died from other causes. Among the latter group, nine patients (10 percent of the original sample) had died of exhaustion or malnutrition *as a direct result of the mental illness* (agitation and refusal to eat), and five patients had died of cardiovascular disease.

Avery and Winokur (1976) summarized the existing data and presented additional evidence that age-adjusted mortality rates are higher among depressed persons than in the general population, and that ECT is particularly effective in reducing the rates of death from suicide and total deaths.

Efficacy of ECT

The most important application of ECT is in psychotic depressions. Among seven studies comparing ECT to imipramine, three found ECT superior and the remaining four found the two treatments equally effective. Comparisons of recovery rates for different treatments must be interpreted carefully, since the available studies vary in patient population, selection criteria, and definition of recovery. Nevertheless, some broad generalizations may be attempted. For psychotic depressions, recovery rates following ECT are between 80 and 100 percent; for TCAs the rates are lower (60 to 70 percent in retarded depressions, 40 to 60 percent in agitated depressions); and for MAOIs the rates are lower still.

Greenblatt, Grosser, and Wechsler (1964) reported a large-scale investigation among severely depressed patients in three hospitals. They found ECT superior to imipramine, two different MAO inhibitors, and placebo in all age and sex groupings. The superiority of ECT was especially prominent among patients diagnosed as manic depressive or involutional melancholic, and there was a trend (not statistically significant) for ECT to be better among patients with schizo-affective depression. Among neurotically depressed patients there were no differences among the five treatments.

Relatively fewer data are available on the effectiveness of ECT for other mental illnesses. Philip May reported a success rate of 79 percent among acute schizophrenics treated with ECT during their first hospital admission; this was significantly better than treatment with psychotherapy or milieu therapy alone, but significantly worse than treatment with trifluoperazine (Stelazine). McCabe (1976) reported data obtained from hospital charts of 56 manic patients hospitalized between 1931 and 1949. The 28 patients treated with ECT required an average of 6.5 weeks of hospitalization, and 96 percent improved sufficiently to return home when discharged. By contrast, the 28 patients who did not receive ECT required an average of 15.3 weeks in the hospital, and only 44 percent improved sufficiently to be discharged for return home (the remainder being transferred to a chronic-care facility).

As a treatment for severe depression, the two significant disadvantages of ECT are the acute brain syndrome it causes and the tendency for many patients to relapse during subsequent months and years. Exact rates of relapse are controversial, but *there is now considerable evidence that maintenance tricyclic antidepressant medication will significantly reduce relapses,* even among patients whose acute depression had responded poorly to medication.

MISCELLANEOUS PSYCHOPHARMACEUTICALS

Antianxiety Drugs

The effects of *acute anxiety* may be diminished by virtually any sedating drug. However, many such drugs simultaneously impair perception, motor skills, cognitive functions, and other mental abilities. Physiological tolerance may be acquired after a very few doses, and in combination with euphoriant effects may lead to rapid development of psy

chological dependence, physical dependence, and even addiction. There may be interference with the pharmacokinetics of other drugs taken simultaneously, unpleasant effects on sleep patterns, or the risk of major side effects.

These disadvantages are significantly less likely for a few specific classes of drugs, collectively referred to as minor tranquilizers or antianxiety agents. Animal experiments and clinical experience have shown that differences in CNS effects between these drugs and true sedative-hypnotics (e.g., barbiturates) are basically quantitative rather than qualitative. However, both show significant differences from major tranquilizers (antipsychotics). Specifically, the minor tranquilizers (1) have no therapeutic effects against functional psychoses, but are preferred to neuroleptics in the treatment of certain organic brain syndromes; (2) have a much narrower range of side effects, and in particular never cause EPS; (3) may potentiate the effects of certain other drugs, but neither so strongly nor so selectively as do the neuroleptics; (4) have some potential for habituation, tolerance to the therapeutic effects, and addiction, and are therefore abusable drugs that are more carefully controlled by law; and (5) in high doses they may be considered as general CNS depressants.

These are among the most frequently prescribed of all drugs, and most prescriptions are written by nonpsychiatrists. Their significant psychiatric indications are as follows: (1) for short-term relief of acute situational anxiety which interferes with necessary functioning; (2) substitution therapy in certain drug withdrawal syndromes (see Chap. 12); (3) to reduce dangerous hyperactivity or panic in certain acute brain syndromes (e.g., LSD hallucinosis) or nonpsychotic functional disorders when psychological measures alone are inadequate; (4) as adjunctive therapy in the treatment of neurotic disorders or depressions with prominent anxiety (but unjudicious use of these drugs may interfere significantly with psychotherapy); (5) as adjuncts to antipsychotic medication, to reduce certain extrapyramidal reactions (akathisia or acute dystonias).

Propanediol carbamates are the oldest class of minor tranquilizers. The prototype is *meprobamate,* which is available in generic form and under many trade names. It resembles the barbiturates in many respects, including: (1) suppression of REM sleep, possibly followed by a REM rebound (see Chap. 7); (2) possible hepatic microsomal enzyme induction; (3) more rapid development of tolerance than with benzodiazepines, and greater potential for physical dependence and addiction; (4) *relatively low lethal dose,* so that accidental or intentional overdoses are very dangerous; and (5) excessive drowsiness and ataxia occurring at relatively low doses. Meprobamate has muscle relaxing and anticonvulsant properties, but neither property is clinically useful, and in fact the drug may aggravate grand mal seizure disorders. The principal side effects are hypotension and allergic reactions, including rashes of all types. Agranulocytosis and many other blood dyscrasias have been reported.

Tybamate is a related drug with a much shorter duration of action, and thereby reduced potential for physical dependence and addiction, but also less clinical applicability.

Benzodiazepines have several advantages over meprobamate or barbiturates, including: (1) absence of microsomal enzyme induction; (2) wider margin of safety, with excessive drowsiness and ataxia unlikely at therapeutic doses, and suicidal overdoses rarely successful (unless other drugs are involved); (3) absence of REM sleep suppression; (4) clinically useful anticonvulsant effects, especially with intravenous administration; (5) slower development of tolerance and physical dependence.

Animal experiments have demonstrated the ability of these drugs to block conditioned fear responses, including avoidance responses, without preventing escape responses (see Chap. 5). This *disinhibiting* effect is one possible explanation for the "paradoxical" *increase in hostility, anger, and aggressive behavior* sometimes shown by patients taking these drugs. At normal doses other side effects are rare and usually not dangerous; however, agranulocytosis has been reported.

The benzodiazepines currently available are: diazepam (Valium); chlordiazepoxide (Librium); oxazepam (Serax); clorazepate (Tranxene); and flurazepam (Dalmane). The latter is marketed only in high dosages for use as a hypnotic, although there is no impressive evidence that it is better for this purpose than other benzodiazepines. All of these drugs except oxazepam have many active metabolites and relatively long duration of action. Intramuscular injections are poorly absorbed and slower acting than the same dosage administered orally.

Sedative-Hypnotics

Barbiturates are the largest class of these drugs, and their basic pharmacology is well described in many other references. A few significant facts may be summarized as follows: (1) These drugs are potent inducers of hepatic microsomal enzymes, thereby greatly increasing the speed of metabolic deactivation of many other drugs; (2) they are strong suppressors of REM sleep, and are followed by a REM rebound when use is discontinued (see Chap. 7); (3) acquisition of tolerance and physical dependence is rapid, and the withdrawal syndrome may be fatal (see Chap. 12); (4) relatively low doses may be lethal, especially in combination with alcohol or other depressants; and (5) occasional patients (especially children and the elderly) may show a *paradoxical excitation* instead of sedation.

Glutethimide (Doriden) is a hypnotic closely resembling the barbiturates, and having the same significant disadvantages. Ethchlorvynol (Placidyl) has pharmacological effects very similar to those of alcohol (including enzyme induction and REM suppression). Chloral derivatives (chloral hydrate, chloral betaine, and triclofos) are among the oldest hypnotic drugs; their significant disadvantage is displacement of other drugs from protein-binding sites, thereby producing short-term potentiation of the drugs displaced. The pharmacology of methyprylon (Noludar) and methaqualone (Quaalude or Sopor) has not been well studied, but these are drugs of widespread abuse and addiction.

Sedating antihistamines such as hydroxyzine (Atarax or Vistaril) and diphenhydramine (Benadryl) have limited use as antianxiety or hypnotic agents. They have relatively weak CNS effects, with reduced potentiation of depressants. They probably have no anticonvulsant effects and are nonaddicting.

Psychomotor Stimulants

CNS sympathomimetic stimulants include racemic amphetamine (Benzedrine), dextroamphetamine (Dexedrine), levoamphetamine, and methylphenidate (Ritalin). A related drug with reduced sympathomimetic action is pemoline (Cylert). These drugs have two types of clearcut indications: (1) as one aspect of the treatment of certain childhood behavior disorders (e.g., minimal brain dysfunction, hyperkinesis, or attention deficit syndrome; see Chap. 19) the drugs may have a "paradoxical" calming effect that reduces certain target symptoms; and (2) certain sleep disorders, especially narcolepsy (see Chap. 7). In addition, these drugs may provide temporary postponement of fatigue and somnolence, but should be so used very selectively and for the shortest possible period. They were formerly widely used in the treatment of obesity, but this has been severely criticized, and the weight reducing effects at best last only for a few weeks unless dosage is escalated.

These drugs have many side effects. Peripherally the most serious involve the cardiovascular system, especially hypertension and increased heart rate. CNS side effects include insomnia, anorexia, increased anxiety and hostility, and euphoria. Curiously, the latter does not occur in children being treated for behavior disorders, who may take the drug for years without developing tolerance, psychological dependence, or addiction. However, *in adults these are highly abusable drugs,* and invariably produce a paranoid or manic psychosis following use at high dosages for a sufficient period of time. The many aspects of stimulant abuse are discussed in Chapter 12.

Deanol (Deaner) is a *parasympathomimetic* drug with CNS stimulant effects which is also occasionally used in childhood behavior disorders. Currently it is being investigated as a possible treatment for tardive dyskinesias.

REVIEW QUESTIONS

85. Central nervous system properties of chlorpromazine and other synthetic antipsychotic drugs include each of the following *except:*
    - (A) anticholinergic
    - (B) anticonvulsant
    - (C) antidopaminergic
    - (D) antiemetic
    - (E) antihistaminic

86. Electroconvulsive therapy is most effective in reducing:
    - (A) memory impairment
    - (B) affective symptoms
    - (C) conversion symptoms
    - (D) delusions
    - (E) obsessional thinking

87. Which of the following is *not* a sign of lithium toxicity?
    - (A) tremor
    - (B) diarrhea
    - (C) nystagmus
    - (D) euphoria
    - (E) vomiting

88. A drug notorious for causing psychotic depression as a side effect of long-term therapy is:
    - (A) lithium
    - (B) meprobamate
    - (C) protriptyline
    - (D) reserpine
    - (E) tranylcypromine

89. Tardive dyskinesia is:
    - (A) an acute extrapyramidal side effect of neuroleptics
    - (B) best treated with anticholinergic medication
    - (C) easily misdiagnosed as psychomotor retardation
    - (D) usually associated with a large number of ECTs
    - (E) a possible complication of long-term neuroleptic therapy

90. Properties of the minor tranquilizers meprobamate and diazepam include each of the following *except:*
    - (A) anticonvulsant

(B) muscle relaxant
(C) addiction potential
(D) antipsychotic
(E) sedative

91. A 21-year-old man in good physical health is admitted to a psychiatric hospital with florid psychotic symptoms (delusions, hallucinations, loose associations, and psychomotor agitation). The diagnosis is paranoid schizophrenia. Therapy is initiated with trifluoperazine (Stelazine), starting at a dosage of 5 mg three times a day, and gradually increasing to 20 mg three times a day over one week. There is good improvement in all the symptoms except the psychomotor agitation, which initially subsides but appears to be increasing again after one week. The patient spends much time in purposeless motion such as pacing or hand-wringing. He complains of feeling very nervous and jittery, and is unable to remain seated for even a five-minute interview. A reasonable course of action is:
    (A) increase the dosage of trifluoperazine
    (B) discontinue trifluoperazine and prescribe diazepam
    (C) reduce trifluoperazine and prescribe lithium carbonate
    (D) reduce trifluoperazine and prescribe benztropine
    (E) none of the above is reasonable

92. A patient with acute renal shutdown has become severely agitated. A sedating drug that might have special applicability in this case is:
    (A) amitriptyline
    (B) diazepam
    (C) haloperidol
    (D) paraldehyde
    (E) phenobarbital

93. An acute toxic psychosis sometimes associated with tricyclic antidepressants closely resembles that due to poisoning by:
    (A) amphetamine
    (B) atropine
    (C) barbiturates

(D) bromides
(E) lithium

94. An absolute contraindication to ECT is:
    (A) third trimester of pregnancy
    (B) lack of peripheral cholinesterase enzymes
    (C) recent coronary thrombosis
    (D) grand mal epilepsy
    (E) none of the above

95. Irreversible hepatocellular damage is a side effect of:
    (A) phenothiazines
    (B) hydrazine MAO inhibitors
    (C) lithium carbonate
    (D) tricyclic antidepressants
    (E) amphetamines

96. Thioridazine (Mellaril) should not be prescribed in dosages exceeding 800 mg daily because there is greatly increased probability of:
    (A) agranulocytosis
    (B) cardiac arrhythmias
    (C) epileptic seizures
    (D) pigmentary retinopathy
    (E) hyperpyrexia

97. Muscle relaxants in electroconvulsive therapy:
    (A) may cause sensations of suffocation if the patient is conscious
    (B) reduce the incidence of fracture
    (C) may prolong apnea following treatment
    (D) all of the above
    (E) none of the above

98. The *most important* reason that glutethimide (Doriden) should not be stopped abruptly if the patient has taken large doses for a long period of time is that he may:
    (A) develop psychosis
    (B) have convulsions
    (C) hallucinate
    (D) become suicidally depressed
    (E) become comatose

99. The most dangerous side effect of neuroleptic drugs is:
    (A) agranulocytosis
    (B) parkinsonism
    (C) jaundice

(D) seizures
(E) retinitis pigmentosa

Summary of Directions

A	B	C	D	E
1, 2, 3	1, 3	2, 4	4	All are
only	only	only	only	correct

100. Known side effects of chlorpromazine include:
(1) orthostatic hypotension
(2) hyperpigmentation
(3) oculogyric crisis
(4) peripheral neuropathies

101. Psychomotor stimulants such as dextro-amphetamine and methylphenidate have established therapeutic value in the treatment of:
(1) narcolepsy
(2) involutional melancholia
(3) attention deficit disorders in children
(4) opiate abstinence syndrome

102. Action of the reticular activating system is altered by therapeutic doses of:
(1) chlorpromazine
(2) reserpine
(3) phenobarbital
(4) diazepam

103. During a conventional course of bilateral ECT, patients commonly develop:
(1) anxiety about future treatments
(2) headaches
(3) temporary amnesia
(4) increased insomnia

104. Contraindications to lithium carbonate therapy include:
(1) hyponatremia
(2) diabetes mellitus
(3) thyroid disturbance
(4) renal impairment

105. Major advantages of benzodiazepines over meprobamate for the treatment of short-term situational anxiety include:
(1) financial cost
(2) reduced potential for addiction
(3) superior antianxiety effects
(4) increased safety if an overdose is taken

106. At serum levels below 1 mEq/L, side effects of lithium may include:
(1) nephrogenic diabetes insipidus
(2) hypothyroidism
(3) leukocytosis
(4) EKG abnormalities

107. Addition of benztropine (Cogentin) to a patient's medication regimen may have an ameliorative effect on which of the following side effects of chlorpromazine?
(1) dryness of mouth
(2) urinary retention
(3) blurred vision
(4) akathisia

108. When the drug is taken chronically, patients may develop tolerance to:
(1) the antipsychotic effects of haloperidol
(2) the anxiolytic effects of diazepam
(3) the antidepressant effects of imipramine
(4) the sedative effects of secobarbital

109. Neuroleptics potentiate:
(1) the sedative effects of barbiturates
(2) the anticonvulsant effects of diphenyl-hydantoin
(3) the analgesic effects of opiates
(4) the antiparkinsonian effects of levodopa

110. Imipramine and other tricyclic antidepressants:
(1) are most effective in retarded depressions
(2) may temporarily increase the danger of suicide
(3) may require three weeks of therapy at adequate dosage before mood improvement is apparent
(4) should not be prescribed for children under age 12

111. Significant microsomal enzyme induction is caused by:
(1) barbiturates
(2) benzodiazepines
(3) glutethimide
(4) chlorpromazine

SELECTED REFERENCES

1. American College of Neuropsychopharmacology — Food and Drug Administration Task Force (1973). Neurological syndromes associated with antipsychotic drug use. *Archives of General Psychiatry*, vol. 28, pages 463–467.

2. American Psychiatric Association — Task Force on Lithium Therapy (1975). The current status of lithium therapy: Report of the A.P.A. Task Force. *American Journal of Psychiatry*, vol. 132, pages 997–1001.

3. Anderson, W.H., and Kuehnle, J.C. (1974). Strategies for the treatment of acute psychosis. *Journal of the American Medical Association*, vol. 229, pages 1884–89.

4. Appleton, W.S., and Davis, J.M. (1973). *Practical Clinical Psychopharmacology*. New York: Medcom Press.

5. Avery, D., and Winokur, G. (1976). Mortality in depressed patients treated with electroconvulsive therapy and antidepressants. *Archives of General Psychiatry*, vol. 33, pages 1029–37.

6. Ayd, F.J. (1961). A survey of drug-induced extrapyramidal reactions. *Journal of the American Medical Association*, vol. 175, pages 1054–60.

7. Ayd, F.J. (1972). Once-a-day neuroleptic and tricyclic antidepressant therapy. *International Drug Therapy Newsletter*, vol. 7, pages 33–40.

8. Ayd, F.J. (1976). Psychotropic drug therapy during pregnancy. *International Drug Therapy Newsletter*, vol. 11, pages 5-12.

9. Ayd, F.J., and Blackwell, B. [Eds.] (1970). *Discoveries in Biological Psychiatry*. Philadelphia: J. B. Lippincott Co.

10. Ban, T.A. (1969). *Psychopharmacology*. Baltimore: Williams & Wilkins Co.

11. Beresford, H.R. (1971). Legal issues relating to electroconvulsive therapy. *Archives of General Psychiatry*, vol. 25, pages 100–102.

12. Byck, R. (1975). Drugs and the treatment of psychiatric disorders. In *The Pharmacological Basis of Therapeutics* (5th ed.), edited by L.S. Goodman, A. Gilman, et al. New York: Macmillan. Chapter 12.

13. Clark, W.G., and del Giudice, J. [Eds.] (1970). *Principles of Psychopharmacology*. New York: Academic Press.

14. Davis, J.M. (1975). Overview: Maintenance therapy in psychiatry. I. Schizophrenia. *American Journal of Psychiatry*, vol. 132, pages 1237–45.

15. Davis, J.M. (1976). Overview: Maintenance therapy in psychiatry. II. Affective disorders. *American Journal of Psychiatry*, vol. 133, pages 1–13.

16. Davis, J.M. (1976). Recent developments in the drug treatment of schizophrenia. *American Journal of Psychiatry*, vol. 133, pages 208–214.

17. Davis, J.M. (1976). Comparative doses and costs of antipsychotic medication. *Archives of General Psychiatry*, vol. 133, pages 858–861.

18. Fink, M., Kety, S., McGaugh, J., and Williams, T.A. [Eds.] (1974). *Psychobiology of Convulsive Therapy*. Washington, D.C.: V. H. Winston and Sons.

19. Gardos, G., and Cole, J. (1976). Maintenance antipsychotic drug therapy: Is the cure worse than the disease? *American Journal of Psychiatry*, vol. 133, pages 32–36.

20. Granacher, R.P., and Baldessarini, R.J. (1975). Physostigmine. *Archives of General Psychiatry*, vol. 32, pages 375–380.

21. Greenblatt, D.J., and Shader, R.I. (1974). Benzodiazepines. *New England Journal of Medicine*, vol. 291, pages 1011–15 and 1239–43.

22. Greenblatt, M., Grosser, G.H., and Wechsler, H. (1964). Differential response of hospitalized depressed patients to somatic therapy. *American Journal of Psychiatry*, vol. 120, pages 935–943.

23. Groves, J.E., and Mandel, M.R. (1975). The long-acting phenothiazines. *Archives of General Psychiatry*, vol. 32, pages 893–900.

24. Hollister, L.E. (1973). *Clinical Use of Psycho-*

therapeutic Drugs. Springfield, Illinois: Charles C Thomas.

25. Huston, P.E., and Locher, L.M. (1948). Involutional psychosis. *Archives of Neurology and Psychiatry,* vol. 59, pages 385–394.

26. Kalinowski, L.B., and Hippius, H. (1969). *Pharmacological, Convulsive and Other Somatic Treatments in Psychiatry.* New York: Grune & Stratton.

27. Klein, D.F., and Davis, J.M. (1969). *Diagnosis and Drug Treatment of Psychiatric Disorders.* Baltimore: Williams & Wilkins Co.

28. Longo, V.G. (1972). *Neuropharmacology and Behavior.* San Francisco: W. H. Freeman and Co.

29. Man, P.L., and Chen, C.H. (1973). Rapid tranquilization of acutely psychotic patients with intramuscular haloperidol and chlorpromazine. *Psychosomatics,* vol. 14, pages 59–63.

30. May, P.R.A. (1968). *Treatment of Schizophrenia.* New York: Science House.

31. McCabe, M.S. (1976). ECT in the treatment of mania: A controlled study. *American Journal of Psychiatry,* vol. 133, pages 688–691.

32. Orlov, P., Kasparian, G., DiMascio, A., and Cole, J. (1971). Withdrawal of antiparkinson drugs. *Archives of General Psychiatry,* vol. 25, pages 410–412.

33. Shader, R.I. [Ed.] (1975). *Manual of Psychiatric Therapeutics.* Boston: Little, Brown and Co.

34. Shader, R.I., DiMascio, A., et al. (1970). *Psychotropic Drug Side Effects.* Baltimore: Williams & Wilkins Co.

35. Shepherd, M., Lader, M., and Rodnight, R. (1968). *Clinical Psychopharmacology.* Philadelphia: Lea & Febiger.

36. Singer, I., and Rotenberg, D. (1973). Mechanisms of lithium action. *New England Journal of Medicine,* vol. 289, pages 254–260.

37. Snyder, S., Greenberg, D., and Yamamura, H.I. (1974). Antischizophrenic drugs and brain cholinergic receptors. *Archives of General Psychiatry,* vol. 31, pages 58–61.

38. Squire, L.R., and Chace, P.M. (1975). Memory functions six to nine months after electroconvulsive therapy. *Archives of General Psychiatry,* vol. 32, pages 1557–64.

39. Tourney, G. (1970). Psychiatric Therapies: 1880–1968. In *Changing Patterns in Psychiatric Care,* edited by T. Rothman. New York: Crown Publishers, Inc. Chapter 1.

9. Community and Social Psychiatry

In Boston they ask, How much does he know?
In New York, How much is he worth? In
Philadelphia, Who were his parents?
Mark Twain

COMMUNITY AND PREVENTIVE PSYCHIATRY

It is more than two hundred years since the Virginia legislature became the first in this country to vote public funds to help in building a hospital devoted exclusively to the insane. The second such hospital for the mentally ill was the Friends Asylum at Frankford, Pennsylvania, which was opened in 1817 by the Philadelphia Society of Friends. During the latter part of the nineteenth century, many large custodial institutions were built that tended to be located in rural areas, where land was cheap and many patients might contribute to their upkeep by working the farm that was operated by the hospital.

During the first half of the present century, continuing immigration and declining mortality contributed to rapid growth of our population. However, there was an even more dramatic growth in the resident population of state and county mental hospitals, due to a variety of factors such as the following: (1) an increase in the proportion of dependent older persons (with relatively high rates of mental illness); (2) urbanization of the population, with emphasis on small and geographically mobile families, no longer able or willing to care for confused or dependent members; (3) increased recognition of psychiatric disorder; and (4) some increased prospect of improvement with somatic therapies introduced shortly prior to World War II (convulsive therapy, insulin coma therapy, and lobotomy).

In any event, by midcentury half of all the hospital beds in the country were mental-hospital beds, and half of the latter were occupied by persons with a diagnosis of schizophrenia. The third quarter of the present century has witnessed a dramatic reversal of the previous growth in mental hospital population. At the present time mental hospital beds constitute little more than one-quarter of all hospital beds in the country.

In large measure this turnabout is due to the advent of effective antipsychotic medications, discussed in the previous chapter. Other important factors have been the increased availability of skilled professional therapy, willingness to spend public funds for mental health facilities and education, and recognition that impairment from chronic mental illness might be compounded by the depersonalizing impact of life in large custodial institutions.

Immediately following World War II, state hospitals tended to have several times as many patients in residence as admissions during the course of a given year. The reverse is now the case, but the much shorter length of stay and the increased emphasis on voluntary admission have been accompanied by rapid escalation in the cost of active treatment programs. This escalation in cost is even more marked in general hospital settings than in public and private mental hospitals.

In addition to emphasis on smaller institutions and general hospital psychiatric units, the community psychiatry movement fosters the development of outpatient treatment resources and facilities for partial hospitalization. There is a focus on the total population residing within a *catchment area,* defined on the basis of location of residence and ideally including roughly 100,000 members of the general population. Federal funds were made available through the Community Mental Health Centers Act of 1963. In order to qualify for such federal funds, each program must accept responsibility for prevention, treatment, and rehabilitation in the community served. In addition, federal funding of a comprehensive community mental health center is contingent on provision of the following five basic psychiatric services for all age groups: (1) inpatient care; (2) emergency services (24 hours a day); (3) community consultation; (4) day care (including partial hospitalization programs and outpatient services); and (5) research and education.

In addition to treatment and rehabilitation of the mentally ill and retarded, the community mental health center is expected to assume responsibility for prevention at three levels: (1) **Primary prevention** programs are intended to lower the rate of onset of emotional disorders by counteracting the stressful social conditions that may produce mental illness or retardation. (2) **Secondary prevention** consists of early identification and prompt treatment of mental disorder. (3) **Tertiary prevention** is intended to reduce the rate of defective functioning produced by the mental disorder. All forms of prevention imply some knowledge of causation, however primitive, and the remainder of this chapter will be concerned with the analysis of social and cultural factors in the causation and development of psychiatric disorder.

EPIDEMIOLOGY OR MEDICAL ECOLOGY

Epidemiology has been described as the diagnostic discipline of mass disease, or as the basic science of public health. Data on the epidemiology of mental disorders started to accumulate more than 50 years ago, but much was provided by social scientists interested in ecology. John Gordon and his colleagues interpreted the relationship between these disciplines as follows: "Ecology is a biologic and social discipline concerned with the general phenomena of mutual relationships between living organisms and their reaction to animate and inanimate surroundings. That part of human ecology relating to health and disease is medical ecology, and medical ecology as it concerns communities of people is epidemiology."

There are four general **measures of frequency** that may be used to compare the distribution of various characteristics (e.g., illness) in the population or in selected groups of the population: (1) *Relative frequency* may be used to outline the proportions of selected diagnoses among specified groups of patients, or the age and sex distribution of selected diagnostic groups. Relative frequencies are expressed as ratios by means of percentages, decimal fractions, rates per unit of population size, etc. The denominator of such ratios is always the total size of the population under study. (2) *Prev-*

alence rates consist of the relative frequency of *all* persons having the selected diagnoses at a specified point in time. (3) *Incidence rates* are defined as the relative frequency of *new* cases of the selected diagnoses; i.e., of persons having onset of illness within a specified period of time. (4) *Expectancy rates* may be regarded as the lifetime incidence or as the probability of developing the disorder during a lifetime, provided the person lives long enough to pass through the period of risk during which he may develop the disorder.

Since prevalence and incidence may vary for each sex and for different age groups, they are frequently expressed as *age-sex-specific rates,* each consisting of the relative frequency of cases within that portion of the population having the specified age and sex. Sometimes a single statistic known as an *age-sex-adjusted rate* (or *age-sex-standardized rate*) of prevalence or incidence may be calculated from the age-sex-specific rates for all groups by applying these to a standard population. Overall comparisons are then possible between segments of the population having dissimilar age distributions. Lifetime expectancy is already a single figure expressing the risk at all ages, so expectancy rates are not described as being age specific or age standardized, but may still be computed separately for the two sexes.

All these measures of frequency vary from one year to another, from one place to another, and among various social groups in the population — according to educational or marital status, etc. We shall therefore look at each a little more closely.

Relative Frequency

The proportions of specific diagnoses among various samples of patients depend on such factors as diagnostic criteria and the setting from which the sample is obtained. For example, the diagnosis of manic-depressive psychosis became relatively less frequent in this country after World War II, while the relative frequency of schizophrenias was increasing (due partly to the new category of schizo-affective psychosis, which is classified with the latter group). In the United Kingdom the diagnosis of manic-depressive psychosis is now relatively more frequent than in this country, since the criteria permit inclusion of some patients with hallucinations and delusions, who would tend to be diagnosed schizophrenic in the United States.

Family physicians and psychiatrists practicing in general hospitals are likely to see and diagnose a high proportion of patients with neurotic anxiety, depression, and various psychophysiological disorders. Those engaged mainly in psychoanalytic therapy with outpatients are likely to see a high proportion of patients with character neurosis. Those who work in state hospitals or community mental health centers will see a relatively high frequency of patients with schizophrenias and organic brain syndromes.

Table 9-1 shows the percentage distribution of various diagnoses among patients newly admitted during the year, and total patients resident at the end of the year, for state and county mental hospitals in the United States. Schizophrenic disorders represent about 30 percent of all admissions to such institutions, but about one-half of all patients resident in such institutions, due to relatively lower rates of death or permanent remission than for other diagnoses. Relatively high discharge rates and low readmission rates among patients with acute brain syndromes, neurotic disorders, and personality disorders result in a lower proportion of these diagnoses among chronic resident patients than among admissions to state hospitals.

During the past few decades, the proportions of various diagnoses among admissions to state hospitals have changed. Relatively few patients now have psychoses due to syphilis (once responsible for 10 percent of male admissions), but admissions have included more patients with organic brain syndromes of senility, with neurotic and personality disorders, and with alcoholism and drug abuse.

Most physicians are aware of some association between psychiatric diagnosis and age and sex of patients. For example, patients with severe mental retardation are likely to be recognized during preschool years, but those with mild retardation are likely to be recognized only through their school performance. About two-thirds of patients with schizophrenias and with antisocial personality are first recognized between the ages of 20 and 40 years. About two-thirds of those with paranoid

Table 9-1. Percentage Frequency of Selected Diagnoses among Total Admissions and Resident Patients in State and County Mental Hospitals, United States, 1973

Diagnosis	Total admissions during 1973 (percent)	Resident patients at end of 1973 (percent)
Mental retardation	2.9	11.7
Alcoholism	23.7	6.1
Drug dependency/intoxication	5.3	0.9
Organic brain syndromes	7.3	18.4
Depression	9.8	5.4
Schizophrenia	30.8	47.6
Other psychoses	0.9	1.3
Other neuroses	2.0	0.6
Personality disorders	5.3	2.1
Preadult disorders	2.5	1.4
Other mental disorders	1.7	0.7
Social maladjustments	0.4	0.2
No mental disorder	0.7	0.1
Undiagnosed	6.8	3.5
Totals percent	100.0	100.0
numbers	442,525	248,522

Data from the National Institute of Mental Health.

psychoses, involutional psychoses, and chronic alcoholism are identified between the ages of 40 and 70 years, while two-thirds of those with organic brain syndromes of senility are over the age of 70 years. The two groups of patients likely to be seen for the first time with equal frequency at any period of adulthood are those with manic-depressive psychoses and those with various forms of neuroses.

The *sex distribution* also varies according to diagnosis and treatment setting. There is a relatively higher frequency of affective psychoses and neurotic disorders among females, whereas male patients are more likely to have diagnoses of anti-social personality, alcoholism or drug dependence, and sexual deviation. General hospital psychiatric units and some private institutions are relatively more likely to attract female patients, while state, county, and Veterans Administration hospitals have relatively more male patients. Such relative frequency distributions provide crude information about patterns of distribution and treatment, but tend to be less informative than rates of prevalence, incidence, and expectancy.

Prevalence of Total Cases at a Given Time

Incomplete or partial estimates of prevalence may be derived from the rate per 100,000 general population of patients resident in various institutions at any given time. Overall rates of psychiatric hospitalization (for all ages combined) roughly doubled during the first half of the present century, but decreased by half during the next quarter century. The earlier increase reflected a number of factors including the increasing age of the population (since elderly persons have higher rates of admission), diminished family size and cohesiveness, and an increasing tendency for voluntary or involuntary hospitalization for relatively milder forms of psychiatric disorder. By contrast, the decreased numbers currently in hospitals reflect more effective treatment, improved community resources, and a trend towards treatment in the least restrictive environment compatible with safety.

The numbers of patients resident in hospitals at a given time now represent a very incomplete picture of total prevalence, corresponding with the tip of the iceberg of psychiatric disorder in the community. Many attempts have been made to estimate overall prevalence in various communities by means of census investigations and surveys of general population samples. Cross-cultural comparisons of frequency have been concerned mainly with such estimates of prevalence, which is one of their major weaknesses. However, some of the best data on prevalence were obtained during the course of studies of social class differences in psychiatric disorder. These showed a differential prevalence of psychiatric disorders among various social classes, with psychosis tending to be most frequent and most chronic at the lower end of the socioeconomic spectrum. Several of these studies will be described below.

Incidence of New Cases during a Given Time

Incomplete or partial estimates were traditionally based on annual rates of first admissions to psychiatric hospitals, often simply public state hospitals. Extensive data were reported during the first half of the present century, and some expressed a high degree of confidence that these data represented an accurate estimate of true incidence for the major functional psychoses. However, this was never likely, even in European countries having low geographic mobility, limited numbers of hospitals, and long-established reporting practices.

The age and sex distribution of first admission rates to mental hospitals with various diagnoses do not represent an accurate picture of all new cases. Such figures are influenced by many factors like the following: social judgment of what constitutes mental illness; social demand for hospital care; availability of psychiatric hospital accommodation (including distance from place of residence); availability of alternative resources for psychiatric treatment; and variations in diagnostic practices. A few attempts have been made to estimate the total incidence of new cases more completely by including data from other treatment facilities. As in the case of prevalence, the best such studies are probably those concerning socioeconomic status, which will be reviewed next.

Lifetime Expectancy

Expectancy corresponds with lifetime incidence, or the total probability of developing a psychiatric disorder during one's lifetime. Estimates of expectancy in various classes of relatives of persons already diagnosed (especially in the two types of co-twins) may be compared to such estimates for the general population to provide important data for the study of heredity, as discussed at the beginning of Chapter 7.

It may be of some interest to estimate the lifetime expectation or probability of ever being admitted to a psychiatric hospital (with or without some specific diagnosis). This has been done by applying age-sex-specific first admission rates to a life table for the population, which gives the proportion of persons remaining alive at successive ages. On the basis of such computation, the expectation of admission to New York state mental hospitals (1940–1941) was estimated as about 8.5 percent. Based on rates immediately following World War II, the probability by now has substantially exceeded 10 percent.

Various Scandinavian studies attempted to establish lifetime expectation by direct enumeration. One of the best-known studies is that by Karl Fremming, who succeeded in tracing more than 92 percent of 5,500 persons born on the Danish island of Bornholm during the years 1883–1887, up to the time of their deaths or of his inquiry conducted in 1947. By the start of their eleventh year, 4,130 remained available, and 2,710 were still living in Bornholm at the time of their death or of Fremming's retrospective study. The figures he computed for the expectation of mental disorders in this sample applied only to the age range 10 through 54 years. His estimates by diagnosis were roughly as follows: psychoses, 4 percent; mental retardation, 3 percent; psychopathy, 3 percent; alcoholism, 2 percent; neurosis, 2 percent. The cumulative expectation of mental disorders in this sample (allowing for multiple disorders in the same person) was about 12 percent, which would be increased by the relatively high frequency of disorders having their onset after the age of 55 years.

Clearly, definitions of psychiatric disorder are crucial in establishing its frequency, and wider categories of abnormality have led to much higher estimates. Psychiatric disorder, like beauty, is in the eye of the beholder, and "significant psychopathology" was reported among 80 percent of the population resident in midtown Manhattan at the time of the well-known survey that will be mentioned below.

DEMOGRAPHIC AND ECOLOGICAL STUDIES

Rates of psychiatric disorder and suicide have been studied according to *time, place,* and *demographic characteristics,* such as age, sex, marital status, race, country of birth, religion, education, occupation, economic status, and residence. The major differences in age and sex distribution have already been reviewed.

Rates of psychiatric disorder are also correlated with *marital status.* Most disorders are least frequent among the married, next among the widowed, then the single, and highest among the divorced. Typical ratios between age-sex-adjusted first admission rates according to marital status (taking a standard value of 100 for the married group) are as follows: married, 100; widowed, 150; single, 200; divorced, 500.

Such variations in frequency have long been attributed to either (1) *protection* against precipitating stresses (for members of those groups having *low* frequencies), or (2) *selection* on the basis of predisposition or existing psychiatric disorder (for those groups having *high* frequencies). The relatively high rates among single persons have been largely attributed to selection by marriage, particularly against males with mental retardation and latent or overt schizophrenias. The higher rates among widowed than married (for several disorders) have been attributed partly to loss, but also partly to some selection against remarriage by vulnerable persons. The very high rate of psychiatric disorder among the divorced is usually attributed to divorce resulting from overt psychiatric disorder (particularly schizophrenia, mania, antisocial personality, and alcoholism). However, since the statistics referred to those who remain divorced, they may also reflect the same two factors as in the case of the widowed (a reaction to loss, and selection against remarriage by some persons with above-average vulnerability).

The distribution of psychiatric disorder according to race, country of birth, and religion is extremely difficult to disentangle from the socioeconomic status of these groups. After corrections have been made for the age and sex composition of each group, psychiatric hospital admission rates in this country remain relatively higher than average among blacks, the foreign born, and members of other minority groups. Similar explanations have been proposed as in the case of marital status. Thus a higher frequency of schizophrenia among immigrants has been attributed to a selective vulnerability among those choosing to migrate. However, recent studies have distinguished between a relatively high frequency among former immigrants of low socioeconomic status, and a relatively lower frequency among more recent immigrants of higher socioeconomic status.

Marked differences in both hospital admission rates and community prevalence of psychiatric disorder have been found to exist within different areas of the same city, and are highly correlated with various indices of overall socioeconomic status. The surveys of the British sociologist Charles Booth (carried out during the years 1886 to 1901) originated the idea of a "submerged tenth" of the population, particularly evident in the large cities that developed after the industrial revolution. Subsequent studies led to the recognition of social dependency among certain families having relatively high frequencies of mild mental retardation, antisocial behavior, and sometimes psychosis. By mid-century it was recognized that multiproblem families, numbering 6 percent of the community's families, might absorb more than 50 percent of the social services provided by the numerous agencies in a large city.

Between 1929 and 1942, Shaw and McKay stimulated a number of sociologists to undertake ecological studies of high delinquency areas in various cities. They found high correlations in Chicago between rates of male juvenile delinquency and zones or areas of the city; these correlations remained the same despite changes in the demographic composition of the populations residing in these areas over a period of time. In Baltimore, Lander observed high positive correlations between juvenile delinquency and overcrowding or substandard housing conditions. He also reported high negative correlations between delinquency and median rentals and median years of schooling. However, he hypothesized that these were only surface relationships, and that high delinquency rates were best interpreted in terms of *anomie,* according to which the group norms of behavior are no longer binding or valid in an area or for a population subgroup. However, within *high* delinquency areas, there are certain streets and families with *low* rates of delinquency, so that within underprivileged neighborhoods it may be that family characteristics are more important than location of residence.

Faris and Dunham analyzed the distribution of mental hospital admission rates for various diagnoses from different areas within the city of Chicago. They found that overall admission rates per 100,000 population increased progressively from the periphery of the city (residential zone of single family dwellings) to the central areas of social disorganization and slum dwellings. The distribution of admissions with schizophrenia, alcoholism, drug addiction, and general paresis (CNS syphilis) all corresponded to the overall distribution of admissions. By contrast, manic-depressive psychosis was randomly distributed throughout the city. Different patterns of distribution were found for various subtypes of schizophrenia, with high rates of paranoid and hebephrenic types being recorded for communities in which the populations were highly mobile, whereas high rates of catatonic schizophrenia were related principally to immigrant slum areas. A similar distribution of schizophrenia and other mental disorders has been reported in other cities.

The *drift hypothesis of schizophrenia* was advanced by Faris and Dunham as one possible explanation of their findings. According to this hypothesis, the concentration of admission rates in the geographic center of the city might be due to *downward drift* of mentally abnormal persons who had failed in economic competition. However, many of the patients with schizophrenia had been born and had always lived in deteriorated areas, suggesting an alternative hypothesis that *social isolation* and other conditions of life in these areas combined to produce mental abnormality. Some authors continue to speculate that *vertical* (socioeconomic) or *horizontal* (geographic) *drift* may be at least as important as social isolation or stress in determining this distribution.

SOCIOECONOMIC STATUS

Certain rights and obligations are inherent in a person's position, or status, within the social structure. Sometimes status is *ascribed* on the basis of such factors as sex, age, and kinship. Sometimes it is *achieved* on the basis of success in an occupation valued by the society, or of marriage to a person of high status. In a *closed society,* exemplified by the medieval European feudal system or by the Indian caste system, opportunities for achieving status are relatively small. In an *open society* such as the United States, opportunities for achieving status are much greater than elsewhere.

There are many yardsticks by which status may be measured, as illustrated in the words of Mark Twain quoted as the beginning of the chapter. When asked the single most important indicator of status, many persons at first respond by saying "income," by which they mean the *quantity* of income. In fact the latter appears to be less important than several other indicators. Even the *source* of income is more relevant than its reported quantity — i.e., whether it is derived from: (1) inherited wealth; (2) wealth accumulated during the person's lifetime; (3) fees for professional services; (4) salary; (5) wages; (6) social agencies, etc.

In the vast majority of cases in this country, the single most important indicator of social status is *occupation,* and the next most helpful indicator is formal *education* (when weighted in a ratio of 7:4, these combine into Hollingshead's two-factor Index of Social Position). A third significant factor is *locality of residence,* but the

latter is by no means obvious, and may require careful sociological mapping of each community.

Although socioeconomic status represents a continuum, there is clustering of our population into five or six identifiable groups or classes (depending on whether the upper two classes are combined into one, as is usual on the basis of small numbers). Among the five social classes generally recognized, the largest is Class IV (semiskilled, or working, class). Class V (unskilled and often unemployed) constitutes about 10 percent of the population, but otherwise the classes decrease in size as one ascends the social pyramid.

Life experiences vary greatly among members of different social classes, and are reflected in their predominant *time-orientation.* For upper-class private-school children the important time dimension is the *past,* whereas for middle-class public-school children the significant time dimension is the *future.* By contrast, people in lower classes are predominantly oriented to the *present.* Studies to be outlined below suggest that the time orientation of the major social classes is related to the form and frequency of psychopathology most typical of their members. Upper-class orientation toward the past involves preservation of the status quo, and may lead to dissatisfaction with the present and a sense of failure that accompanies *depression and suicide* (the highest frequencies of which may be found at this level). Middle-class orientation towards future achievement involves postponement of impulse gratification, often accompanied by *anxiety and neurotic conflict.* Orientation to the present among members of the lower social class is accompanied by tendencies to hedonistic impulse gratification, with sexual and aggressive behavior that may be regarded as *delinquent or antisocial.*

In their important study of social class and mental illness, Hollingshead and Redlich extensively analyzed a census of all psychiatric patients (at a given time) from the city of New Haven, Connecticut, and all new patients admitted to treatment during a period of six months in 1950. Their enumeration included patients receiving treatment outside the city of New Haven, such as those currently residing in state or private psychiatric hospitals and those commuting to New York for psychoanalysis. Their data permitted estimates of *prevalence* at a given time and *incidence* of new cases, for both psychoses and neuroses, each according to social class membership, as shown in Table 9-2. This table shows that the incidence of new cases of neurosis was fairly evenly distributed, whereas the total prevalence of neurotics receiving treatment was highest among members of the upper classes. The incidence of new cases of psychosis was highest among the lowest social class, and the total prevalence of patients with psychoses (receiving treatment or custodial care) was relatively higher yet in the lowest class. The latter reflects a tendency to chronicity, as illustrated by the final column of the table. This column was computed by dividing the prevalence rates by twice the six-month incidence rates. Since both rates were based solely on patients receiving treatment, the resulting quotient may be interpreted as average years of duration of treatment. Hollingshead and Redlich attributed the differences for psychosis to the inadequate treatment received by members of the lowest class and they did, in fact, document social class differences in prevailing patterns of psychiatric treatment — but the tendency toward chronicity may have existed prior to hospitalization. For example, one may mention a strong correlation between socioeconomic status and

intelligence ($r = + 0.5$, which is as high as the intelligence correlation between parent and child, or between siblings, or between husband and wife). Moreover, members of the lowest social class are apt to have the greatest mistrust of helping agencies, including physicians, and to resist involvement in psychiatric treatment until some crisis intervenes. In the case of neuroses, patients of high socioeconomic status are selected into longer-term treatment through such factors as intelligence, verbal ability, similar cultural background, and ability to pay. Neurotic patients of lower socioeconomic status are offered less adequate treatment and are less motivated to accept or persist in the treatment that is available.

A few years later Srole and his colleagues reported the results of the Midtown Manhattan Study, which involved both a census of psychiatric patients and a home survey among the population. This permitted estimates of the prevalence of both treated and untreated psychopathology, but the latter was presented only in global terms, and not according to psychiatric diagnoses. However, the study included some interesting data on upward and downward social mobility during the course of the person's lifetime. These data provide evidence that good mental health is most frequent among those with parents of superior socioeconomic status, and also tends to be associated with occupational stability or upward mobility. Psychi-

Table 9-2. Incidence and Prevalence Rates per 100,000 and Average Duration in Treatment for Neuroses and Psychoses (New Haven, Connecticut, receiving treatment, 1950)

Class	Six-month incidence	Prevalence	Average years duration of treatment
		Neuroses	
I-II	69	349	2.5
III	78	250	1.6
IV	52	114	1.1
V	66	97	0.7
		Psychoses	
I-II	28	188	3.4
III	36	291	4.0
IV	37	518	7.0
V	73	1505	10.3

Adapted from Hollingshead, A. B., and Redlich, F. C. *Social Class and Mental Illness.* Copyright 1958 by John Wiley & Sons, Inc., p. 235.

atric impairment is most frequent among those with parents of low socioeconomic status, and also among those with downward occupational mobility. The relative frequency of psychiatric impairment was more than twice as high among all downwardly mobile persons as among all upwardly mobile persons.

SOCIAL STRESS: UNEMPLOYMENT AND WAR

Members of different groups experience different types and degrees of psychological and biological stress. During the past two hundred years there have also been repeated expressions of profound concern over the supposed adverse effects of civilization on mental stability.

Comparisons of hospital admission rates over a prolonged period of time present serious problems, but the best long-term study provides little support for the preceding thesis. Goldhamer and Marshall carefully examined all available data for Massachusetts for the 100-year period from 1840 to 1940. They found there had been a very marked increase

in hospital admission rates for the older age groups. However, when appropriate comparisons were made (equating the class of patients received and conditions affecting hospitalization), admission rates for persons under the age of 50 were just as high during the last half of the nineteenth century as at the termination of the period studied. While nineteenth-century admissions to hospitals contained a larger proportion of psychotic and severely deranged patients, there was no long-term increase during the century in the frequency of the psychoses of early and middle life.

Although no overall escalation in psychiatric disorder has been evident, there have been substantial fluctuations in rates of suicide and hospital admissions increasing in times of economic depression (with high unemployment) and decreasing in times of war (with low rates of unemployment).

Annual average rates of unemployment in this country have been published since 1929, and the two-year moving average of unemployment has ranged from a high of 24.25 percent for the years 1932–33 to a low of 1.55 percent during the years

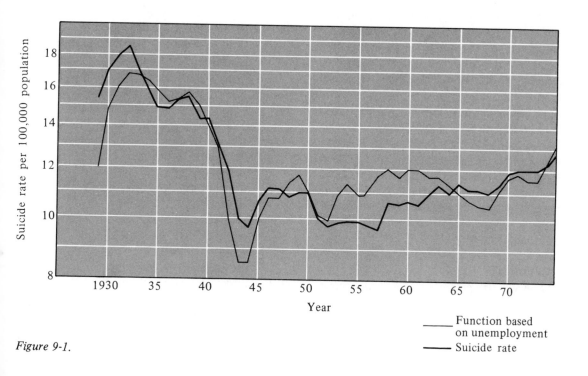

Figure 9-1.

1943–45. During the same period of time, an overall annual suicide rate (adjusted for changes in age, sex, and racial composition of the population) has ranged from a high of 18.6 per 100,000 (in 1932) to a low of 9.6 per 100,000 (in 1944 and again in 1957). The high figure for unemployment is approximately sixteen times the low figure, whereas the high figure for suicide is roughly twice the low figure. If plotted on semilogarithmic graph paper, the vertical range of unemployment on four cycle paper corresponds roughly with the vertical range of suicide rates on one cycle paper. Indeed, the fourth root of the two-year moving average of unemployment bears a fairly constant relationship to the suicide rate, the correlation being about + 0.9 over the period of nearly fifty years. This suggests that roughly 80 percent of the observed variation in suicide rates for the total population of the United States was attributable to the same factors as unemployment. However, all of the variation in suicide rates is attributable to less than 25 percent of the total cases (Fig. 9-1).

Rates of suicide and hospital admission have decreased in times of war when most people are employed and united against the common enemy. However, in countries that have been defeated and occupied by the enemy, there have been marked increases in rates of suicide among vulnerable segments of the population. Moreover, during wartime, the decreased rates of admission apply only to civilian mental hospitals, whereas high rates of breakdown have been reported among the vulnerable combatant military personnel. The more remote effects of war and its aftermaths (mediated through such situations as illegitimacy, widowhood, orphanhood, physical disability, difficulties in vocational readjustment) are impossible to separate from the precipitating stresses reflected in the statistics of later years.

REVIEW QUESTIONS

112. *Secondary* prevention of mental illness is defined as:
    (A) efforts made to reduce the likelihood of mental illness in the children of the mentally ill

(B) early identification and prompt treatment of mental illness
(C) efforts made to modify community prejudices and discriminatory practices against the mentally ill
(D) efforts made to prevent relapse by persons whose mental illness is in remission
(E) activities of persons who are not mental health professionals that serve to prevent mental illness

113. In order to receive federal funds, a community mental health center is required by law to provide five basic services. Each of the following is one of the five required services *except:*
    (A) inpatient psychiatric treatment
    (B) emergency psychiatric treatment
    (C) day-care services
    (D) methadone maintenance program
    (E) research and education

114. Which of the following would most clearly and directly serve the *primary* prevention of mental illness?
    (A) improvement of the early social environment of children
    (B) more trained psychiatrists
    (C) increased use of behavior modification therapy
    (D) mental health screening programs for school children
    (E) increasing psychiatric training of pediatricians

115. According to recent statistics, a person living in the United States has approximately what chance of being hospitalized for a psychiatric disorder at some time during his lifetime?
    (A) 10%
    (B) 5%
    (C) 2%
    (D) 1%
    (E) 0.1%

116. The *drift hypothesis* postulates that certain mental disorders:
    (A) tend to result in downward social mobility
    (B) tend to result from downward social mobility

(C) result in an absence of significant relationships

(D) can be attributed to our increasingly hectic way of life

(E) are associated with forced mass emigrations in wartime

117. The largest single diagnostic group of inpatients currently being treated in state and county mental hospitals are patients with:

(A) schizophrenia

(B) depression

(C) alcoholism

(D) chronic brain syndromes

(E) mental retardation

Summary of Directions

A	B	C	D	E
1, 2, 3 only	1, 3 only	2, 4 only	4 only	All are correct

118. Community mental health centers receiving federal funds are required to serve:

(1) both adults and children

(2) only persons unable to afford psychiatric care

(3) a specific geographic region

(4) according to guidelines determined primarily at the local level

119. In comparison with the rest of the United States population, groups which have greater rates of psychiatric impairment include:

(1) the divorced

(2) the elderly

(3) those whose socioeconomic status is declining

(4) those living in rural areas

SELECTED REFERENCES

1. Caplan, G. (1964). *Principles of Preventive Psychiatry*. New York: Basic Books.

2. Faris, R.E.L., and Dunham, H.W. (1939). *Mental Disorders in Urban Areas* (Reprinted 1960). New York: Hafner Publishing Co.

3. Goldhamer, H., and Marshall, A.W. (1949). *Psychosis and Civilization*. Glencoe, Illinois: The Free Press, Division Macmillan Co.

4. Hollingshead, A.B., and Redlich, F.C. (1958). *Social Class and Mental Illness*. New York: John Wiley and Sons.

5. Joint Commission on Mental Illness and Health (1961). *Action for Mental Health*. New York: Basic Books.

6. Langner, T.S., and Michael, S.T. (1963). *Life Stress and Mental Health*. Glencoe, Illinois: The Free Press, Division Macmillan Co.

7. Myers, J.K., and Roberts, B.H. (1959). *Family and Class Dynamics in Mental Illness*. New York: John Wiley and Sons.

8. Pasamanick, B. [Ed.] (1959). *Epidemiology of Mental Disorder*. Washington, D.C.: American Association for the Advancement of Science (Publication No. 60).

9. Rubin, B. (1969). Community psychiatry. *Archives of General Psychiatry*, vol. 20, page 497.

10. Srole, L., Langner, T.S., Michael, S.T., Opler, M.K., and Rennie, T.A.C. (1962). *Mental Health in the Metropolis*. New York: McGraw-Hill.

10. Psychiatry and the Law

It may not be amiss to observe that this matter of the testimony of experts, especially in cases of alleged insanity, has gone to such an extravagance that it has really become of late years a profitable profession to be an expert witness, at the command of any party and ready for any party, for a sufficient and often exorbitant fee.
From the 1873 annual report to the legislature by the managers of the New York State Lunatic Asylum.

The present chapter is concerned with four major areas of interaction between psychiatry and the law: (1) hospital admission or commitment procedures, and the rights of involuntary patients; (2) competency to enter into contracts or manage property; (3) competency to stand trial and responsibility for criminal behavior; (4) professional liability of the physician.

COMMITMENT PROCEDURES AND PATIENTS' RIGHTS

Early laws were more concerned with preserving the property of the mentally ill or retarded than with the custody of the individual. The latter was generally assumed to be the responsibility of the family, unless the patient was too disturbed, in which case he was detained in jail and perhaps later in an asylum. Often the procedures for taking him into custody were quite informal. Some persons were detained for years on a brief order written by the person in charge of the custodial institution and based only on verbal allegations by members of the community. During the nineteenth century, public concern was aroused over the legality of detaining mildly disordered persons against their will, and states enacted a wide variety of commitment laws.

At least five general issues may be covered by legislation governing the hospitalization or confinement of the mentally disordered:

1. *Who may be admitted:* the mentally ill (sometimes with the stipulation that they must be dangerous to themselves or others); the mentally retarded; epileptics, with or without mental illness or retardation; alcoholics and drug addicts; psychopathic sexual offenders or other criminals with mental illness.

2. *Where they may be admitted:* to jail, state hospitals, or other state institutions such as training schools for the retarded; to private psychiatric hospitals; to university-affiliated psychiatric hospitals; to psychiatric units in general hospitals; to community mental health centers; etc.

3. *How long they may be detained:* indefinitely, meaning until the hospital authorities or court considers that discharge is appropriate; or for a temporary period, ranging from several days to several months, and sometimes specified as being a period of observation and evaluation rather than treatment.

4. *How the patient shall be admitted and discharged:* on his own voluntary application; involuntarily on the application of some member of the community; involuntarily on the basis of medical certificates; or involuntarily by court order — with or without court hearing, sometimes entailing trial by jury.

5. *What rights the patient has after admission to hospital:* these may include the rights to accept or refuse recommended treatment; to retain control over property and enter into legal contracts and to communicate with family or attorney; to initiate proceedings for release from hospital. The latter rights are much more likely to be preserved in the case of a voluntary patient than an involuntary one, and are more likely to be preserved for short-term involuntary patients than for long-term involuntary (or custodial) patients.

During the years immediately following World War II there were very few voluntary admissions to state mental hospitals in the United States, In 1949 such voluntary admissions constituted only 10 percent of all admissions in this country (as contrasted with about two-thirds of all such admissions in the United Kingdom). At the same time there was often undue emphasis on legal formalities, so that patients with medical emergencies were not infrequently taken to jail pending commitment procedures, where many committed suicide or died from other causes.

Major efforts on the part of the American Psychiatric Association, the United States Public Health Service, and many legislators resulted in widespread modernization of the commitment laws. There was particular emphasis on voluntary, rather than involuntary, hospitalization — and on medical certification and involvement in the commitment process. In recent years, however, there has once more been an emphasis on judicial commitment and due process of law rather than simple certification by physicians or other professionals.

At the present time the four admission procedures most likely to be preserved are as follows:

1. **Informal voluntary admission.** At present there are believed to be over two thousand psychiatric units in general hospitals for which this admission procedure may be used. It implies that the patient is free to leave hospital at any time, and that he is not restrained from doing so by locked doors.

2. **Formal voluntary admission.** This requires the patient to make written application for admission on a specified form, and is the usual procedure for admission to those psychiatric units where doors are sometimes locked. Laws governing such procedures often stipulate that a voluntary patient whose release is requested in writing shall be permitted to leave hospital forthwith, except under certain specified circumstances; for example, prompt application for court order in the case of a patient who is believed to be suicidal or homicidal.

3. **Temporary or emergency admission.** In some states this procedure involves one or more medical certificates, which may be valid for a period of several weeks (provided the emergency situation remains unchanged). However, the recent trend for such emergency admissions is away from medical certificates, and from involuntary detention for any period longer than about three court days.

4. **Involuntary or compulsory admission.** Often this has been accomplished on the certificates of two physicians (not on the staff of the hospital to which the patient was committed), which might

then be valid for a period of about three months, or even indefinitely. The recent trend has been to eliminate such procedures where they existed, and to require all such involuntary detention (or incarceration) to be made on the basis of court order, sometimes including the right to jury trial. However, although all involuntary patients should have the right to a court hearing, they should also retain the right to later change their own status and become voluntary patients, and to receive treatment in the least restrictive environment compatible with safety.

In June 1975, for the first time in this century, the Supreme Court of the United States handed down a decision on the constitutional rights of civilly committed mental patients. The Supreme Court ruled unanimously that "A state cannot constitutionally confine without more a non-dangerous individual who is capable of surviving safely in freedom by himself or with the help of willing and responsible family members or friends." In this case, *O'Connor v. Donaldson,* the landmark decision recognized that mental illness alone is not a sufficient basis for denying a person his fundamental right to liberty. The phrase "without more" may constitute the basis for further litigation and judicial interpretation, but has generally been assumed to mean "without more than custodial care."

The immediate impact of this decision was limited to patients who, like Kenneth Donaldson, were: (1) involuntarily committed; (2) receiving only custodial care; (3) not dangerous to themselves or to others; and (4) capable of surviving safely in the community alone or with available help. The Court did *not* recognize a constitutional "right to treatment," but reserved the right for courts to judge the adequacy of treatment (in cases for which this constituted the basis for commitment). The Court also maintained that an initial determination was insufficient, and that there must be a continuing basis for detention in a hospital over long periods of time.

While leaving "dangerousness" undefined, the Court noted that even where there is no "foreseeable risk of self-injury or suicide a person is literally 'dangerous to himself' if for physical or other reasons he is helpless to avoid the hazards of freedom . . . ." These "hazards of freedom" were not specified, but would presumably include a substantial risk of death from neglect, accident, or homicide. It is doubtful that they would be extended to the less dramatic but very real consequences of rejection by family and employers who may be alienated by a severely disturbed patient.

A legal analysis published by the National Institute of Mental Health (1976) stated: "Among the issues most likely to be raised in litigation or the legislative process following the Donaldson decision are: (1) constitutionally acceptable procedures and criteria for involuntary commitment; (2) the definition of 'dangerous,' as established by statute and as applied in practice; (3) the existence and implementation of a right to treatment; (4) the right to the 'least restrictive alternative' setting for treatment; and (5) the constitutional and functional distinction between voluntary and involuntary commitment."

INCOMPETENCY, GUARDIANSHIP, AND TESTAMENTARY CAPACITY

It has long been recognized that some persons may need hospital care and yet remain capable of handling their business affairs. Others may be incapable of managing their property but able to live in society with varying degrees of supervision or nursing care. Historically, laws concerning the property of the mentally incompetent long preceded laws concerning the care of his person. In the *Twelve Tables* of Rome (449 B.C.) it was provided that: "If a person is a fool, let his person and goods be under the protection of his family or his paternal relatives, if he is not under the care of anyone." In thirteenth-century England, the king was granted custody of all property throughout the lifetime of an idiot (retaining the profits after providing for his maintenance) — but only temporary custody in the case of a lunatic (returning the profits to him after the recovery of his reason).

Incompetency consists of inability to care for one's property or person due to some form of mental disability. A court determination of mental incompetency may be undertaken to protect a person's estate from dissipation, and to provide protection for one unable to care for himself. The issue of incompetency has increasingly been regarded as independent from that of commitment, although both determinations may be made during a single court hearing. However, hearings to determine incompetency are often held for persons who are not being admitted to hospital. In this case, it is not sufficient to demonstrate symptoms of mental illness (such as disorientation, hallucinations, or delusions), but it must be shown that the patient has a *disorder of thinking that causes impaired judgment and results in squandering, hoarding, or self-injurious gullibility.*

When the patient has been declared incompetent, it is necessary for the court to appoint a guardian, trustee, curator, or committee to manage his estate and protect his interests. In some jurisdictions this may be an autonomous public body specifically established for this purpose and which remains responsible for the patient's affairs as long as the latter is considered incompetent. In those states where incompetency is implicit in involuntary hospitalization, legal competency is usually automatically restored on complete discharge from the hospital, but *not* when he is absent from the hospital on leave, parole, probation, or trial visit (which may sometimes be prolonged for an undesirably long period of time, and include loss of other rights than control over property). When incompetency has been established separately from involuntary hospitalization, however, another court hearing will usually be necessary to restore the patient's competency and discharge his guardian.

The legal status of the incompetent person is comparable with that of a minor, and he usually loses other rights than simply the power to dispose of his property, such as the right to drive an automobile, to enter into contracts, to vote, to marry or divorce, and to practice a profession. Most courts distinguish between the contracts of an incompetent person made prior to the adjudication of his condition, and those executed after such an adjudication. Most courts hold that contracts made prior to an adjudication of incompetency are voidable, and may be disaffirmed by the incompetent under certain conditions, but that they remain in full force until disaffirmed. Legal transactions made by an incompetent person after a guardian has been appointed are usually considered void, except that in some jurisdictions they may be enforced for the benefit of the incompetent.

Among other rights lost by the incompetent person are the rights to authorize release of confidential information and to give informed consent for special treatment procedures. Some legislation provides that the court-appointed guardian may give informed consent for certain special procedures (for example, surgery or convulsive therapy) but *not* for other procedures (e.g., aversion therapy, sterilization, experimental procedures, or psychosurgery).

Testamentary capacity is defined as mental competency for making a will, and is usually dependent on "sound mind and memory." In order to make a valid will the testator must be able to comply with the following:

1. Know, without prompting, the nature and extent of the property of which he is about to dispose;

2. Know the nature of the act he is about to perform (i.e., what it means to make a will);

3. Know the names and identities of the persons who are to be the objects of his bounty;

4. Know his relation toward them;

5. Have sufficient mind and memory to understand all of these facts;

6. Appreciate the relations of these factors to one another;

7. Recollect a short time later the decision which he has formed.

A will may be declared invalid if mental disorder interferes with any one of these criteria. However, the mentally retarded may make valid wills if they understand what they mean and what they are distributing; and psychotic patients with delusions may make valid wills provided the delusions do not materially affect the disposition of property. In upholding any will made during or shortly after a period of known mental disorder, it will be necessary to prove that the patient had testamentary capacity at the time the will was made. This is best accomplished by having the patient examined separately by two competent psychiatrists on the same day and preferably within the same hour that the patient signs his will.

THE INSANITY DEFENSE

There are at least two separate major issues involved in defending a person with mental illness or retardation who has committed a criminal offense. The first issue concerns his competency to stand trial (based on his actual condition at the time of his pretrial examination). The second concerns the possibility of diminished responsibility for the alleged criminal behavior due to mental disorder (at the time of the alleged offense).

Competency to Stand Trial

In order to be competent to stand trial the defendant must be able: (1) to understand the nature and object of the proceedings against him; (2) to understand his position in relation to those proceedings; and (3) to advise and assist counsel in his own defense. To elaborate on these criteria, it is necessary for the person to understand the charge against him, the possible outcome of the trial, the roles and identities of the persons involved in the proceedings, the fact that the alleged act is a criminal offense, his rights to legal counsel and protection against self-incrimination, the need to account for his movements in detail, and the necessity of cooperating with and assisting his own legal counsel.

The determination of competency to stand trial is made by the court, which considers the advice of one or more psychiatrists who have examined the defendant. In the event that he is considered incompetent to stand trial, the person is usually hospitalized (as required by more than forty states), although he may be imprisoned or released for treatment as an outpatient. In the event of a minor offense, the charge is often dismissed and the patient referred for treatment. In the event of a major offense, however, the outcome is frequently indefinite commitment to a mental institution, with trial at a later date if there is sufficient improvement in the person's psychiatric condition.

Diminished Criminal Responsibility

Responsibility for criminal behavior is generally disavowed in the case of a small child and for certain psychotic patients. It should also be diminished in a larger intermediate group (mentally retarded and neurotic) who cannot be fitted into conventional legal definitions of sane and insane. However, it has been remarked that judicial utterances of "not guilty by reason of insanity" are rarer than poisonous snake bites in Manhattan. There were reportedly only 11 successful verdicts of not guilty by reason of insanity in New York State during the entire decade of the sixties, although many persons never came to trial at all because of obvious continued incompetency to do so. Nevertheless, the issues involved are matters of widespread concern.

Insanity first became a defense against a criminal charge in England during the fourteenth century, but the degree of insanity required to absolve the person was extreme, and in 1724 Judge Tracey instructed a jury that for an accused to escape punishment he must "not know what he is doing, no more than . . . a wild beast."

THE M'NAGHTEN TEST. The M'Naghten test of criminal responsibility has been the most widely accepted in American courts during the past century. It was based on the opinions of fifteen English judges following the M'Naghten trial of 1843, in which the accused was acquitted of murder on grounds of insanity. The House of Lords subsequently posed five questions to the judges of England whose relevant answers can be reduced to two rules for determining the responsibility of a person who pleads insanity as a defense against criminal prosecution.

1. To establish a defense on the ground of insanity it must be clearly proved that, at the time of committing the act, the party accused was laboring under such a defect of reason, from disease of the mind, as not to know the nature and quality of the act he was doing; or if he did know it, that he did not know he was doing wrong.

2. Where a person labors under partial delusions only and is not in other respects insane (and commits an offense in consequence thereof) he must be considered in the same situation as to responsibility as if the facts with respect to which the delusion exists were real.

IRRESISTIBLE IMPULSE TEST. The M'Naghten Test remains the sole test in less than half of the states, but an additional fifteen states rely on a combination of this rule supplemented by an irresistible impulse test. According to the latter, an offender may know the difference between right and wrong but find himself under the influence of an overwhelming impulse that forces him to commit the criminal act. A defense of irresistible impulse may therefore be based on the impulsive act of a psychotic patient, compulsive neurotic behavior, or rage reactions in otherwise normal people.

THE DURHAM TEST. According to the Durham decision, "An accused is not criminally responsible if his unlawful act was the product of mental disease or mental defect . . . . We use 'disease' in the sense of a condition which is considered capable of either improving or deteriorating. We use 'defect' in the sense of a condition which is not considered capable of either improving or deteriorating and which may be either congenital, or the result of injury, or the residual effect of a physical or mental disease."

The preceding rule originated in the District of Columbia Court of Appeals (1954), but was later rejected in the same court. It has since been adopted by statute in Maine and the Virgin Islands. The rule is based on a much earlier New Hampshire test, whose intent was to permit the jury to formulate the standard of insanity.

THE AMERICAN LAW INSTITUTE (ALI) TEST. This was first presented in 1955 and has since been adopted by statute or decision in about ten states. It reads as follows:

1. A person is not responsible for criminal conduct if at the time of such conduct as a result of mental disease or defect he lacks substantial capacity either to appreciate the criminality of his conduct or to conform his conduct to the requirements of law.

2. As noted in the Article, the terms "mental disease or defect" do not include an abnormality manifested only by repeated criminal or otherwise antisocial conduct.

PROFESSIONAL LIABILITY OF THE PHYSICIAN

The Physician-Patient Relationship

The physician-patient relationship constitutes a legal contract, involving a promise or set of promises by the physician, the performance of which the law considers to be a duty, and for breach of which the law gives remedy to the patient. The physician should therefore recognize his obligations to the patient, and the rights of the patient to confidentiality and privacy, to self-determination, to competent evaluation and treatment, and to information regarding the probable outcome of treatment, including any known potential hazards.

The physician should distinguish between the therapeutic communication of realistic optimism, and unwarranted promises of a cure, which may lead to subsequent disillusionment and hostility on the part of the patient, and to possible litigation. On the other hand, the physician should avoid undue defensiveness that will be communicated verbally or nonverbally to the patient and may well invite or provoke a hostile patient to bring legal action.

The physician should recall that verbal transactions are subject to retrospective falsification, and should therefore keep adequate written records. He should routinely obtain the written consent of the patient to release confidential information, to seek admission to the hospital, or to undertake special treatment procedures. Apart from such safeguards, however, the physician's professional security rests in the integrity of his relationship with the patient — his genuine interest in the welfare of the patient, his competence and self-confidence, and his honesty in communicating with the patient.

A *contract* between two persons may be either expressed or implied, depending on whether the parties have specifically set forth (orally or in writing) the terms of their agreement, or whether the conditions are to be inferred or deduced from the conduct of the parties rather than from any definite language. The contract between doctor and patient is usually implied by the patient's visit to the doctor's office or the doctor's response to a call from the patient. There is no legal obligation for a physician to accept a request to attend the patient even though no other physician is available. The mere rendering of such services as may be necessary in an emergency does not automatically result in a contract for subsequent services, although the physician is required to use due skill and care in administering emergency treatment. By special agreement with the patient, the physician may limit his contract to treating the patient in one particular time or place, or by means of one particular procedure. Once a physician has accepted responsibility for the patient's evaluation and treatment, however, his obligation continues for the duration of the patient's illness, and until the physician's services are no longer necessary — unless the physician is relieved of this obligation by the patient, or unless he gives the patient reasonable notice of his intention to withdraw and allows the patient an adequate opportunity to secure the services of another physician.

The physician is obligated to possess the same degree of skill and learning possessed by other members of his profession at the time and place he renders services. He should exercise ordinary and reasonable care and diligence in applying this knowledge and skill, should employ such available remedies as experience has shown to be most beneficial, and, in case of doubt, he should recommend consultation with a colleague who has special skill and experience with patients with similar problems or disorders. A psychiatrist or other specialist must possess that degree of additional skill and

145

knowledge possessed by physicians who devote appropriate study and attention to a particular field of specialization.

Negligence and Malpractice

The omission or failure of a physician to perform his duties to the patient constitutes negligence, and he or she may be considered guilty of malpractice if injury or damage to the patient results directly therefrom. Malpractice has been defined as the treatment of a patient in a manner contrary to accepted rules and with injurious results to the patient and, hence, any professional misconduct or any unreasonable lack of skill or fidelity in the performance of professional or fiduciary duties. The elements constituting a cause of action based on negligence are as follows: (1) The physician has not fulfilled his legal duty, or obligation, to conform to a reasonable standard of care in order to protect his patients from unreasonable risk. (2) The physician has failed to adhere to the standard required. (3) Actual loss or damage has resulted to the person or property of another. (4) There has been a reasonably close causal connection between the substandard conduct involved and the resulting injury.

Consent of the Patient

A physician requires the *consent* of a patient or of his legal guardian in order to undertake either examination or treatment. Failure to obtain such consent may constitute assault, which is punishable even though no actual harm has been done. If asked to examine a person by a third party (e.g., employer, police officer, or judge), the physician should tell the person concerned that he has the right to refuse, and that if he consents the results of the examination will be conveyed to the third party. The patient's signed consent to examination and release of information should be obtained before these are undertaken. It is also necessary to obtain the patient's signed consent for certain special treatment procedures such as those involving loss of consciousness (including electroshock treatments).

The patient must give intelligent and *informed*

consent, with full understanding of what is to be done and of any risks involved, in order for consent to be legally valid. Informed consent for treatment should *not* be incorporated into a routine application form for admission to hospital, but should involve a separate form to be signed only when the treatment has been recommended and planned for the immediate future. Involuntary patients are sometimes given a statutory right to refuse specified forms of treatment (particularly psychosurgery, sterilization, or aversive conditioning procedures). Even when an involuntary patient consents to such procedures, the law may specify that consent must also be obtained from the patient's guardian or from the court. Regardless of what procedures have been appropriately authorized by informed consent, the signing of such forms does *not* absolve the physician from carrying out appropriate investigations beforehand, or from exercising reasonable skill and care during and after the treatment procedure.

Information and Instructions

The physician is also required to give the patient and others responsible for his care (e.g., his guardian or nursing attendants) such information and instructions as will enable them to comply with recommended treatment or act intelligently on behalf of the patient. Often information about diagnosis and prognosis has been withheld from patients having incurable disease, but some patients seek such information directly. It has sometimes been held that the physician has an obligation to volunteer such information to the patient (e.g., so that he may make a valid will), and in other circumstances that the responsible next of kin must be informed. However, the law has distinguished between passive concealment (mere silence) and active concealment (the deliberate suppression of fact, or deceit). Some courts have held that the physician is not required to volunteer such information, but has a duty to disclose it if asked. In the case of psychiatric diagnosis and prognosis, the patient or responsible next of kin has a right to a truthful interpretation of such information as is within their comprehension.

Confidentiality

It is a general principle that information obtained from the patient is to be kept *secret and confidential.* In the event that the physician reveals confidential information to a third party, and thus harms the patient, he is liable to be sued for damages. However, disclosure is permissible with the explicit, signed consent of the patient (or legal guardian). The physician may be required by law to report certain situations or conditions (e.g., child abuse or infectious diseases). In most situations, physicians may also disclose the medical condition of a patient to his or her spouse without breaking the rules of confidential communication.

Privileged communication is a statutory right, recognized in more than thirty states, whereby a patient may bar his doctor from testifying about his medical treatment and the disclosures that are an integral part of it. Privileged communication between patient and physician was recognized by the State of New York in 1828. The New York Civil Rights Law of 1972 extends privileged communication to include psychologists, nurses, and social workers. However, it must be recognized that the confidential information belongs to the patient, and not to the physician or mental health practitioner. Hence, if the patient consents to having information brought out in a court proceeding, the practitioner may not refuse the patient's request.

REVIEW QUESTIONS

120. Testamentary capacity consists of being legally competent to:
     (A) testify in a legal proceeding
     (B) make a will
     (C) enter into binding contracts
     (D) stand trial for an alleged criminal act
     (E) conduct one's own business affairs

121. Which of the following is *not* a legal criterion related to determination of a defendant's legal responsibility for an alleged crime?
     (A) involuntary commitment law
     (B) M'Naghten rule
     (C) Durham decision
     (D) American Law Institute rule
     (E) irresistible impulse rule

122. If it were the only allegation that could be substantiated, each of the following would be sufficient grounds for a court to declare a man's will invalid *except:*
     (A) he did not understand that he was making a will
     (B) he did not understand or remember what property he had to bequeath
     (C) he did not remember the names and identities of certain close relatives (the "natural objects of his bounty")
     (D) he could not recall major provisions of the will a short time after signing it
     (E) he was suffering from psychotic depression

Summary of Directions				
A	B	C	D	E
1, 2, 3 only	1, 3 only	2, 4 only	4 only	All are correct

123. Competency to stand trial for an alleged criminal offense requires that the accused be able to:
     (1) cooperate with his defense counsel
     (2) understand the nature of the legal proceedings and the possible outcomes
     (3) understand his legal rights during the proceedings
     (4) remain free of psychotic symptoms during the course of the trial

124. According to the M'Naghten rule, a person would be "not guilty by reason of insanity" if it were adequately proved that he:
     (1) was unaware of the nature, quality, and consequences of his act
     (2) acted on the basis of a delusional belief which, if true, would have constituted adequate defense
     (3) was incapable of understanding that his act was wrong
     (4) acted as the result of an impulse which he was incapable of resisting

125. A legal declaration of civil incompetency:
    (1) results in an individual's being deprived
        of certain rights
    (2) is based on the person's impairment in
        ability to make sound judgments
    (3) results in the appointment of a legal
        guardian to protect the person's interests
    (4) in most jurisdictions, is independent of
        the fact of being hospitalized for a psy-
        chiatric disorder

SELECTED REFERENCES

1. American Bar Association, Commission on the
   Mentally Disabled (1976). *Mental Disability
   Law Reporter.* Washington, D.C.: American
   Bar Association.
2. Lindman, F.T., and McIntyre, D.M. [Eds.]
   (1961). *The Mentally Disabled and the Law.*
   Chicago: University of Chicago Press.
3. National Institute of Mental Health (1976).
   Analysis and Implications of the Supreme Court
   Decision in *O'Connor v. Donaldson.* Washington, D.C.: U.S. Government Printing Office
   (633-955/71).
4. Redlich, F., and Mollica, R.F. (1976). Overview: Ethical issues in contemporary psychiatry. *American Journal of Psychiatry,* vol. 133,
   pages 125–136.
5. Stone, A.A. (1975). *Mental Health and Law:
   A System in Transition.* Washington, D.C.:
   National Institute of Mental Health. D.H.E.W.
   Publication No. (ADM) 75-176.
6. Tancredi, L.R., Lieb, J., and Slaby, A.E. (1975).
   Legal Issues in Psychiatric Care. Hagerstown,
   Maryland: Harper & Row.

11. Organic Mental Disorders (Organic Brain Syndromes)

Body and mind, like man and wife, do not always agree to die together.
Charles Caleb Colton

COMMON DENOMINATORS OF ORGANIC MENTAL DISORDERS

Organic mental disorders, or brain syndromes, are caused by impairment of brain tissue function. They may develop rapidly or slowly, may be of brief or prolonged duration, may be completely reversible, or progressive and even fatal.

Their manifestations are extremely diverse and variable, but may be better understood if they are considered as resulting from interaction between: (1) *increased or decreased neural function* resulting from a pathological process affecting specific areas of brain tissue, precipitating primary symptoms of impaired intellectual functioning; and (2) *symptoms based on lifelong personality and predisposition,* that have sometimes been referred to as secondary, or functional, symptoms. The latter may include the whole range of psychopathology, and lead to prominent signs of neurotic anxiety, depression or euphoria, paranoid misinterpretation of reality, or various forms of antisocial behavior.

These interactions may lead to prominence of any one or more of the following groups of symptoms in a given patient with a specific organic mental disorder:

1. Disturbances in *consciousness* and level of arousal, with possible agitation or somnolence and stupor;

2. Impairment of *orientation,* most marked for time, less so for place and person;

3. Impairment of *memory,* most marked for recent events, less so for events of the remote past. Sometimes there is unconscious fabrication (confabulation) to compensate for memory gaps.

4. Impairment of other *intellectual functions* — including comprehension, calculation, general knowledge, ability to learn, and abstract reasoning. Ideation tends to be impoverished and concrete, and may be expressed in stereotyped repetition (perseveration) of words or actions.

5. Shallowness or lability of *affect* (emotional response);

6. *Personality changes,* that may represent intensification of preexisting character traits, or release of hitherto latent characteristics and behavior.

Mild or selective organic mental impairment may be revealed or measured by means of special psychological tests, as outlined briefly in Chapter 4. Two test instruments frequently employed are the Bender-Gestalt Visual-Motor Test, and the Graham-Kendall Test for memory and reproduction of geometric designs. Impairment of various intellectual functions may also be evident on specific subtests of the Wechsler Adult Intelligence Scale, and many other tests have been designed to reveal or quantify various intellectual consequences of organic brain damage.

Neurological tests and other laboratory procedures may be essential in evaluation and diagnosis. The electroencephalogram (EEG) is particularly helpful in demonstrating the diffuse slow wave activity that reflects the cerebral metabolic insufficiency found in acute or symptomatic organic mental disorders (stupor or delirium). However, it should not be overlooked that cerebral insufficiency may be cumulative, and result from interaction of two or more processes (e.g., hypoxia, vitamin-B deficiency, and electrolyte imbalance). Effective therapy depends on early and accurate identification of all such significant processes.

ACUTE SYMPTOMATIC PSYCHOSES vs CHRONIC ORGANIC DEMENTIAS

Psychiatrists have long distinguished between acute and chronic brain syndromes on the basis of their potential *reversibility,* whether it be spontaneous or contingent on rapid medical intervention. This distinction represents less of a dichotomy than a continuum, since reversibility is often partial in cases when some neurons have been damaged too badly to permit full recovery. Initially, however, many processes cause temporary reversible changes in brain cell function (or biochemical lesion) rather than permanent irreversible damage leading to changes in brain structure (or morphological lesion).

Acute (i.e., reversible) brain syndromes are most frequently *symptomatic or exogenous psychoses,* due to generalized processes originating outside the central nervous system such as drug or poison intoxications, systemic infections, endocrine, metabolic, and nutritional disorders. *Chronic* (i.e., irreversible) brain syndromes may result from any of the preceding processes, but more often originate from *local intracranial processes* such as degenerative diseases, local infections, trauma, and tumors.

The symptomatic psychoses, or acute brain syndromes, usually take one of two alternative forms, depending on whether there is increased or decreased arousal, perception, and psychomotor activity. When the latter are decreased there is an *acute confusional state,* with clouding of consciousness, often proceeding to stupor or coma. By contrast, increased arousal and psychomotor activity are more typical of *delirium,* in which there is also perceptual distortion (particularly visual or tactile hallucinations), together with changing delusions and often extreme apprehension and agitation.

The clinical syndrome most typical of chronic, irreversible organic mental disorders is that of *dementia,* with progressive disorientation, amnesia, and gross impairment of intellectual functions. However, there may be prominent functional symptoms of associated personality disorder, neurosis, or psychosis (e.g., depression or paranoia). Some of the main characteristics of patients with these major forms of organic brain syndromes are summarized in Table 11-1.

SENILE, PRESENILE, AND CEREBRO-VASCULAR DEMENTIAS

Senile Dementia

Senile dementia is associated with diffuse atrophy of the cerebral cortex beginning after the age of 60 years. The symptoms have a gradual, progressive onset over a period of several years. In this age range, women outnumber men in the population by a ratio of roughly 2:1, and there is a corresponding preponderance of female patients with senile dementia.

Case Report. One typical patient was a 78-year-old widow, brought to the state hospital by her children, with a five-year history of gradual deterioration of memory, other intellectual functions, and social behavior. She had a high school education and had made a career of being a housewife and mother. After her husband's death, she had lived with one or another of her children until the time of her admission to hospital. There was no history of psychiatric disorder until she was more than 70 years old. The first time her family noticed anything wrong was when she was given some money to visit a friend in a nearby city but lost the money. Shortly after this, she set out from her home to visit one of her other children, but failed to arrive, and the police were called to help find her. From this time on she gradually lost her former interest in reading, writing letters, knitting, and other pastimes. For a year before her admission to hospital she did not recognize her children most of the time, and her conversation was often unintelligible to them. She was able to eat without assistance, but for six months before admission she had to be dressed and undressed, and taken to the toilet to avoid incontinence.

On arrival at the hospital she was pleasant and cooperative, but showed gross impairment in comprehension. She misinterpreted everyday situations, and when given her first bath in the hospital, she said, "I don't want to get in the boat; the current is too swift." Much of her spontaneous speech was unintelligible, and there was gross impairment of memory for both recent and remote events. She was able to give her name correctly, but when asked her age she replied, "I am 21 to 22 anyway, every minute." She was unable to state her birthday, the year of her birth, or any other information about her previous life. However, she remained pleasant and cooperative until the time of her death from pneumonia six months later.

The brains of such patients show generalized atrophy, particularly of the cerebral cortex, with widening of the sulci and enlargement of the ventricles. Microscopically, there is widespread degeneration of ganglion cells, which are shrunken or vacuolated and often contain lipid deposits.

Table 11-1. Characteristics of Acute Symptomatic and Chronic Organic Mental Disorders

Acute Symptomatic Brain Disorders	Chronic Organic Mental Disorders
Usual clinical syndrome acute confusional state (sometimes stupor or coma), or delirium with agitation	Usual clinical syndrome dementia
Impairment of orientation, memory, and other intellectual functions. Associated with disturbances of consciousness, perception, and psychomotor activity	Progressive impairment of orientation, memory, and other intellectual functions. May be prominent associated functional symptoms due to intensification or release of latent personality characteristics — psychotic, neurotic, or behavioral (e.g., depressed, paranoid, anxious, or antisocial)
Due to temporary reversible changes in brain cell function (biochemical lesion). Cerebral metabolic insufficiency accompanied by diffuse slow waves on EEG	Due to permanent irreversible damage to brain structure (often with morphological lesion)
Usually *symptomatic* of generalized toxic, infective, or metabolic disorder also affecting other parts of the body	May result from all the same pathological processes as acute reversible disorders, but also from insidious localized intracranial lesion or degenerative process (sometimes hereditary)
Commonly encountered on general medical and surgical, pediatric, or obstetric wards of general hospitals	Commonly encountered on neurological services of general hospitals or in psychiatric hospitals
Course brief, and may terminate in death, complete remission, or chronic (irreversible) organic mental disorders	Course may be chronic or progressive (resulting in death)

There are apt to be many senile plaques in older patients, and neurofibrillary tangles among patients at the younger end of the age range.

Alzheimer's Presenile Dementia
The presenile age range has been traditionally regarded as ages 40 to 60 years. This earlier age of onset is the basis on which Alzheimer's form of presenile dementia was distinguished from the senile dementia described above. Alzheimer's disease shows the same diffuse cortical atrophy, with gradual onset of dementia, progressing to profound regression and usually death within 5 to 10 years. Microscopic examination of the brain shows relatively more neurofibrillary tangles (in the forms of whirls and baskets), and relatively fewer senile plaques. However, *the process appears to be essentially identical with that of senile dementia.*

Pick's Presenile Dementia
Pick's disease also has its onset during the pre-

senile age period but differs from the preceding in that it is a localized rather than a generalized process. Areas of atrophy involve both gray and white matter in one or more lobes of the brain. Microscopically there is a loss of nerve cells, but none of the other characteristic signs of Alzheimer's presenile or senile dementias. In addition to progressive dementia, Pick's disease results in symptoms of focal cortical lesions that include aphasias, apraxias, and agnosias. There is a strong familial tendency, with hypothesized hereditary transmission as a simple mendelian autosomal-dominant characteristic.

Cerebrovascular Dementias
Cerebral arteriosclerosis is most likely to produce symptoms of a chronic but fluctuating organic mental disorder during the senile age period, but may also lead to cerebral insufficiency in the presenile age range. Although the process itself is chronic, there are often dramatic changes in the

severity of symptoms, related to episodes of reduced blood supply to various parts of the brain. There may be sudden onset following occlusion of the middle cerebral artery or other major source of blood supply. In some cases there is a history of repeated minor strokes, with several focal areas of softening found at autopsy.

There may be a history of hypertension, but there is relatively little correspondence between cerebral arteriosclerosis and systemic or even retinal arteriopathy. Moreover, cerebral arteriosclerosis often coexists with Alzheimer's disease or diffuse senile cortical atrophy.

Cerebrovascular insufficiency due to localized extracranial arterial occlusive disease may be correctible by surgery. Diffuse intracranial arteriosclerosis is not amenable to any such specific treatment, and management is directed towards maximization of recovery of function after anoxic episodes.

ALCOHOLIC PSYCHOSES

Acute Alcohol Intoxication

The term *acute alcohol intoxication* has been applied to all acute organic mental disorders (brain syndromes) of psychotic proportions due to alcohol, with the exception of three more specific diagnoses: pathological (idiosyncratic) intoxication, delirium tremens, and alcoholic hallucinosis. The degree of impairment is more severe than that seen in simple drunkenness, and the mildest form of acute alcohol intoxication probably consists of the recurrent episodes of amnesia (i.e., blackouts or palimpsests) that occur in most patients with established alcohol addiction.

Pathological (Idiosyncratic) Intoxication

Pathological intoxication is an acute brain syndrome that occurs in vulnerable persons following relatively minor provocation (minimal or short-term alcohol intake). The symptoms usually include both confusion (with disorientation, hallucinations, illusions, and sometimes delusions) and disturbed behavior (with agitation, rage, and violent behavior). The duration may be from a few minutes to a few days. Similar episodes may be observed in the absence of alcohol intake among those with hysterical (dissociative) or epileptoid personality disorders.

Delirium Tremens

Delirium tremens is the most widely recognized form of acute organic mental disorder (brain syndrome) associated with alcoholism. The symptoms are of psychotic intensity with delirium, involving amnesia, disorientation, and visual or tactile hallucinations (seeing snakes or pink elephants). There is hyperarousal of the central nervous system, with psychomotor agitation, coarse tremors of the extremities, and sometimes spontaneous epileptic convulsions (particularly when there is associated hypoglycemia). The latter represent one form of *withdrawal seizures* (occurring within a few hours after withdrawal of chronic alcohol intake, with its sedating effects). The psychosis itself has been largely attributed to abrupt withdrawal from prolonged alcohol intake, and is therefore rare in persons under the age of 30 years and those who do not have a history of several years of copious alcohol use. It most commonly occurs in such persons after a short-term increase to a higher-than-usual level of alcohol consumption ("binge"), even when this is followed by a return to the previous level and not by total abstinence. It may also be provoked by an acute infection or injury to an alcoholic whose level of consumption is not interrupted.

The disorder may be life-threatening, particularly in older persons and those with associated medical problems such as cardiac decompensation or gross hepatic insufficiency. The immediate treatment should include: (1) sedative and anticonvulsive medication, one of the most appropriate being diazepam (Valium); (2) parenteral administration of vitamin B complex (not thiamine alone, since there may be deficiency of other constituents); (3) hydration, restoration of electrolyte balance, and other appropriate supportive measures. The preceding forms of therapy may be referred to under the general term *detoxification,* which may then be followed by administration of *deterrents* to further alcohol intake (e.g., disulfiram or

Antabuse), and *psychotherapies* or other measures directed towards reduction of alcohol abuse.

Antipsychotic medications such as chlorpromazine were formerly widely used in the treatment of delirium tremens, both for sedation and for the antipsychotic effects against fear, agitation, and hallucinations. This practice is no longer recommended, since the drugs have serious adverse effects on blood pressure, seizure threshold, temperature regulation, and liver function, to which the withdrawing alcoholic may be especially vulnerable. Moreover, several of the minor tranquilizers (chlordiazepoxide, diazepam, or hydroxyzine) have proved to be quite satisfactory substitutes for the indications mentioned, and involve none of the above risks. A more controversial agent is diphenylhydantoin (Dilantin). Its use as a prophylactic anticonvulsant during delirium tremens is generally recommended when the patient is epileptic. However, there is no evidence that it has any value for preventing withdrawal seizures if the patient is not epileptic, and most authorities advise against its routine use in this case.

Alcoholic Hallucinosis

Alcoholic hallucinosis is an acute reversible psychosis precipitated by prolonged excessive drinking of alcohol. It is characterized by *auditory* hallucinations and relatively mild impairment of intellectual functions, in contrast with the visual hallucinations and profound confusion that are characteristic of delirium tremens. Alcoholic hallucinosis has been viewed as very similar to an acute schizophrenic episode, and tends to respond to antipsychotic medication within a period of a few weeks. Although it has also been attributed to withdrawal from alcohol, this relationship is less well established than in the case of delirium tremens.

Alcohol Paranoid State (Alcoholic Paranoia)

Alcoholic paranoid state is a form of paranoid psychosis associated with chronic alcoholism in which there is excessive jealousy and delusions that the spouse is unfaithful. Patients are usually middle-aged men whose alcoholism has led to impairment of various somatic functions, including adrenocortical insufficiency and impotence. Paranoid ideation may improve with antipsychotic medication, but the prognosis is poor when there is significant impairment of intellectual functions.

Wernicke's Encephalopathy

Wernicke's syndrome is an *acute* life-threatening brain syndrome, with hemorrhages into the brain stem, particularly in the region of the mamillary bodies. The triad described by Wernicke consists of clouding of consciousness, ophthalmoplegia, and ataxia. The ophthalmoplegia is due to a deficiency of thiamine and responds to therapy with this vitamin. The clouding of consciousness may respond specifically to thiamine in some cases, and to niacin in others, but may require large doses of the entire vitamin B complex in some patients. The latter should always be administered, since delay may lead to death or permanent residual organic dementia, which takes the form of Korsakoff's syndrome. About 90 percent of patients with Wernicke's encephalopathy are alcoholics.

Korsakoff's Syndrome

Korsakoff's syndrome is a *chronic* organic mental disorder, which is often preceded by one or more episodes of delirium tremens, or sometimes by Wernicke's syndrome. The triad described by Korsakoff consisted of amnesia, confabulation, and peripheral neuropathy, but other signs of organic intellectual impairment are also present. The polyneuropathy is attributable to thiamine deficiency, and is likely to respond slowly to administration of this vitamin. However, other aspects of the brain syndrome may be attributable to deficiency of other constituents of the vitamin B complex, which should be administered for a period of about three months. Although the syndrome is partly reversible, there is a strong tendency for some permanent residual impairment.

Alcoholic Deterioration

The term *alcoholic deterioration* has been applied to all forms of *chronic* organic psychoses resulting from alcoholism that do not show the characteristic features of Korsakoff's psychosis. As in the case of senile and presenile dementias, there is likely to be diffuse atrophy of the cerebral cortex, but the clinical manifestations are variable.

PSYCHOSES WITH INTRACRANIAL INFECTIONS

General Paralysis (Dementia Paralytica)

General paralysis is a chronic organic psychosis due to progressive syphilitic infection of the brain. Prior to World War II, general paresis was responsible for roughly 5 to 10 percent of all admissions to state hospitals, and 10 to 20 percent of all admissions of men (since the frequency in men was roughly three times as high as the frequency in women). The psychosis usually became evident in middle age, about 5 to 15 years after the initial infection, and affected roughly 5 percent of all patients with neurosyphilis.

The classical symptoms of this psychosis include euphoria, with delusions of grandeur, and extravagant behavior based on convictions of great power or wealth. This may include indiscriminate gifts of money, automobiles, or yachts. However, some patients may show evidence of depression or paranoid suspiciousness with delusions of persecution. As the condition progresses there is increasing confusion and apathy, accompanied by tremor and paralysis and leading to profound regression and death within five years of onset. Neurological examination often reveals irregularity or inequality in size of pupils, with an Argyll-Robertson response to accommodation but not to light. Blood serology is usually positive, and the spinal fluid usually shows a paretic gold curve.

The prognosis was changed dramatically when Wagner von Jauregg introduced malaria therapy in the treatment of paresis. This and other forms of fever therapy led to arrest of the disease process in roughly two-thirds of all patients, with partial reversal and significant clinical improvement in roughly half of those in whom the disease process was arrested (i.e., one-third of all patients). The prognosis was improved somewhat further by means of penicillin therapy, but the dramatic decrease in frequency of general paresis since

World War II is due to antibiotic therapy of primary and secondary infections.

Creutzfeldt-Jakob Disease

Creutzfeldt-Jakob disease is a diffuse, degenerative process of both pyramidal and extrapyramidal systems that usually develops during the presenile age range (40 to 60 years). The symptoms of dementia are usually associated with ataxia and impairment of speech. The course is progressive and rapid with death after about a year. One form of this disease has now been definitely attributed to a transmissible viral infection.

Other Intracranial Infections

Acute or chronic organic mental disorders may result from many forms of encephalitis or meningitis, the characteristics of which depend partly on the infecting organism (bacterial, mycotic, viral, rickettsial, or protozoal). Even when specific antibiotic therapy is available, it must be instituted promptly, and there is still a danger of residual organic brain damage. The consequences of the latter may vary greatly, depending on its degree and location, as well as on the age of the patient at the time of the infection. Severe infections occurring in childhood may be followed by lifelong mental retardation, or by increased vulnerability to various forms of personality disorder.

PSYCHOSES WITH OTHER INTRACRANIAL DISORDERS

Epilepsy

A single grand mal epileptic seizure (whether idiopathic or secondary) proceeds through five phases. The first four consist of aura, tonic contraction, clonic contraction, and coma. The fifth phase, which may not be recognized, consists of *postconvulsive confusion*. Following a single seizure, the latter is apt to be minimal, with mild and brief disorientation for time together with impairment of memory for events immediately preceding the seizure. Following a series of several uncontrolled seizures within a short space of time, there is likely to be evidence of an acute brain syndrome of moderate degree and duration. If there is associated impairment of brain metabolism (as in children with high fevers) or status epilepticus, the brain syndrome may be much more severe and prolonged. A sufficient number of uncontrolled seizures will, in fact, lead to the development of marked and permanent organic intellectual impairment that may be severe enough to require chronic institutional care. In any event, epileptic seizures should never be ignored nor taken lightly. Every effort should be made to control idiopathic epilepsy by means of appropriate anticonvulsant medication. A search should also be made for hidden brain lesions that might constitute the basis for the development of secondary or symptomatic seizures.

Intracranial Neoplasm

The three most common forms of intracranial tumor are as follows: (1) meningioma (roughly 20 percent); (2) glioma (33 to 50 percent of most series); and (3) secondary metastatic carcinoma (roughly 20 percent). Although presenting symptoms are usually neurological, they are likely to be accompanied by intellectual impairment and other evidence of a brain syndrome that may be fully reversible if surgical intervention is prompt and successful.

Brain Trauma

Acute brain syndromes develop immediately following head injury or brain surgery. Although neurons destroyed at this time will not regenerate, there may be considerable recovery of function in damaged tissues during ensuing weeks, and some continuing transfer of function to undamaged cells through a process of learning that continues for many months afterward. In some instances, belated improvement in intellectual functions on specific tests has been noted more than a year after an initial traumatic or anoxic episode.

Degenerative Diseases Involving the Brain

In addition to senile and presenile dementias outlined in a previous section, there are many degenerative diseases of the central nervous system that include chronic brain disease and symptoms of organic dementia as a part of the total neurological

syndrome. In some cases the mental disorder may be more prominent and in others the associated forms of neurological impairment will predominate. The following forms of brain disease are particularly important:

1. *Friedreich's ataxia*, or *hereditary spinal ataxia*, usually begins during the first two decades of life, with primary involvement of the spinal cord and secondary changes in the cerebellum. Lesions are progressive, and there may be variable cerebral involvement, with associated mental retardation or symptoms that may be precipitated by an organic brain syndrome developing in adult life.

2. *Diffuse cerebral sclerosis* is a generic term that includes various degenerative conditions involving widespread subcortical demyelinization. All forms are rare, but Schilder's disease is the most frequent, with onset any time from infancy to young adult life. Intellectual deterioration may be rapid and is irreversible.

3. *Huntington's chorea* is a well-known hereditary disease that is transmitted by a single autosomal-dominant gene. There is degeneration of the basal ganglia leading to involuntary *choreiform movements* of the limbs, and degeneration of the cerebral cortex, leading to *dementia*. Either of these two forms may predominate, but both are likely to become more obvious with the passage of time, and progress to death within 5 to 20 years after onset (which usually occurs in the fourth or fifth decade of life).

4. *Amyotrophic lateral sclerosis* also usually develops in the fourth or fifth decade, and results in destruction of the pyramidal tract from cortex to spinal cord. The severity of dementia is variable, but progress of the disease is rapid, with death occurring within about three years of onset.

SYMPTOMATIC PSYCHOSES WITH GENERAL SYSTEMIC DISORDERS

Endocrine Disorders

Acute, reversible brain syndromes may be associated with hormonal insufficiency or excess, particularly involving adrenal cortex, thyroid, parathyroid, anterior pituitary, and pancreatic islet cells. The type of syndrome precipitated by *ACTH* or *cortisone* is likely to involve euphoria or even an overt manic episode. Abrupt withdrawal of these steroids may be followed by severe depression, but the latter may be related partly to the increased severity of arthritis or other disability for which the steroids were being administered.

Hypothyroidism leads to a typical generalized impairment of cellular function that includes brain, heart, skeletal muscles, and bone marrow. The person becomes lethargic and overweight, with hypochromic anemia, impaired cardiac function (low voltage ECG with reduced or absent T waves) and diffuse slowing of the EEG. Laboratory tests of thyroid function confirm the diagnosis, and constitute part of a routine admission screening battery in a number of psychiatric facilities. Congenital hypothyroidism leads to mental retardation *(cretinism),* and is initially at least partly reversible, with degree of improvement dependent on early diagnosis and prompt therapy. Hypothyroidism occurring later in life is known as *myxedema,* which was long known to progress to psychosis before thyroid extract was available for treatment. At that time, about half of such patients were reported to have hallucinations and delusions, but simple confusion and intellectual impairment is more typical of milder degrees.

In recent years *psychiatric* patients with hypothyroidism have often shown symptoms of functional psychoses, particularly paranoid schizophrenia. They should *not* be regarded as typical of all patients with hypothyroidism, and the symptoms that bring them to psychiatric treatment may well persist after appropriate treatment renders them euthyroid. They will therefore usually require additional antipsychotic medication or other appropriate psychiatric treatment.

Hyperthyroidism is invariably accompanied by anxiety and tremor. Hyperarousal may precipitate or aggravate various forms of functional psychopathology. An acute brain syndrome is not likely to develop except in severe life-threatening hyperthyroid crises, in which there may be associated delirium.

Hypoglycemia may result from various disorders, and may be sufficiently severe to produce acute brain syndromes, with or without epileptiform seizures. A high dosage of insulin (sometimes self-administered with suicidal intent) may lead to coma. Prolonged coma may result in a residual chronic brain syndrome with some persistent intellectual impairment.

Diabetes mellitus may result in repeated acute brain syndromes when the blood sugar is labile and poorly controlled. There is also an increased vulnerability to the development of chronic brain syndromes associated with generalized arteriosclerosis and other complications.

Metabolic or Nutritional Disorders

Uremia results from renal failure, and is probably the most frequent metabolic basis for organic brain syndromes. When uremic episodes are of brief duration, particularly in relatively young patients, the associated confusional state is likely to be completely reversible. However, with advancing age, and if uremia is recurrent or chronic, there is irreversible damage to cortical neurons and chronic dementia.

Porphyrias result from inborn errors of metabolism, usually transmitted by single autosomal-dominant genes. There may be acute intermittent organic brain syndromes, with or without epileptiform seizures. Certain drugs, notably barbiturates, may precipitate or aggravate an attack and should therefore never be given. However, there may be considerable benefit from antipsychotic medications.

Wilson's disease consists of hepatolenticular degeneration due to chronic copper intoxication. There is usually cirrhosis of the liver and atrophy of the lenticular nuclei, with involuntary movement and onset of a chronic brain syndrome. There is typically a greenish-brown Kayser-Fleischer ring in the cornea. Onset is usually between the ages of 20 and 50 years, with progressive increases in intellectual impairment. Treatment has been attempted with chelating agents such as dimercapral (BAL) or penicillamine to promote the excretion of copper.

NUTRITIONAL DEFICIENCIES. Nutritional deficiencies may lead to either acute or chronic brain syndromes, particularly deficiencies of three constituents of the vitamin B complex: thiamine, niacin, and vitamin B_{12}.

Beriberi results from deficiency of *vitamin B_1*, or *thiamine*, and leads to generalized impairment of cellular functions similar to that caused by hypothyroidism. Thiamine deficiency has already been mentioned as a significant component of Wernicke's and Korsakoff's syndromes.

Pellagra is due to deficiency of *niacin*, and the classic symptoms and outcome begin with the letter *D*: dermatitis, diarrhea, delirium, dementia, and death. The diarrhea is not only a result of pellagra, but may also be a *cause* of further deficiencies of B vitamins that are usually absorbed and may be synthesized in the intestine. Hence, deficiency of these vitamins in industrialized countries is most likely to occur among elderly or alcoholic patients with diarrhea and various debilitating diseases.

Vitamin B_{12} deficiency leads to three related syndromes that may be present in varying degrees: (1) pernicious anemia, which is a chronic macrocytic megaloblastic anemia; (2) subacute combined degeneration of the spinal cord; and (3) encephalopathy, resulting in acute or chronic brain syndromes that have been referred to as *megaloblastic madness*. As in other brain syndromes, the latter are accompanied by diffuse slowing of the EEG.

Systemic Infections

Systemic infections may sometimes produce acute brain syndromes, particularly when they are severe and accompanied by electrolyte imbalance or high fever. Such infections include malaria, pneumonia, typhoid fever, and acute rheumatic fever. However, they may occur with a variety of other conditions, and at any age, although the very young and very old appear the most vulnerable.

Drug or Poison Intoxication

In recent years there has been a rapid escalation of potent drugs and chemicals with the potential for adverse effects on the brain. They may precipitate a tremendous variety of acute or chronic brain syndromes, some of which closely resemble naturally occurring schizophrenic or affective psychoses. In the case of sedative drugs (e.g., barbiturates) and antianxiety agents or minor tranquilizers (e.g., diazepam), the psychosis may result from either *acute intoxication* or from *abrupt withdrawal* after prolonged high dosage, in which event there is also a danger of epileptic seizures, with a possibility of status epilepticus and death. The particular form of brain syndrome is likely to depend on such factors as: (1) the nature of the drug or drugs; (2) the route of administration; (3) the duration of administration or exposure; (4) the magnitude and frequency of recent dosage; (5) individual vulnerability and response.

The following represents an incomplete list of substances that may lead to acute or chronic brain syndromes:

1. *Anesthetic gases,* such as nitrous oxide, ether, or trichlorethylene. Although these agents may precipitate excitement and delirium, persistent postsurgical brain syndromes are attributable largely to relative *oxygen deficiency,* or *hypoxia.* A person may survive brief periods of total *anoxia* from cardiac arrest, but hypoxia may result from a variety of situations, and some patients are much more vulnerable than others (for example, older patients with cerebral arteriosclerosis or various forms of metabolic insufficiency).

2. *Other gases,* including oxygen itself (at pressures greater than 2 atmospheres), carbon dioxide, carbon monoxide (for which the treatment is administration of oxygen under a pressure of two atmospheres), gasoline, and various *solvents,* including carbon tetrachloride, carbon disulfide, and solvents used in making glue.

3. *Metals,* including mercury, manganese, and lead. The latter usually results in a chronic brain syndrome with neuromuscular defects (e.g., wrist drop), and may be helped by administration of chelating agents such as dimercapral (BAL) followed by calcium disodium edetate.

4. *Sedatives.* Bromide psychosis tends to be chronic, with a time lag in onset and resolution of psychosis. The organic brain syndrome may not

develop until a blood level of 300 mg has been attained, but may continue after the blood level has dropped as far as 75 mg/100 cc. Treatment of bromide psychosis consists of administration of sodium chloride from 6 to 12 gm a day. Bromide excretion may be speeded up if patients also receive deoxycorticosterone.

Barbiturates may produce an organic brain syndrome when taken alone or in combination with alcohol (which potentiates their effects). Abrupt termination of barbiturates may result in withdrawal psychoses and/or seizures that may be fatal. They should therefore be withdrawn gradually over a period of about three weeks.

5. *Minor tranquilizers or antianxiety agents* may precipitate a brain syndrome, and all of these agents may be abused with resulting dependence, increased tolerance, and potential for withdrawal seizures and psychoses. They should be withdrawn gradually for the same reason as in the case of barbiturates.

6. *Stimulants.* Single large doses of cocaine or amphetamines may result in delirium, but the typical amphetamine psychosis results from chronic drug abuse and takes the form of a paranoid schizophrenic or schizo-affective psychosis. Major tranquilizers or antipsychotic agents are usually the immediate treatment of choice.

7. *Hallucinogens* include mescaline, psilocybin, and LSD-25, all of which are stimulants and produce delirium that is usually of brief duration but may sometimes result in persistent organic intellectual impairment. Antipsychotic agents are usually helpful in the acute stages and in schizophrenic patients whose psychosis has been exacerbated by drugs.

8. *Antipsychotic and antidepressant drugs.* MAO inhibitors, tricyclic antidepressants, and antipsychotic drugs may precipitate delirium when taken in excessive dosage.

9. *Antimanic agents.* The toxic effects of lithium include an acute brain syndrome.

10. *Anticholinergic or antihistaminic drugs,* including atropine, scopolamine, and benztropine (Cogentin).

11. *Analgesic drugs,* including salicylates and opioids such as meperidine (Demerol) and pentazocine (Talwin).

12. *Miscellaneous drugs,* such as disulfiram (Antabuse), levodopa (used in treatment of parkinsonism), thiocyanates (used for hypertension), atabrine (used in treating malaria), sulfonamides and other antibiotics, and also hormones (previously mentioned in the section on endocrine disorders).

Organic Psychoses with Childbirth (Antepartum or Postpartum Organic Brain Syndromes)

It is important to emphasize that this is a residual category, which includes a very small proportion of all psychiatric disorders associated with pregnancy, delivery, and the immediate postpartum period. By far the majority of such psychiatric problems involve *neurotic* anxiety, grief, or depression. Moreover, most patients with *postpartum psychoses* are likely to be suffering from schizophrenias or major affective psychoses, which should be treated accordingly.

Even those *organic brain syndromes* that do occur among women who are pregnant or immediately postpartum may be readily attributable to one or more of the many processes already described in this chapter, and should be so diagnosed. These include those syndromes clearly related to infection or drug intoxication, as well as hypoxic episodes resulting from such agents as general anesthesia or severe postpartum hemorrhage.

There remains a very small group of organic brain syndromes for which the primary basis appears to be toxemia of pregnancy or preeclampsia without other established basis — in the absence of eclamptic convulsive seizures or toxicity from medication administered to prevent the latter. This small subset of organic brain syndromes associated with childbirth may then appropriately be diagnosed as such.

REVIEW QUESTIONS

126. Wrist drop, ataxia, and irritability, followed by increased intracranial pressure, basophilic stippling of erythrocytes, and possible coma characterize the acute brain syndrome due

to the toxic influence of:
(A) mercury
(B) bromides
(C) lead
(D) carbon tetrachloride
(E) carbon monoxide

127. Among hospitalized patients, the two most common metabolic disorders that may produce an organic brain syndrome are diabetes mellitus and:
(A) pellagra
(B) hyperthyroidism
(C) pernicious anemia
(D) uremia
(E) porphyria

128. Which of the following is always due to inadequate metabolic support of the brain?
(A) loss of memory
(B) disorientation
(C) dementia
(D) delirium
(E) none of the above

129. An organic brain syndrome associated with aging and often having abrupt onset consisting of a delirious episode (with confusion, restlessness, incoherence, and hallucinations) which gradually subsides is:
(A) senile dementia
(B) diffuse cerebral arteriosclerosis
(C) Pick's disease
(D) Alzheimer's disease
(E) Creutzfeldt-Jakob's disease

130. Focal cortical lesions and atrophy largely restricted to frontal and temporal lobes are commonly found in:
(A) Pick's disease
(B) Alzheimer's disease
(C) senile dementia
(D) cerebrovascular dementia
(E) Huntington's chorea

131. A chronic brain syndrome associated with long-term alcoholism and characterized by amnesia, confabulation, and peripheral neuropathy is:
(A) Alzheimer's disease
(B) Pick's disease
(C) Wernicke's encephalopathy
(D) Wilson's disease
(E) Korsakoff's syndrome

Summary of Directions

A	B	C	D	E
1, 2, 3 only	1, 3 only	2, 4 only	4 only	All are correct

132. *Reversibility* is always characteristic of:
(1) organic brain syndromes due to drugs
(2) organic brain syndromes in young, otherwise healthy individuals
(3) organic brain syndromes in which amnesia and disorientation are not severe
(4) acute brain syndromes

133. Psychological tests helpful in differentiating between organic and purely functional mental disorders include:
(1) Bender-Gestalt
(2) WAIS
(3) Graham-Kendall
(4) MMPI

134. Huntington's chorea:
(1) produces amnesia
(2) in early stages may resemble schizophrenia
(3) is transmitted by a single dominant gene
(4) has early onset and rapid course

135. Typical of Alzheimer's disease is:
(1) atrophy limited to frontal lobes
(2) onset before age 60
(3) destruction of caudate nucleus
(4) impairment of judgment and loss of inhibition

136. In acute intermittent porphyria, the patient:
(1) commonly experiences colicky abdominal pain
(2) may show a variety of psychopathological symptoms with few or absent physical symptoms
(3) produces an excess of uroporphyrin
(4) should not receive phenothiazines

137. The delirium associated with bromide intoxi-

cation responds to treatment with:
  (1) sodium chloride
  (2) phenobarbital
  (3) phenothiazines
  (4) naloxone

138. *Dementia* is always:
  (1) irreversible
  (2) psychotic
  (3) due to structural changes in brain tissue
  (4) accompanied by EEG abnormalities

139. Pathological intoxication is characterized by:
  (1) extremely hyperactive behavior, often assaultive or destructive
  (2) subsequent amnesia for the episode
  (3) onset following minimal intake of alcohol
  (4) clear consciousness and correct orientation

140. Which of the following are *common to both* Wernicke's syndrome and Korsakoff's syndrome?
  (1) due to vitamin deficiency
  (2) usually begin with an episode of delirium
  (3) amnesia
  (4) tissue deterioration in the cerebrum and peripheral nerves

141. General Paralysis of the Insane is:
  (1) often accompanied by an Argyll-Robertson pupillary response
  (2) usually best treated with penicillin
  (3) usually first manifested by insidious personality changes
  (4) an inevitable result of untreated tertiary syphilis

142. Hallucinations are primarily auditory rather than visual in:
  (1) delirium tremens
  (2) alcoholic hallucinosis
  (3) cocaine intoxication
  (4) functional psychoses

143. Recommended treatment for extremely agitated behavior (assaultive or homicidal) by a person who is grossly intoxicated with alcohol is an intravenous or intramuscular injection of:
  (1) phenobarbital
  (2) diazepam
  (3) chlorpromazine

  (4) hydroxyzine

144. Psychiatric symptoms which suggest a diagnosis of acute or chronic brain syndrome include:
  (1) disorientation
  (2) impairment of judgment
  (3) lability of affect
  (4) neologisms

145. An organic brain syndrome with moderate impairment (of which the patient is partially aware) may lead to:
  (1) regressed behavior
  (2) catastrophic anxiety
  (3) rapidly increasing impairment during testing or interviewing
  (4) greater confusion in daytime than at night

SELECTED REFERENCES

1. Asher, R. (1949). Myxoedematous madness. *British Medical Journal,* vol. 2, pages 555–562.
2. Blachly, P.H., and Starr, A. (1964). Post-cardiotomy delirium. *American Journal of Psychiatry,* vol. 121, pages 371–375.
3. Connell, P.H. (1956). *Amphetamine Psychosis.* London: Chapman and Hall, Ltd. (Maudsley Monograph No. 5).
4. Dewan, J.G., and Spaulding, W.B. (1958). *The Organic Psychoses.* Toronto: University of Toronto Press.
5. Engel, G.L., and Romano, J. (1959). Delirium — A syndrome of cerebral insufficiency. *Journal of Chronic Diseases,* vol. 9, pages 260–277.
6. Gregory, I. (1955). The role of nicotinic acid (niacin) in mental health and disease. *Journal of Mental Science,* vol. 101, pages 85–109.
7. Kalinowski, L.B. (1958). Withdrawal convulsions and withdrawal psychoses. In *Problems of Addiction and Habituation,* edited by P. H. Hoch and J. Zubin. New York: Grune & Stratton. Pages 48–56.
8. Kety, S.S. (1952). Cerebral circulation and metabolism. In *The Biology of Mental Health and Disease.* New York: Hoeber Medical Division, Harper & Row. Pages 20–31.

9. McFarland, R.A. (1952). Anoxia: Its effects on the physiology and biochemistry of the brain and on behavior. In *The Biology of Mental Health and Disease.* New York: Hoeber Medical Division, Harper & Row. Pages 335–355.

10. Slaby, A.E., Lieb, J., and Tancredi, L.R. (1975). *Handbook of Psychiatric Emergencies.* Flushing, New York: Medical Examination Publishing Co.

11. Smith, A.D.M. (1960). Megaloblastic madness. *British Medical Journal,* vol. 2, pages 1840–45.

12. Drug Use Disorders

*O thou invisible spirit of wine! if thou hast no
name to be known by, let us call thee devil!
O God! that men should put an enemy in their
mouths to steal away their brains!
That we should, with joy, pleasance, revel and
applause, transform ourselves into beasts!*
Shakespeare, Othello

DRUG DEPENDENCE AND ABUSE

Drug abuse, or **substance abuse,** consists of the
self-prescribed use of a drug or toxic substance for
nonmedical purposes. The terms are sometimes
contrasted with *misuse* of a drug by a physician,
through excessive or inappropriate administration
to his patient.

Some patterns of drug abuse are accompanied by the development of **tolerance,** which
may be defined as an adaptive state characterized
by diminished response to the same quantity of
the substance, or by the fact that a larger dose is
needed to produce the same degree of pharmacodynamic effect. The concepts of *drug dependence*
and *addiction* have been defined in various ways.
An Expert Committee of the World Health Organization (1957) proposed the following definitions:

Drug addiction is a state of periodic or chronic
intoxication produced by the repeated consumption of a drug (natural or synthetic). Its characteristics include: (1) an overpowering desire or
need (compulsion) to continue taking the drug and
to obtain it by any means; (2) a tendency to increase the dose; (3) a psychic (psychological) and
generally a physical dependence on the effects of
the drug (the latter being defined as the appearance of an **abstinence syndrome** if the drug is
abruptly discontinued); and (4) a detrimental
effect on the user and/or society.

Drug habituation was defined as a condition
resulting from repeated use of a drug. Its characteristics include: (1) a desire (but not a compulsion) to continue taking the drug for the sense of
improved well-being which it engenders; (2) little
or no tendency to increase the dose; (3) some
degree of psychic dependence, but absence of

physical dependence; and (4) possible detrimental
effects on the user.

Drug dependence, defined as a state of psychic or
physical dependence that develops after a substance
is periodically or continuously administered, is
viewed as encompassing both habituation and addiction. The Committee pointed out that the characteristics of such dependence vary with the agent
involved in each specific case. Others have observed
that both drug dependence and drug abuse may
occur without the demonstration of tolerance.

The analysis of each form of drug abuse or
dependence should include consideration of interaction between at least three different sets of variables: (1) pharmacological effect and potential
for physical or psychological dependence of
specific drugs; (2) sociocultural prohibition versus
acceptance among various peer groups; and (3)
psychological vulnerability among various individuals within each peer group (based on both
psychosocial and biological variables). These factors will now be discussed briefly.

Pharmacological Characteristics

Pharmacological characteristics of various groups
constituted the basis for the World Health Organization to establish a continuum, from drugs with
strong addictive potential to those that are only
habit-forming, with many drugs intermediate
between these two extremes.

Some drugs, particularly opiates, will always
produce compulsive craving, physical dependence,
and addiction under appropriate conditions of
dosage and prolonged duration. Such addiction
may develop sooner among those with psychological vulnerability. However, pharmacological
action is a more significant factor than psychological makeup. Such addictive drugs result in
both individual and social damage, leading to
efforts at rigid control by legislation and law
enforcement.

At the other extreme of the continuum are
drugs that never produce compulsive craving, but
whose pharmacological action is so desirable to
some persons that their use readily leads to habituation. Termination or withdrawal of such drugs

does not lead to a physiological abstinence syndrome, so that psychological factors are paramount in their use. Such drugs do not need legal control.

Between these two extremes are other drugs whose use may lead to compulsive craving, physical or psychological dependence, and addiction among persons with sufficient individual vulnerability. Alcohol and cannabis (marijuana) are generally considered within this intermediate group, which may be the subject of state or national regulation, but rarely international control.

Sociocultural Differences

Sociocultural differences in peer group acceptance or prohibition of drug abuse or dependence have long been recognized. The World Health Organization has published annual mortality rates from specific disorders among various developed countries. Reliable comparisons have been made between deaths from cirrhosis of the liver and the frequency of alcoholism in various countries. Countries consistently at the top of this list have included France and the United States, whereas countries consistently at the bottom of the list have been Italy and the United Kingdom. Two of these countries (France and Italy) are both wine-producing and wine-drinking countries in close geographic proximity to each other. These profound differences have been attributed to contrasting patterns of alcohol use among the people. In Italy less than 1 percent of the adult population has been estimated to be alcoholic, and less than 1 percent of the population consumes alcoholic beverages apart from meals. In France, the incidence of alcoholism has been estimated as more than 5 percent of the adult population, and the dominant pattern of excessive drinking has traditionally consisted of continual drinking throughout the day without obvious signs of intoxication. The diagnosis of alcoholism in France was therefore reserved for those heavy drinkers who developed an organic complication such as cirrhosis of the liver or one of the alcoholic psychoses (see Chap. 11).

Marked differences have also been noted in the sex ratio for alcoholism in various countries.

Although this is now changing, the traditional ratio reported in the United States was about five male alcoholics to one female alcoholic. This contrasted with a ratio as low as two males to one female alcoholic in the United Kingdom, but as high as twenty males to one female alcoholic in certain Scandinavian countries. These differences have been attributed to varying cultural approval of drinking and tolerance of intoxication. They reflect a double standard of drinking behavior for males and females, comparable to what has been the traditional double standard of sexual behavior.

Studies within the United States have documented relatively high frequencies of alcoholism among certain groups (notably Irish Catholics), and relatively low frequencies among certain other groups (notably Jews, Moslems, and Mormons). These may be related to four different attitudes towards drinking behavior, as follows: (1) a calling for complete abstinence (e.g., Moslems and Mormons); (2) a ritual attitude usually associated with religious observances (e.g., Orthodox Jews); (3) a convivial attitude in which drinking is social rather than religious; and (4) a utilitarian attitude, whereby the effects of alcohol are intended to promote self-interest and personal satisfaction, as is typical among those abusing alcohol (or other drugs).

Psychological Differences

Psychological differences in individual vulnerability show some degree of statistical correspondence with the two other major groups of interacting variables considered above. Those drugs that are most strongly addictive (e.g., opiates) tend to invite the strongest sociocultural censure and prohibition among most peer groups. Persons who voluntarily initiate exposure to the established addictive potential of such forbidden drugs therefore tend to be those persons who most strongly reject normal adult roles of independence, performance, productivity, and economic competition. Many persons who use such street drugs have a life history characterized by deprivation, underachievement, nonconformity, rebellion, and antisocial behavior of other kinds.

Hence, it is not surprising that scale 4 on the MMPI (Minnesota Multiphasic Personality Inventory) is usually elevated among those addicted to hard drugs, since such addiction reflects antisocial attitudes and behavior. Moreover, such attitudes and behavior appear to be *ego-syntonic,* as reflected by a tendency to concurrent *high* scores on scales 8 and 9 (schizoid and manic) versus *low* scores on the three inhibitor scales, scales 2, 5, and 0 (depression, femininity, and social introversion).

This corresponds with observations that most young drug users have engaged in delinquent activities for some time prior to beginning their drug use.

Three further observations have been made about the *effects of addiction on the delinquent behavior* of a person: (1) The need for money to support the drug habit leads the user to commit offenses with greater frequency and less caution than previously; (2) after becoming addicted to opiates, delinquents do not engage in types of antisocial behavior in which they are not already experienced; (3) there is often a *lower* frequency of violent behavior *after* the onset of addiction, which may be attributable to several factors such as (a) the sedative effects of the drug; (b) desire to present a low profile and avoid attracting attention of the police; and (c) the tendency for many adolescents to become quieter as adults.

Alcohol is less strongly addictive than narcotics, and its social use has been widely accepted and institutionalized. Those who greatly exceed normal patterns of social use may be distinguished statistically from the majority of the population by relative elevation on scale 4 of the MMPI. However, in contrast with narcotic addicts, their underachievement, rebellion, and antisocial attitudes are often *ego-alien,* involving considerable intrapsychic conflict, anxiety, and guilt. Hence the typical MMPI profile among those alcoholics who enter psychiatric treatment may show elevation on scales 2, 7, and 0 (depression, "psychasthenia," and social introversion) in addition to elevation on scale 4 (psychopathic deviate).

Samuel Johnson remarked, "In the bottle, discontent seeks for comfort, cowardice for courage, and bashfulness for confidence." Alcohol and other drugs meet various emotional needs for different persons. Escape from fear and misery into temporary disinhibition and pleasure constitute powerful motivation for many neurotic persons to become involved in drug abuse and dependence. If experimental proof were necessary, it has been demonstrated that animals (cats and monkeys) may develop learned dependence on alcohol or other drugs when these agents are found to relieve fear (and other "neurotic" behavior) resulting from previously induced motivational conflicts.

There is a tendency for like to marry like, so that there are often similarities in intelligence, experiential background, and personality characteristics of husband and wife. Sometimes both spouses may be alcoholic or addicted to the same drug. Even when this was not the case, Rae (1972) reported that the MMPI of the *wife* bore a relationship to the outcome of therapy for her alcoholic husband. While depression in the wife often led to early divorce, the prognosis for the husband's alcoholism was far worse if the wife's MMPI was elevated on scale 4.

Eric Berne characterized alcoholism as a *life game,* in which the alcoholic plays the primary role of Victim. The primary supporting role is that of Persecutor, which is typically played by a member of the opposite sex, usually the spouse. A third role is that of Rescuer, usually played by someone of the same sex, often an inexperienced therapist. A fourth role is that of Patsy (or dummy) often played by an overindulgent mother who provides secondary gains and reinforcement of drinking behavior. The fifth role of Connection is the direct source of supply, who is usually a professional and may be more significant in other addictions than alcoholism. Steiner later elaborated on three variants of the alcoholic game, which he termed "Drunk and Proud," "Lush," and "Wino" — together with the corresponding games played by other drug-dependent persons. "HIP (High and Proud)," "Speed Freak," and "Drug Fiend." All of these games are assumed to have the common denominator that the individual has been programmed for joylessness and is engaging in transactions from an existential position exemplified by the sentence, "I'm no good and you're OK (ha, ha)." The value of these constructs may have severe limitations in analyzing the causes and development of drug dependence. However, group therapy based on principles of transactional analysis has compiled a promising record in the treatment of persons dependent on alcohol or other drugs.

Treatment of Drug Abuse and Dependence

The following is a summary of therapeutic approaches appropriate to various forms of drug dependence, which will be considered further in the following sections of this chapter concerning different specific types of dependence: (1) *detoxification,* involving supportive measures to minimize effects of the drug and of its withdrawal; (2) *substitution* of related drugs, which may be temporary (as in withdrawal of sedatives) or long-term (as in substitution of methadone for heroin); (3) *deterrents* to further ingestion of alcohol (e.g., by disulfiram or Antabuse) or of opiates (e.g., by cyclazocine or other opiate antagonists); (4) *antianxiety or antidepressant medication;* and (5) *group and individual psychotherapies* intended to eliminate psychological dependence.

ALCOHOL DEPENDENCE

Alcoholism is the term applied to the state of those persons whose alcohol intake is great enough to damage their physical health or their personal or social functioning, or when it has become a prerequisite to normal functioning. Three degrees of severity have been officially recognized in the APA Diagnostic and Statistical Manual:

Episodic excessive drinking refers to alcohol abuse to the degree of intoxication at least four times a year. *Intoxication* has been defined as a state in which the person's coordination or speech is noticeably impaired or his behavior clearly altered. This would probably correspond with a blood alcohol level of at least 100 mg/100 ml (i.e., 100 mg %), which in most states is defined by law as sufficient evidence of being under the influence of alcohol. Levels above 250 mg/100 ml usually

result in coma, while levels above 400 mg/100 ml are usually lethal.

Habitual excessive drinking is the diagnostic term applied to the behavior of those persons who become intoxicated more than 12 times a year, or who are noticeably under the influence of alcohol more than once a week (even if not to the extent of becoming intoxicated). This degree of severity is often accompanied by the onset of *blackouts,* which consist of amnesic episodes while the person is drinking excessively (also known as alcoholic *palimpsests*).

Alcohol addiction corresponds with the term *alcohol dependence,* the best evidence for which is the appearance of an abstinence syndrome following abrupt withdrawal. Dependence also corresponds with an inability of the person to go without drinking for at least 24 hours, or with the continuation of habitual excessive drinking for a period of more than three months.

Alcohol is always a *sedative* drug, although in low doses it appears to be a stimulant because of selective removal of cortical inhibition, with consequent euphoria and often increased psychomotor activity. As in the case of other acute brain syndromes, a person's behavior at a given blood alcohol concentration results from interaction between: (1) release of latent functional personality characteristics ("in vino veritas"), and (2) vulnerability to organic intellectual impairment, which is one factor affecting tolerance of a given dose of alcohol.

Other factors affecting tolerance include total body weight (i.e., a person weighing 200 pounds presumably should tolerate twice the amount of alcohol as a person weighing 100 pounds), *habituation* resulting in *increasing* tolerance with frequent exposure, and *medical complications* (such as chronic gastritis and hepatic cirrhosis) which result in *a decrease* in tolerance in advanced stages of chronic alcoholism.

Blood alcohol concentration shows a statistical correlation with individual behavior, and is affected by a variety of factors. Alcohol is absorbed rapidly when the stomach is empty, particularly if moderately diluted with water or if there is also some intake of carbon dioxide (as contained in sparkling wines or soft drinks). It is absorbed more slowly from beer, after food, and as the concentration in the stomach rises. The blood concentration is reduced gradually through metabolism at a fairly constant rate (which, unlike with most drugs, is independent of the actual level of concentration). The average rate of oxidation is sometimes stated as about 18 mg/100 ml (about three-quarters of an ounce of whiskey) per hour, but this is a rough approximation that varies according to such factors as body weight and metabolic efficiency.

The *life-time expectancy* (cumulative frequency) of alcoholism among the general population of the United States is roughly 5 percent. Overall death rates from cirrhosis of the liver roughly doubled during the 20-year period beginning in 1950, and are currently about twice as high among blacks as whites. They are also roughly twice as high among males as females, so that black males have a rate roughly four times as high as white females.

The *self-destructive nature of alcoholism* has both chronic and acute aspects. In addition to cirrhosis of the liver and other medical complications, chronic self-destructive behavior includes disruption of family and other social relationships, and employment and other economic factors. *Acute* self-destructive behavior consists of accidents and suicide. In some reported series of suicides, alcoholism constituted the second most frequent retrospective psychiatric diagnosis (after psychotic depression).

There is a significantly increased *family frequency* of alcoholism among the first-degree male relatives (fathers, brothers, and sons) of male alcoholics. The life-time expectancy of alcoholism in all three groups has been estimated as roughly 25 percent, which has led some to speculate about a possibility of hereditary predisposition. This speculation is supported by at least one study of twins in which the concordance rates for drinking among monozygotic co-twins was 65 percent, and among same-sexed dizygotic co-twins was only 30 percent (resulting in a Holzinger Index of Heritability of roughly 50 percent). However, there is

no indication that any genetic predisposition would involve a simple mendelian (monogenic) mechanism, and many persons attribute the sex-specific familial findings to psychosocial relationships, emphasizing *identification* with a father and older brothers who are already in severe conflict with the boy's mother.

Treatment

Treatment begins with detoxification and normalization of metabolic processes, and with prevention of withdrawal psychoses or seizures. The latter is best accomplished by immediate administration of one of the benzodiazepines (50 to 100 mg of chlordiazepoxide or 10 to 20 mg of diazepam). This should be accompanied by appropriate hydration and correction of any electrolyte imbalance, and by administration of intravenous fluids with glucose and possibly normal saline. At the same time, every patient should receive a parenteral dose of 5 ml of vitamin B complex (not thiamine alone), which may be conveniently included in the intravenous glucose solution. Dilantin may be indicated when the patient has a history of grand mal seizures, and it will be necessary to continue both giving vitamin B complex and gradually reducing doses of minor tranquilizers (benzodiazepines) during the ensuing week or two.

Disulfiram (Antabuse), to be taken voluntarily by the patient for as long as a year, is recommended by many therapists as part of the initial contract for participation in other forms of psychiatric treatment. The initial dosage of disulfiram is 0.5 gm per day for the first week, which may usually then be reduced to a daily maintenance level of 0.25 gm. This drug blocks the normal oxidation of alcohol so that if it is ingested there is accumulation of acetaldehyde, which results in unpleasant symptoms such as tachycardia and vomiting. The patient is warned about various side effects of disulfiram and its interaction with alcohol, but there is no deliberate aversive conditioning process.

Other psychiatric treatment will depend on the presence of obvious psychiatric disorder (e.g., depression or schizophrenia), as well as the age and environmental reality situation of the patient. A significant proportion of patients are sufficiently depressed to require antidepressant medication, preferably with a mildly sedative tricyclic such as amitriptyline. Others with alcoholic or schizophrenic psychoses may require antipsychotic medication.

Group or family therapy should be considered as a primary approach to treatment, whether or not the patient is also likely to benefit from individual psychotherapy. Transactional analysis is one form of group therapy that has shown considerable promise in effecting substantial changes in interpersonal relationships, and, it is hoped, the "life-script." As with other patients, the therapist must avoid being trapped into overreacting as Persecutor or Rescuer, and may be able to help the spouse and other intimates of the patient to avoid the same pitfalls.

Alcoholics Anonymous (AA) is a self-help organization of "nonpracticing" as well as "practicing" alcoholics that has the overriding goal of sobriety for its members. The approach is both inspirational and spiritual, and members are expected to assist in rehabilitating other alcoholics whom they bring to regular group meetings. This approach has considerable appeal for a number of alcoholics, who are thereby enabled to maintain sobriety and recover their self-esteem, as well as to rebuild relationships with families and employers. However, many members of Alcoholics Anonymous tend to be antimedical and antipsychiatric, thereby rejecting certain types of treatment that have proved effective for appropriate patients.

OPIOID DEPENDENCE

Commonly used derivatives of opium include morphine, heroin, codeine, dihydromorphinone (Dilaudid), and oxymorphone (Numorphan). Various synthetic opioids without a phenanthrene nucleus include meperidine (Demerol), methadone (Dolophine), phenazocine (Prinadol), pentazocine (Talwin), and dextropropoxyphene (Darvon).

The preceding drugs are all narcotic, sedative, and analgesic, with a strong potential for habituation, increasing tolerance, and psychological and physiological dependence. Users may have symptoms of acute overdosage, which may be deliberate or accidental (sometimes related to unknown strength of the illicit supply they have purchased). Alternatively, they may have symptoms of opioid withdrawal (the abstinence syndrome).

In the United States, the majority of addicts reside in the poorest slum areas of large cities, where illicit supplies of hard drugs are readily available, and where antisocial attitudes and behavior become the prevailing social norm. According to records of the federal government, roughly half of all narcotics addicts in this country reside in New York State, mainly in New York City. Nearly all are below the age of 40 years, and males tend to outnumber females in a ratio of about 4:1. There has also been substantial overrepresentation of blacks and members of other minority groups. The overall frequency of addiction to narcotics increased roughly tenfold during the decade from 1963 to 1973. However, during the next few years there was a relative decrease in addiction to hard drugs, with corresponding increases in *addiction to multiple drugs,* including barbiturates and other sedatives.

Acute overdosage results in impaired consciousness or coma, with depressed respiration and usually pinpoint pupils. There is likely to be a history of drug abuse, and evidence such as recent needle tracks. *Emergency management* consists of supporting vital functions (including administration of a 50% glucose solution) and administration of an opioid antagonist.

The **opioid antagonist** of choice for reversal of respiratory depression is naloxone (Narcan), given intravenously in a usual initial adult dose of 0.4 mg. Restraints should be in place or other preparations made before the drug is given, since patients may become agitated as they emerge rapidly from coma. Excessive administration of naloxone may precipitate withdrawal symptoms (an abstinence syndrome) if the patient is addicted, but this is unlikely to last longer than one-half hour to two hours. The effects of the naloxone itself may wear off much more rapidly than those of the narcotic drug (particularly in the case of an oral overdose of methadone, which may last for up to 48 hours). The patient must therefore be hospitalized and observed closely, with repeated administration of naloxone if indicated. The possibility of multiple-drug effects should also be borne in mind since the situation may be complicated by the development of a barbiturate withdrawal syndrome.

Naloxone is practically an ideal drug for the treatment of opiate overdoses. It has been found to have no agonist properties (unlike such drugs as pentazocine which have both agonist and antagonist effects) and is apparently pharmacologically inert in the absence of opiates. It is therefore diagnostic of the presence of opiates, and will produce no complications if administered when the diagnosis is doubtful. Its only disadvantage appears to be the relatively short duration of action.

Withdrawal from heroin or morphine leads to the onset of an abstinence syndrome about 8 to 12 hours after the last dose. Symptoms include psychomotor restlessness, irritability, increased rate of respiration, yawning, lacrimation, rhinorrhea, sweating, piloerection, tremor, anorexia, and dilated pupils. Within two to three days, the patient develops more severe symptoms, with insomnia, diarrhea, vomiting, painful abdominal cramps and muscle spasms, tachycardia, and hypertension. The syndrome of abrupt withdrawal (cold turkey) is extremely unpleasant but *not* life-threatening, except in patients with cardiac decompensation or other debilitating disease.

Substitution Therapy with Methadone (Detoxification)

Withdrawal is much more likely to be accepted, and effective, if accomplished by using oral methadone to reduce the severity of the abstinence syndrome. The patient should be admitted to the hospital, and an initial dose of 10 to 20 mg of methadone should be given by mouth after the appearance of withdrawal symptoms. No more than 20 mg of methadone should be required during any 12-hour period, and the dose is rapidly adjusted to the minimum level that will suppress symptoms of withdrawal. Regulations of the Food and Drug Administration (1972) require that

detoxification must be completed within 21 days, but this is usually accomplished within half this time by reducing methadone by 5 mg (or not more than 20 percent of the total dose) per day. *It is illegal* to prescribe methadone or any other narcotic for a known addict who is not an inpatient unless a license is obtained to operate a methadone maintenance program. The 21-day limitation for withdrawal of addicts who are inpatients may be exceeded only "for the maintenance treatment of an addict who is hospitalized for medical conditions other than addiction and who requires temporary maintenance during the critical period of his stay, or whose enrollment has been verified in a program which has approval for maintenance treatment with methadone." *Violations of these regulations carry criminal penalties.* Authorized hospital pharmacies are permitted to dispense methadone to nonaddicted inpatients or outpatients for analgesia for severe pain.

Outpatient methadone maintenance programs provide a daily oral dose of methadone, in order to reduce a person's craving for heroin or morphine. Any such outpatient methadone maintenance program *must* be licensed by the federal government and is subject to strict regulation by the Food and Drug Administration. Current regulations set criteria for acceptance of patients in methadone maintenance programs, limit the maximum daily dose to 120 mg, and the maximum supply that may be taken home by the addict to 100 mg for 48 hours. The regulations also require the keeping of adequate records, regular urinalysis, and other supportive services.

Other long-acting opioid derivatives are in process of development, and may be widely adopted if superiority to methadone maintenance programs can be demonstrated. One such drug is LAAM (L-alpha-acetyl-methadol), which has a duration of action up to three days after an oral dose, so that it may be taken less frequently than methadone (only three times a week). However, the contrary approach may be taken, whereby a former addict, who has been withdrawn from opioids, is kept drug-free through prolonged administration of an opioid *antagonist,* as described below.

Administration of long-acting opioid antagonists such as naltrexone may be regarded as a form of *deterrent therapy,* since such substances prevent the effects that may otherwise be sought through self-administration of opioid drugs. Promising results have been reported, with successful prevention of relapse in up to two-thirds of former opioid addicts participating in the drug-free programs initiated by withdrawal and prolonged voluntary administration of opioid antagonists.

Psychotherapies have received relatively less emphasis in the treatment of opioid addiction than alcoholism because of a higher rate of recidivism associated with such factors as prevailing antisocial personality characteristics, and an adverse reality situation, in addition to the very strong addiction potential of the drugs involved. However, group and family therapies are strongly recommended adjuncts to both drug-free and long-term maintenance programs. In addition, there are a number of therapeutic communities and self-help programs.

DEPENDENCE ON BARBITURATES AND SEDATIVE-HYPNOTICS

During the early 1970s there was some reduction in the prevalence of addiction to opioid drugs, accompanied by escalation in the frequency of addiction to multiple drugs, including the barbiturates. The latter are often used in combination with alcohol or opioid drugs, and are a frequent cause of death from deliberate or accidental overdosage, or from the uncontrolled seizures that may follow abrupt withdrawal.

Barbiturates, other sedatives or hypnotics, and minor tranquilizing (antianxiety) drugs such as meprobamate or the benzodiazepines are readily available to adolescents and young adults and are known commonly as downers. They may also be known more specifically by the colors of their capsules as redbirds, red devils, blue angels, blue heavens, rainbows, yellow jackets, and so on. There is a strong tendency for the development of psychological dependence among vulnerable individuals, followed by increasing tolerance and physical dependence, associated with a potential for dangerous withdrawal symptoms.

The withdrawal symptoms (abstinence syndrome) involve generalized hyperarousal of the central nervous system, with insomnia, anxiety, tremors, and vulnerability to convulsions, with or without the development of delirium or other organic brain syndromes. Spontaneous seizures are relatively infrequent unless the daily dose of pentobarbital or secobarbital exceeds about 600 mg. Similarly, delirium is infrequent, unless the daily doses of these drugs exceed 900 mg. In such an event, the abrupt withdrawal of such drugs is much more life-threatening than the abrupt withdrawal of opioid drugs. Hence, the sedative or hypnotic must be withdrawn gradually over a period of roughly three weeks. The maximum daily reduction should be no more than 10 percent of the established daily intake. When a person is dependent on both an opioid and a sedative-hypnotic drug, the latter should first be withdrawn gradually with the opioid maintained at a constant level.

Substitution therapy with pentobarbital or phenobarbital is usually the most convenient when initiating *detoxification* of a patient with an established dependency on barbiturates or similar agents. The appropriate initial dose of pentobarbital may be established by administration of a 200 mg test dose, which may be repeated every hour until symptoms of withdrawal have disappeared and mild sedation or intoxication is noted. This dosage should then be repeated for two days, followed by a reduction of no more than 10 percent per day. If withdrawal symptoms appear during this program, the dose should be increased and subsequent decreases should be at a lower rate.

There may be some advantage to using phenobarbital during a program of withdrawal, since there is less variation in the blood barbiturate level, and hence both less danger of undesirable side effects and less reinforcement of psychological dependence associated with rapidly increasing blood level.

Among the middle-aged persons dependent on such drugs are substantial proportions of neurotic persons who have become dependent through excessive medical prescription, and of alcohol-dependent persons who also abuse sedative-hypnotics. Regardless of age, it is likely that such drug-dependent persons will benefit from group or family therapy, whether or not they receive concurrent psychotherapy. However, the prognosis is likely to be better in those with a basis of neurotic anxiety or depression, than in those with antisocial personality characteristics or complicating organic brain syndromes.

ABUSE OF AMPHETAMINES, COCAINE, HALLUCINOGENS, AND ANTICHOLINERGICS

There is a strong tendency toward psychological dependence on "uppers" or "mind-expanding drugs," with development of tolerance and a tendency to increase dosage, but *not* toward true physiological dependence, leading to an abstinence syndrome following withdrawal. However, there are several types of unpleasant consequences that may occur. Among these are "bad trips," caused by excessive dosage, idiosyncratic vulnerability of the individual (including precipitation or exacerbation of functional psychoses), or inappropriate circumstances of administration. There is also an increasing tendency in recent years for users to combine these drugs with various sedative-hypnotics having true addictive potential. Group and family therapy approaches are usually more successful for treating abusers of these drugs than is one-to-one psychotherapy.

Amphetamines

Amphetamines and certain related central sympathomimetic amines such as methylphenidate (Ritalin) and phenmetrazine (Preludin) generally produce a typical toxic delirious state when a single overdose is taken. However, chronic use of amphetamines is likely to produce a syndrome that is very hard to distinguish from paranoid schizophrenia, and which should be treated in a similar manner. Signs such as bruxism (teeth grinding), stereotyped or repetitive behavior, preoccupation with mechanical objects (such as taking apart and reassembling a watch), formication, and hypersexuality are somewhat more typical of amphetamine psychoses. Toxicology tests may confirm

the diagnosis, but it should be noted that this psychosis often has a prolonged or chronic course, persisting long after ingestion of amphetamines has stopped. Psychoses due to these drugs respond preferentially to antipsychotic medication.

Sudden withdrawal from stimulant drugs following prolonged or high dosage administration produces a marked *decrease* in central nervous system activity, sometimes described as "crashing." The principal symptoms are somnolence, fatigue, apathy, and severe depression of mood which may lead to suicidal ideation. REM sleep may be greatly increased and lead to nightmares. There is a gradual normalization of these functions several days after withdrawal, so the best approach to treatment is to permit the patient to sleep and to provide physical and emotional support and protection. Antipsychotic drugs are indicated if symptoms of amphetamine psychosis are apparent, and attention should be given to nutrition if there has been prolonged anorexia and weight loss.

Psychiatric problems caused by abuse of **cocaine** are quite similar to those described for amphetamines, and should be treated in an identical manner.

Psychedelics

Psychedelics, also known as *hallucinogens, psychotomimetics,* and *psychotogenics,* are centrally acting drugs which have been somewhat arbitrarily grouped together for legal or quasi-descriptive purposes. The prototype and most potent of these agents is D-lysergic acid diethylamide (LSD), which was first synthesized in the 1940s but later found to occur naturally in the seeds of the herb *Rivea corymbosa.* Other drugs included under this label are mescaline (from peyote cactus), psilocybin (from the mushroom *Psilocybe mexicana*), diethyltryptamine (DET), dimethyltryptamine (DMT), and 2, 5-dimethoxy-4-methylamphetamine (DOM or STP). These agents share the property of producing altered states of awareness, encompassing perceptual, cognitive, and affective changes that resemble those of natural psychoses. Signs and symptoms of hallucinogenic intoxication include alteration of mood (usually euphoria), increased vividness of real or fantasized sensory perceptions, illusions and hallucinations (predominantly visual), synesthesia ("overflow" from one sensory modality to another), and a confusional syndrome. There are also often peripheral sympathomimetic changes such as pupillary dilation, sweating, and increases in body temperature, pulse, and blood pressure. Unless the drug aggravates or precipitates a functional psychosis, the syndrome is time-limited to 24 hours or less. Treatment of the acute episode is therefore conservative, and consists of frequent reorientation, reassurance, and protection to prevent panic (which may lead to dangerous or suicidal behavior). Medication, if needed, should be a benzodiazepine or other sedating drug. Antipsychotics were formerly used, but carry greater risks, and are now only recommended when amphetamines have also been used or the length of the episode is unduly long and a functional psychosis may be involved.

Cannabinoids

Cannabinoids such as marijuana and hashish are euphoriants that are, in some settings, used in much the same manner as alcohol. The behavioral effects of these drugs are difficult to predict since they depend on many factors, such as dosage, route of administration, environment, and the experience and expectations of the subjects. In Asian countries, where dosages used may be several hundred times as great as dosages used here, prolonged psychotic states and syndromes resembling chronic brain syndromes have been reported. However, it is clear that these drugs are substantially different from the psychedelics and amphetamines, and the medical and behavioral results of usage patterns common in the United States are controversial. Psychiatric emergencies related to use of cannabinoids should therefore be viewed as functional illnesses and diagnosed and treated accordingly; many of these cases may in fact represent an attempt at self-medication for a preexisting illness.

Anticholinergics

Anticholinergic drugs are increasing subjects of abuse by adolescents because of their ready avail-

ability from wild plants (e.g., jimsonweed) and in nonprescription drugs. Symptoms of toxicity include a confusional state or delirium, with visual hallucinations and restlessness. There may be signs of peripheral parasympathetic blockade, such as dryness of mouth and other mucous membranes, hoarseness, urinary retention or difficulty, dysphagia (difficulty swallowing), intense thirst, burning of eyes and throat, and inability to sweat. Pupils may be widely dilated and inactive; the skin is hot, dry, or flushed; pulse is rapid and weak; and there may be a high fever. Death may result from coma and circulatory collapse. Some authorities state that *scopolamine* differs from other anticholinergics by producing slow pulse and signs of central nervous system depression.

Treatment consists of withdrawal or reduction in dosage of anticholinergic medications, gastric lavage if there has been an orally administered overdose, and attention to symptomatic relief (e.g., moistening of eyes and mucous membranes). Catheterization may be necessary, as may respiratory support. *Physostigmine salicylate* (Antilirium) is a specific antidote that can cross the blood-brain barrier and thereby relieve centrally mediated symptoms (delirium, coma, etc.) as well as peripheral ones. The usual adult dosage of 0.5 to 2.0 mg intramuscularly or intravenously (the latter injected very slowly) may need to be repeated at 30-minute intervals if symptoms persist. This agent is so effective that it is a useful diagnostic test in doubtful cases. Side effects of physostigmine are usually mild (e.g., nausea, vomiting, excessive sweating) but are an indication to reduce the size of subsequent doses. There are also a number of relative contraindications to use of physostigmine; they include asthma, mechanical bowel or bladder obstruction, diabetes, heart block, and pregnancy.

The wide variety of drugs that may cause this syndrome include over-the-counter "sedatives" (Compoz, Excedrin-PM, Sleep-Eze, Sominex, etc.); antihistamines such as chlorpheniramine, diphenhydramine (Benadryl), and promethazine (Phenergan); atropine; prescription sedatives such as gluthethimide (Doriden); cough mixtures containing scopolamine; eye drops (even when administered locally); anticholinergic antiparkinson drugs such as benztropine (Cogentin) and trihexyphenidyl (Artane); tricyclic antidepressants; and even antipsychotics, especially the ones with marked anticholinergic activity such as chlorpromazine and thioridazine.

REVIEW QUESTIONS

146. Each of the following statements about naloxone (Narcan) is true *except:*
    (A) administration of naloxone to an opiate addict will abruptly induce an abstinence syndrome
    (B) naloxone completely inhibits the analgesic and euphoriant effects of opiates taken concurrently
    (C) naloxone has addiction potential
    (D) intravenous naloxone is the treatment of choice for an overdose of opiates by a nonaddict
    (E) intravenous naloxone is the treatment of choice for an overdose of opiates by an addict

147. The blood ethanol level of an automobile accident victim was 150 mg/100 ml. At this level, a typical healthy young adult would be:
    (A) without grossly apparent defect
    (B) acutely intoxicated
    (C) unconscious, but arousable by painful stimuli
    (D) deeply comatose without response to painful stimuli
    (E) very likely to die

148. In detoxification treatment for barbiturate addiction:
    (A) abrupt cessation of barbiturates is indicated
    (B) the same drug *must* be used and gradually reduced
    (C) short-acting barbiturates should be substituted and gradually withdrawn
    (D) symptoms of withdrawal can be controlled with chlorpromazine
    (E) diazepam is the most effective agent for replacement therapy

149. In amphetamine addiction, as contrasted

with heroin addiction:
    (A) no tolerance develops
    (B) withdrawal symptoms do not involve hyperarousal
    (C) there is no insomnia or restlessness
    (D) all of the above
    (E) none of the above

150. Of the following drugs, the one that is most effective in suppressing the opiate withdrawal syndrome is:
    (A) methadone
    (B) dextroamphetamine
    (C) diphenylhydantoin
    (D) naloxone
    (E) phenobarbital

Summary of Directions

A	B	C	D	E
1, 2, 3 only	1, 3 only	2, 4 only	4 only	All are correct

---

151. In chronic drug usage involving increased tolerance and escalating dosage, which of the following produce a *life-threatening* withdrawal syndrome?
    (1) amphetamines
    (2) minor tranquilizers
    (3) opiates
    (4) barbiturates

152. Absorption of orally ingested alcohol:
    (1) is not appreciably affected by food in the stomach
    (2) is increased in rate by carbon dioxide, as in champagne
    (3) takes place only in the small intestine
    (4) is slowed as the concentration of alcohol in the stomach increases

153. A syndrome clinically resembling paranoid schizophrenia is associated with prolonged high dosage use of:
    (1) cocaine
    (2) amphetamines
    (3) phenmetrazine (Preludin)
    (4) jimsonweed *(Datura stramonium)*

154. The injection of naloxone into a comatose

patient resulted in a marked improvement in respiration and other vital signs. The patient could have had an overdose of:

(1) phenobarbital
(2) meperidine
(3) meprobamate
(4) morphine

155. Antipsychotic drugs such as chlorpromazine have therapeutic advantages over benzo-diazepines such as diazepam and similar drugs for the treatment of brain syndromes due to the acute toxic effects of:

(1) anticholinergics
(2) LSD
(3) alcohol
(4) amphetamines

SELECTED REFERENCES

1. Chafetz, M.E., and Demone, H.W. (1962). *Alcoholism and Society*. New York: Oxford University Press.

2. Chein, I., Gerard, D.L., Lee, R.S., and Rosen-feld, E. (1964). *The Road to H*. New York: Basic Books.

3. Glasscote, R., Sussex, J.N., Jaffe, J.H., Ball, J., and Brill, L. (1972). *The Treatment of Drug Abuse*. Washington, D.C.: American Psychi-atric Association.

4. Goodman, L.S., and Gilman, A. [Eds.] (1975). *The Pharmacological Basis of Therapeutics* (5th ed.). New York: Macmillan. Chapter 16.

5. Hoch, P.H., and Zubin, J. [Eds.] (1958). *Problems of Addiction and Habituation*. New York: Grune & Stratton.

6. Longo, V.G. (1972). *Neuropharmacology and Behavior*. San Francisco: W. H. Freeman and Co. Chapter 4.

7. Rae, J.B. (1972). The influence of the wives on the treatment outcome of alcoholics: A follow-up study at two years. *British Journal of Psychiatry*, vol. 120, pages 601–613.

8. Shader, R.I. [Ed.] (1976). *Manual of Psychi-atric Therapeutics*. Boston: Little, Brown and Co.

9. Slaby, A.E., Lieb, J., and Tancredi, L.R. (1976). *Handbook of Psychiatric Emergen-cies*. Flushing, New York: Medical Examina-tion Publishing Co.

10. Steiner, C. (1971). *Games Alcoholics Play*. New York: Ballantine.

13. Schizophrenic and Paranoid Disorders

Babylon in all its desolation is a sight not so awful as that of the human mind in ruins.
Scrope Davies, Letters to Thomas Raikes

DEMENTIA PRAECOX, OR THE GROUP OF SCHIZOPHRENIAS

The term *démence précoce* was introduced in 1856 by the French psychiatrist Benedict-Augustin Morel to describe a severe mental illness in a 14-year-old boy who had previously been a good student but underwent rapid deterioration of intellect and behavior. In 1870 Hecker used the term *hebephrenia* to describe malignant mental illnesses of this type with onset around the time of puberty (Hebe was the Greek goddess of youth), which led to permanent dementia with profound disorganization of personality.

A few years earlier, Kahlbaum (1863) had distinguished between *dementia paranoides,* in which there were prominent delusions and gross disorganization of behavior, and *paranoia,* characterized by well-systematized delusions, with relative preservation of intellect and behavior. In 1868 he introduced the term *catatonia,* or "tension insanity," to describe a form of mental illness in which the patient remained mute and motionless.

It remained for Emil Kraepelin (1896) to note certain similarities in the preceding syndromes, and apply the term *dementia praecox* to all three forms (hebephrenic, catatonic, and paranoid). He subsequently accepted a fourth group, characterized by gradual onset and lack of initiative, for which Diem (1903) proposed the term *dementia praecox simplex.* For Kraepelin, the common denominators of these four syndromes were onset in adolescence or early adult life and irreversible progression to a permanent state of dementia. While neither of these characteristics is essential to these descriptive syndromes, the overall term *dementia praecox* was preserved as part of the official nomenclature in the United States until 1950. Unresponsiveness to treatment often led to chronic care in custodial institutions, and half of all patients in state hospitals had this diagnosis.

In his classic text, *Dementia Praecox or The Group of Schizophrenias,* the Swiss psychiatrist Eugen Bleuler (1911) pointed to considerable variation both in age of onset (typically between 15 and 45 years) and in spontaneous outcome or prognosis, with partial or temporary remissions most characteristic of catatonic or paranoid forms with acute onset after the age of 30 years. The term *schizophrenia* has generally been interpreted as meaning "splitting of the mind," and there is a popular misconception that this involves having a split, or multiple, personality, with alternation of conflicting characteristics as in Dr. Jekyll and Mr. Hyde. However, the latter represents a form of hysterical dissociation that will be referred to again in Chapter 15. In schizophrenias, on the other hand, the split consists of *fragmentation* or *incongruity* between various mental functions, as between thought content and emotional response or motor behavior.

Bleuler distinguished between certain symptoms of schizophrenia that he regarded as primary or essential characteristics of the process, and others that he regarded as secondary elaborations present only in certain persons at certain times. *Bleuler's primary symptoms* are known as the four A's: *association defects* – loosening and fragmentation of thinking; *affect* – inadequate (blunt or flat) and inappropriate; *autism* – peculiar to the self (social isolation, narcissistic preoccupation, and idiosyncratic thinking); and *ambivalence* – coexistence of conflicting feelings, with inconsistent behavior and vacillation.

Bleuler's *secondary symptoms* consisted of manifestations that were not universal but variable in appearance, such as delusions, hallucinations, catatonic and hebephrenic features, and regressive behavior. However, the latter may sometimes appear more characteristic of schizophrenia than certain primary manifestations, particularly ambivalence, which is also frequent in other forms of psychiatric disorder, notably in severe depression.

In recent years, the schizophrenias have been

regarded as a large group of disorders, with a wide variety of manifestations and differing responses to treatment, based on multiple separate or interacting causal factors. To some persons it has seemed that the term *schizophrenia* was at least as broad as the term *blindness,* or that there might be as many forms of schizophrenia as there are forms of mental retardation. However, a number of similarities or common denominators have also been established.

In the early stages of schizophrenia there is usually a hypersensitivity to perceptual and interpersonal stimuli. This is accompanied by hyperarousal of the nervous system and vulnerability to energy depletion (as might be accomplished with amphetamines or sleep deprivation). These symptoms are accompanied by heightened emotionality, apprehensiveness, and avoidance, manifested by social withdrawal and isolation. This leads to increased preoccupation with inner fantasy and symbolism, with egocentricity or narcissism and dependency on others for basic needs, or regression to an oral phase of development.

Disorders of thinking have often been regarded as the most basic and typical manifestations of schizophrenia. These may take several forms, which may often be demonstrated by asking the patient to interpret well-known proverbs such as, "A stitch in time saves nine," or "People in glass houses shouldn't throw stones." A schizophrenic will often respond with a *concrete,* or *literal,* interpretation (as contrasted with an abstract response), but the same kind of concrete, or literal, thinking is also seen in a number of other persons (normal children, mentally retarded adults, or persons with organic brain syndrome). A second form of response that is much more typical of schizophrenia results from *overinclusive thinking.* The latter involves inclusion of irrelevant material, resulting from loosening of associations, so that the response will extend to several sentences. Most characteristic of all, however, is the personalized response based on *autistic thinking,* which follows the person's own idiosyncratic rules of logic. This may be further displayed in the form of delusions, neologisms, and other symptoms discussed in

Chapter 2. Following are descriptions of the major forms of schizophrenic disorder.

Simple Schizophrenia

Simple schizophrenia is characterized mainly by early insidious onset, social isolation or withdrawal, inactivity, passivity, and dependency on others. There is indifference, apathy, and lack of initiative. Neither hallucinations nor delusions are prominent, and the course is chronic. As time passes, there may be increased evidence of schizophrenic thinking, with intellectual impairment and regressive behavior.

Hebephrenic Schizophrenia

Hebephrenic schizophrenia is characterized by disorganized thinking, with a shallow and inappropriate emotional response. The onset tends to occur during adolescence, and the behavior is frequently bizarre. There may be grimacing, mannerisms, strange gestures, silly laughter and giggling, or quick impulsive actions, without any evident relationship to external stimuli.

Catatonic Schizophrenia

Catatonic schizophrenia involves marked disturbances in motor activity, which may be either greatly increased or decreased.

CATATONIC EXCITEMENT. Catatonic excitement consists of excessive and sometimes violent motor activity that may be difficult to distinguish from severe delirium (acute brain syndrome) or acute mania (affective psychosis). The condition was often fatal before convulsive therapies became available, but nowadays the condition usually responds most effectively to large doses of antipsychotic medication (major tranquilizers).

CATATONIC WITHDRAWAL. In catatonic withdrawal there is generalized inhibition or retardation that may be accompanied by various other manifestations such as mutism, negativism, waxy flexibility, or stupor. In fact, such patients are usually *hyperaroused* and *hyperalert* despite their withdrawn appearance. The condition may sometimes be difficult to distinguish from an acute brain syndrome or a severely retarded depressive psychosis. However, there will usually be other evidence of schizophrenia, and the patient may dramatically and unpredictably swing from a state of stupor to one of excitement and vice versa. Antipsychotic medication is often effective in diminishing catatonic withdrawal, but convulsive therapy may be indicated if there is persistent refusal of all fluids or failure to respond to medication.

Paranoid Schizophrenia

Paranoid schizophrenia is characterized by delusions of reference, active or passive control (influence), persecution, or grandeur. The delusions are typically poorly systematized and are usually accompanied by hallucinations, particularly auditory. The average age of onset is slightly greater than for the preceding forms of schizophrenia, and there may have been a more favorable premorbid personality adjustment. The latter would be associated with a relatively favorable prognosis, particularly when the onset of symptoms was acute and there were obvious precipitating stresses. Delusions of persecution tend to be associated with a more favorable prognosis than delusions of grandeur, and auditory hallucinations are associated with a more favorable prognosis than hallucinations of other senses (particularly olfactory).

Schizo-affective Disorders

Schizo-affective disorders are characterized by a combination of schizophrenic thought disorder with prominent and persistent symptoms of mood disorder: *depression* or *mania*, or both. The usual form of schizo-affective disorder represents a combination of paranoid schizophrenia with persistent and severe depression. Unfortunately, these patients have generally been classified and treated as though they were primarily schizophrenic, when the mood disorder should be regarded as equally severe and may be potentially more dangerous. In a study of 420 twin pairs of veterans, one or both of whom had a psychotic diagnosis, Cohen and co-workers (1972) found the monozygotic co-twin concordance rate for schizo-affective disorder to be more than two times higher than that of schizophrenia, but *not* significantly different from that of manic-depressive illness. Monozygotic twins concordant for schizo-affective disorder had affective symptoms equal to those of manic-depressive twins *and* schizophrenic symptoms equal to those of schizophrenic twins. Schizo-affective psychoses were found to have a mean age of onset earlier than both manic-depressive psychosis and schizophrenia. Moreover, 7 of 21 (33 percent) of monozygotic index schizo-affective twins committed suicide, as contrasted with none of the 18 manic-depressive and 3 of the 100 index schizophrenic twins. It is evident that these are severe disorders, and that appropriate treatment should be directed toward both the schizophrenic and the affective manifestations.

Latent Schizophrenia

Latent schizophrenia is also referred to as *borderline, prepsychotic,* or *incipient* schizophrenia, or as *borderline personality.* This category is a controversial one that is used for patients who have clear schizophrenic symptoms but no history of a psychotic episode. The term *pseudoneurotic schizophrenia* is sometimes applied when the underlying psychotic process is (at least initially) masked by complaints ordinarily regarded as neurotic. A wide variety of such symptoms may be apparent in any single patient ("panneurosis"), but the most frequent is excessive diffuse or free-floating anxiety ("pananxiety"). The term *pseudopsychopathic schizophrenia* may be used when the underlying psychotic process is (initially) expressed as delinquent, antisocial, or "acting out" behavior. Such behavior often involves sexual deviations and offenses resulting from a state characterized as chaotic sexuality.

Residual Schizophrenia

Residual schizophrenia refers to a state in which clear schizophrenic symptoms remain following the termination of a full-blown psychotic episode.

Childhood schizophrenia refers to all forms of the illness in children prior to the onset of puberty, and will be discussed in Chapter 19.

Undifferentiated Schizophrenia

Undifferentiated schizophrenia may refer to either an acute episode or to a chronic state of schizophrenic psychosis in which the patient's symptoms show no clear or consistent pattern having a more specific label. *Chronic undifferentiated schizophrenia* is an apparently permanent psychotic state that may remain stable over a long period of time, or that may deteriorate to a terminal stage resembling profound dementia. Many stable chronic patients require permanent institutional care, but some are able to maintain a marginal existence in halfway houses, group homes, or with relatives. Terminal schizophrenia has now become rare, probably because of the availability of partially effective treatments and improvement of institutional environments.

CONTINUUM OF PROCESS SCHIZOPHRENIAS vs REACTIVE SCHIZOPHRENIAS

Process schizophrenia is a term that has been applied to schizophrenias with early onset and poor prognosis based on poor premorbid personality. In summary form the latter implies underachievement, unemployment, being unmarried, and being unsociable. This is regarded by some as the true ("stainless-steel") form of schizophrenia, having an endogenous, biological, or somatic basis. Diagnostically the most likely subtypes of schizophrenia would be simple, hebephrenic, and catatonic. Other significant findings are likely to include a positive family history of chronic psychosis, family history of maternal dominance, and statistical associations with low socioeconomic status and relatively lower intelligence.

Reactive schizophrenia is a term applied to schizophrenias that develop in adult life in response to severe environmental stress or provocation. There is a relatively acute onset with good prognosis based on good premorbid personality, with evidence of appropriate educational achievement, reliable employment, stable marriage, and social interaction. These are sometimes referred to as *schizophreniform psychoses*, which are exogenous and involve psychological or experiential factors in their development. The diagnostic sub-

group is likely to be paranoid or schizo-affective. Other significant factors tend to include absence of family history of schizophrenia, growing up in a father-dominated family, middle or upper socioeconomic status, and at least average intelligence.

The process-reactive continuum of schizophrenias should be regarded as a simplified model that may help our understanding of causation, as well as assisting our assessment of probable response to treatment. However, some of the factors relevant to prognosis in schizophrenias will be found equally relevant to prognosis in major mood disorders or other forms of psychiatric disorder.

BIOLOGICAL DETERMINANTS

Hereditary Predisposition

It has long been established that there is a much increased empirical risk, or *lifetime expectancy,* of schizophrenia among the close relatives of hospitalized patients with this diagnosis. Prior to World War II, the lifetime expectancy for schizophrenia in the general population was estimated as slightly under 1 percent, whereas reported frequencies among full siblings (or dizygotic co-twins) were roughly 10 to 15 percent. The observed frequencies of schizophrenia among parents of schizophrenics were slightly lower (roughly 5 to 10 percent). The estimated frequency in children of one schizophrenic parent was about the same as that in siblings, whereas estimates of expectancy in children of *two* schizophrenic parents ranged from 40 to 65 percent.

Many attempts have been made to force these and similar data to conform with a simple mendelian hypothesis of transmission, usually by a single pair of recessive genes (Kallmann's theory), but sometimes a single dominant gene (Book's theory). This was done by invoking concepts of *partial penetrance* or *expressivity* of the genes, which means that overt schizophrenia would only develop in a certain proportion (perhaps a minority) of the persons assumed to have the necessary genetic predisposition.

When the empirical risk, or lifetime expectancy, of schizophrenia among various classes of relatives is compared with theoretical expectancies under various monogenic hypotheses (including incomplete penetrance or expressivity in homozygote or heterozygote), *no single gene hypothesis is compatible with all the data.* However, both twin studies and foster child studies (summarized below) support the belief that some form of genetic predisposition is necessary (and *may* be sufficient) for the development of at least some forms of schizophrenia. It is possible that this hereditary predisposition might involve *genetic heterogeneity* (several different single-gene mechanisms in different families or subgroups of schizophrenia). An alternative explanation is that hereditary predisposition to schizophrenia is an infinitely variable characteristic that is attributable to the cumulative effect of multiple minor genes at various different loci; i.e., to *polygenic transmission.*

TWIN STUDIES. While they provide no information about possible mechanisms of genetic transmission, twin studies strongly support the existence of some predisposition, particularly among chronic or process schizophrenias. The results of eleven studies of twins with schizophrenia are summarized in Table 13-1, which shows estimated concordance rates in monozygotic and dizygotic co-twins, together with Holzinger's index of heritability. The consistency evident in the first six of these studies is impressive, but the first five of them did *not* involve serological determination of zygosity, and all of them involved hospital samples with a high proportion of chronic patients. On the other hand, most recent studies do employ serological determination of zygosity, and sampling that includes acute and reactive forms of schizophrenia.

Several studies support the belief that heredity is more important in predisposition to chronic or process schizophrenias than to acute or reactive schizophrenias. Rosenthal (1959) examined the case histories of monozygotic twins with schizophrenia, which had been published in detail by Slater. He found an almost total absence of schizophrenia among the families of the discordant twin pairs (in which the co-twin did not develop schizophrenia), in contrast with a positive history among roughly 60 percent of the families of the concordant twins (in which the co-twin also developed schizophrenia). Moreover, the discordant male twins tended to have a later age of onset, with more favorable prepsychotic personality and outcome than the concordant male twins. The diagnostic subtype of the discordant twin tended to be paranoid and of the concordant twin, catatonic.

Another study supporting a genetic distinction between process and reactive forms of schizophrenia was by Inouye (1961), who divided his group of monozygotic schizophrenic twins into three subgroups, the two largest of which each contained 23 twins. Among those with chronic progressive schizophrenia, he found 17 of 23 pairs (74 percent) to be concordant, whereas among those with mild or transient schizophrenias, he found only 9 of 23 pairs (39 percent) to be concordant.

FOSTER CHILD STUDIES. Foster child studies also provide evidence of some form of genetic predisposition. Heston (1966) compared the psychosocial adjustment of 47 adults born to chronic schizophrenic mothers with 50 control adults; all 97 subjects had been separated from their natural mothers within the first few days of life. A significant excess of both schizophrenic and antisocial personality disorders were found among the offspring of schizophrenic mothers (with whom they had never lived). The offspring of these schizophrenic mothers included 5 with schizophrenia, 4 with mental deficiency, 9 with antisocial personalities, and 13 with neurotic personality disorders. The offspring of the normal controls included none with schizophrenia or mental deficiency, 2 with antisocial personalities, and 7 with neurotic personality disorders. These findings suggested both specific and nonspecific genetic predisposition, whereas the following study was more suggestive of specific predisposition only.

In a sample of more than 5,000 adults who had been adopted early in life by persons not biologically related to them, Kety and his associates (1974) identified 33 who had been admitted

Table 13-1. Estimated Concordance Rates in Monozygotic and Dizygotic Co-twins of Schizophrenic Twins

Investigator, Country, and Year	Apparent Zygosity of Twins	Numbers of Pairs	Estimated Concordance Rate (Percent)	Heritability $H = \dfrac{CMZ - CDZ}{100 - CDZ}$
Luxenburger, Germany, 1928	MZ	17	67	0.67
	DZ	33	0	
Rosanoff, United States, 1934	MZ	41	67	0.63
	DZ	101	10	
Essen-Möller, Sweden, 1941	MZ	7	71	0.65
	DZ	24	17	
Slater England, 1953	MZ	41	76	0.72
	DZ	115	14	
Kallmann, United States, 1953	MZ	268	86	0.84
	DZ	685	15	
Inouye, Japan, 1961	MZ	55	76	0.69
	DZ	17	22	
Tienari, Finland, 1963	MZ	16	0	−0.11
	DZ	21	10	
Harvald and Hauge, Denmark, 1965	MZ	7	29	0.25
	DZ	59	5	
Kringlen, Norway, 1966	MZ	50	28	0.23
	DZ	175	7	
Gottesman and Shields, England, 1966	MZ	24	42	0.36
	DZ	33	9	
Cohen et al, United States, 1972	MZ	81	23	0.19
	DZ	113	5	

to mental hospitals with a definite diagnosis of schizophrenia. Matching controls for each schizophrenic index patient were picked from adopted individuals who had never been admitted to a mental hospital. The index group was found to have a total of 63 half-siblings who shared only their biological father, and the control group was found to have a comparable total of 64 biological paternal half-siblings. The frequency of definite schizophrenia among the paternal half-siblings of the schizophrenic group was 8 of 63 (13 percent), whereas the frequency in the control group was only 1 of 64 (1.6 percent). This finding is statistically significant (p = 0.015) and is compelling evidence that genetic factors operate significantly in the transmission of schizophrenias.

Biochemical Correlates

The search for organic, or somatic, bases for schizophrenias has led to numerous reports of positive findings, a majority of which have not been replicated in subsequent studies. Structural anomalies have been reported in the brains and in other parts of the bodies of schizophrenics. Various infectious processes have been implicated (e.g., tuberculous, rheumatoid, and viral). Diverse metabolic findings have been reported, some of which involve significant differences between constitutional, nuclear, or process (e.g., simple, hebephrenic, or catatonic) schizophrenias and acute or reactive (e.g., paranoid) schizophrenias.

Many biochemical theories of schizophrenia, advanced during the decade after World War II, have been grouped by Kety under the following five headings: (1) oxygen, carbohydrates, and energetics; (2) amino acids and amines; (3) epinephrine; (4) ceruloplasmin and taraxein; and (5) serotonin. Early studies suggested that defective carbohydrate metabolism was characteristic of the schizophrenic process. The principal flaws of such studies have been failure to control for important factors that are unrelated to schizophrenia, and failure of other investigators to replicate the findings. For example, an abnormal glucose tolerance and other evidence of liver dysfunction could be explained by incidental hepatic disease or nutritional deficiencies. Similarly, there are numerous mechanisms whereby vitamin deficiencies may cause substantial changes in the complex patterns of metabolism of amino acids. A reported increase in serum copper in schizophrenics, with demonstration that practically all of the serum copper was in the form of ceruloplasmin, led to the development of the color reaction known as the Akerfeldt test, but it was not long before the high ceruloplasmin level in schizophrenics was found to be due to low ascorbic acid levels resulting from dietary insufficiency. A low level of ascorbic acid in the blood is also an important and uncontrolled variable influencing rapid in vitro oxidation of epinephrine in plasma from schizophrenic patients.

Two hypotheses relating to the biological substrates of schizophrenia were reviewed in detail by Kety (1976) and have been summarized in Chapter 7. The first of these is the *transmethylation hypothesis,* according to which there may be an accumulation of hallucinogenic methylated metabolites such as DMPEA (identified as the substance responsible for the pink dot on paper chromatography) in the urine of schizophrenic patients. The other major hypothesis involves an *increase in dopamine activity* accompanied by a *decrease in norepinephrine activity,* both of which might be a result of the "throttling" of a single enzyme (dopamine-beta-hydroxylase).

Consistently replicated biochemical findings would result in reliable identification of schizophrenic subgroups, and permit further evaluation of etiology, including interactions between heredity, nutrition, developmental stress, and insufficient exposure to normal stress. The latter alternatives are implicit in some of the psychosocial studies which are briefly summarized in the next section.

PSYCHOSOCIAL DETERMINANTS

Social isolation has long been recognized as one of the characteristic manifestations and possible causal factors in the development of schizophrenias. As long ago as 1908, Bleuler remarked "The overt symptomatology certainly represents the expression of a more or less successful attempt to find a way out of an intolerable situation."

Some have sought the origin of this withdrawal within the schizophrenic himself, whereas others have sought to find environmental circumstances from which withdrawal was inevitable. Sullivan concluded that the withdrawal represented an avoidance of painful interpersonal relationships characterized by criticism, threats, and inevitable failure. Schilder (1939) interpreted the failure of such patients to differentiate adequately among cues in the environment as follows: "It is as if the schizophrenic would say, 'This fully differentiated world of yours is much too difficult and dangerous and therefore I content myself with a more primitive world.'" Fromm-Reichmann (1950) attributed schizophrenic aloofness to the desire to avoid yet another rebuke in a long row of thwarting rebuffs that the schizophrenic has experienced in childhood and has been conditioned to expect in endless repetition.

Relationships with Parents and Peers

The search for adverse childhood experiences led to many studies of relationships within the nuclear family. The finding most frequently reported among male schizophrenics was that of overprotection by a dominating and manipulative mother. In one such study, Mark (1953) administered an attitude survey to 100 mothers of male schizophrenics and to 100 mothers of male nonschizophrenics. Of 139 items in the survey, 67 differentiated between the two groups of mothers at the 0.05 level of significance or better. On analyzing the content of these items, it appeared that the mothers of schizophrenics were mainly restrictive in their control of the child. When it came to the warmth of the relationship, they showed attitudes of both excessive devotion and cool detachment.

In a later study of the mother-child relationship in schizophrenia, McGhie (1961) found overprotection to be more typical of the early background of the neurotic than that of the schizophrenic. However, the mothers of his schizophrenic patients showed a remarkable capacity for denial in their attitude to the patient's earlier difficulties. "Not only does she distort reality in projecting the cause of the patient's abnormal reactions outside of him, but she also accepts, approves, and actively encourages the deviant features in his development. Her influence on the patient is almost specifically designed effectively to cripple the child's attempts to reach an independent and stable level of adjustment." The mothers themselves tended to report an unhappy early home life that was often disrupted further by parental loss. As children they had been unhappy, insecure, and unable to make good contact with others. They had remained relatively isolated socially throughout their lives, their marriages predestined to failure by their own rejection of their femininity.

Bowen and his associates (1959) reported on intensive observations of three-way relationships within families containing a schizophrenic child. They reported that parents were often separated from each other by an emotional barrier, which had many characteristics of an "emotional divorce." Either father or mother could have a close relationship with the patient when the other parent permitted. The patient's function appeared similar to that of an unsuccessful mediator of the emotional differences between the parents. The most frequent family pattern was an intense twosome between mother and child, which excluded father, and from which he permitted himself to be excluded.

Lidz and Fleck (1960) reviewed a series of intensive analyses of families containing a schizophrenic member. Among the characteristics of *the mothers* of schizophrenic patients were an

imperviousness to what the child seeks to convey, combined with an inordinate intrusiveness; a tendency to confuse the child's needs with the mother's own needs projected onto the child; and disparity between what was expressed verbally and what was demonstrated. Moreover, *the fathers* were as frequently and severely disturbed as the mothers, were often insecure in their masculinity, and needed constant admiration and attention to bolster their self-esteem. Many of the fathers had the same quality of imperviousness to the feelings and sensitivities of others that was typical of so many of the mothers. The adverse influence of father on child might be exerted either directly or indirectly through their relationship with mother.

Some of the relationships between parents were characterized by severe chronic disequilibrium and discord, which Lidz and Fleck termed *marital schism*. In other cases, the serious psychopathology of one marital partner dominated the home, a situation they described as *marital skew*. In comparing the parent-child relationships of male and female schizophrenics, they found that schizophrenic *males* often came from skewed families with passive, ineffectual fathers, and disturbed, engulfing mothers. Schizophrenic *females* typically grew up in schismatic families, with narcissistic fathers who were often paranoid and (although seductive of the daughter) disparaging of women, and with mothers who were emotionally distant.

Relative absence of normal peer relationships is often regarded as inevitable in the childhood of patients with severely disturbed families. Experimental data from studies of monkeys support a hypothesis that *defective peer relationships may be even more significant in producing deviant social development than impaired relationships with parents.* Harlow (1962) reported gross abnormalities of behavior among monkeys reared in isolation from other monkeys, particularly in the absence of play contact with peers of both sexes. As adults, such *isolated* monkeys showed autistic self-preoccupation, stereotyped movements (e.g., catatonic rocking), and extreme apprehensiveness and agitation when confronted with normal adults of the same species. They were *asocial* (failed to participate in grooming or other normal interactions) and were either *asexual* or *autoerotic*. The isolated *males* were never able to learn to interact sexually with a mature and sexually receptive female. Although some of the isolated *females* responded to long and patient education by sexually sophisticated males, and were successfully impregnated, they later rejected and abused their offspring so severely that the latter had to be removed from the deprived mothers in order to survive. In the event of a second pregnancy, the isolated female tended to be more accepting of the demands of her infant, and responded in a less deviant manner.

In a well-controlled biochemical study, developmentally isolated monkeys were the only group that showed serum abnormalities similar to those previously reported by investigators studying human schizophrenics.

Ecology and Socioeconomic Status

Relatively high rates of schizophrenia have been found in central urban areas, among blacks and members of other minority groups, and among those of low educational, occupational, or socioeconomic status. Faris and Dunham (1939) found hospital admission rates for schizophrenia in Chicago to be highest in the central areas of social disorganization, decreasing progressively toward the periphery of the city. The overall distribution of schizophrenia in some cities has been found to correspond with the residential pattern of a minority of patients: single, separated, and divorced men living alone. Sociologists and psychiatrists have debated whether these areas specifically attract schizophrenics (the drift hypothesis) or whether they tend to produce schizophrenia (the breeder hypothesis).

In their extensive study of social class and mental illness, Hollingshead and Redlich (1958) found that the *incidence* of newly diagnosed cases of schizophrenia showed a moderate inverse relationship with socioeconomic status. In Table 13-2 it may be seen that the rate in class V is twice as high as that in class IV, and three times as high as that in classes I and II combined. However, the

same table shows even more dramatically an inverse relationship between social class and total *prevalence* rate for all schizophrenics, whether receiving treatment or custodial care. The rate for class V is three times as high as that for class IV and about eight times as high as that for classes I and II combined. The authors tentatively concluded that the *excess of psychoses from the poorer classes* was a product of the life conditions among the lower socioeconomic strata, and also that the *greater tendency to chronicity among members of the lower classes* was related to the poorer quality of psychiatric treatment they received. The latter was particularly true at the time of this important study (based on an extensive census carried out in 1950), but there have since been many changes in the treatment of schizophrenias, the most important of which are the widespread use of antipsychotic medication and increased emphasis on treatment in the community.

Labelling and Communication of the Schizophrenic Role

Bateson and his associates (1956) advanced the concept of a *double-bind* pattern of communication that provokes behavior characteristic of schizophrenia. Weakland (1960) elaborated the essential characteristics of the double-bind situation as follows: (1) In a double-bind situation, a person is faced with a significant communication involving a pair of messages of different level or logical type which are related but incongruent with each other. (2) Leaving the field is blocked.

Table 13-2. Incidence and Prevalence Rates per 100,000 for Schizophrenia, by Social Class (New Haven, Conn., 1950)

Social Class	Six-month Incidence	Prevalence
I and II	6	111
III	8	168
IV	10	300
V	20	895

Adapted from Hollingshead, A.B., and Redlich, F.C., *Social Class and Mental Illness.* Copyright 1958 by John Wiley and Sons, Inc. P. 236.

(3) It is therefore important to respond adequately to the communication situation, which includes responding to its duality and contradiction. (4) An adequate response is difficult to achieve because of the concealment, denial, and inhibition inherent in or added to the basic contradictory pair of messages.

At about this time, some social scientists become convinced that the behavior of staff members in mental hospitals was largely responsible for the adoption of a chronic role by some patients. Garfinkel (1956) wrote on the conditions of successful "degradation ceremonies" such as the psychiatric examination, and Erving Goffman (1961) emphasized the total loss of civil liberties resulting from imprisonment in an asylum. Thomas Szasz (1961) wrote on the "myth" of mental illness, and many others have come to believe that schizophrenia is merely a convenient label that initiates a self-fulfilling prophecy, through indoctrination of the patient in a process of social alienation and dehumanization.

Ronald Laing (1967) has been one of the most persuasive advocates of the position that there is no such condition as schizophrenia, but that the label is a social fact and political event. According to Laing, "It is a social prescription that rationalizes a set of social actions whereby the labelled person is annexed by others, who are legally sanctioned, medically empowered, and morally obliged, to become responsible for the person labelled. The person labelled is inaugurated not only into a role, but into a career of patient, by the concerted action of a coalition (a 'conspiracy') of family, G.P., mental health officer, psychiatrists, nurses, psychiatric social workers, and often fellow patients . . . ." Toward the end of this interpretation of the schizophrenic, Laing reached the following conclusion: "Perhaps we can still retain the now old name, and read into it its etymological meaning: *schiz* – 'broken'; *phrenos* – 'soul' or 'heart.'"

The preceding view may be more relevant to the significance of *perpetuating* factors in reducing the effectiveness of treatment than it is to *predisposition* and prevention. It does not refute the compelling evidence in favor of a medical model that has been provided by Kety (1974) and others.

TREATMENT OF SCHIZOPHRENIAS

Many attempts have been made to apply modified psychoanalytic techniques and other forms of intensive individual psychotherapy as the primary treatment in schizophrenia. Harry Stack Sullivan pioneered the development of social milieu therapy for young hospitalized schizophrenics, and many private hospitals in this country continue to favor relatively long-term psychotherapies, initiated on an inpatient basis and continued following discharge from hospital. Glick and his associates (1976) compared treatment results for 141 schizophrenic patients randomly assigned to short-term (21 to 28 days) or long-term (90 to 120 days) hospitalization. Test results showed that the long-term group was functioning significantly better one year after admission. However, the differences were modest and may have been confounded by the amount of psychotherapy patients received after hospitalization. These findings appear to conflict with a number of other findings reported in recent years.

Insulin coma treatment was regarded by many psychiatrists as the treatment of choice for physically healthy schizophrenics (under the age of about 40 years) for a period of about 20 years after its introduction by Manfred Sakel (1933). During the same two decades, however, many schizophrenic patients received various convulsive therapies, and a substantial minority were subjected to *psychosurgery (lobotomy)*. The latter was usually reserved for chronic schizophrenic patients who had been psychotic for many years, and the standard lobotomy caused more brain damage than other varieties of psychosurgery. Hence, the results of lobotomy in schizophrenias were generally far less favorable than in disorders characterized by incapacitating depression or anxiety.

Drug Therapy

Both insulin coma therapy and psychosurgery have become largely obsolete since the availability of chlorpromazine (1953) and other *antipsychotic drugs.* The *convulsive therapies* are likely to be reserved for patients with suicidal depression (including schizo-affective psychoses) and patients with catatonic withdrawal to the point of life-threatening dehydration (which fails to respond to adequate dosage and duration of psychotherapeutic medication).

Within a few years after the introduction of phenothiazines, there was a reversal of the previous trend toward accumulation of chronic schizophrenic patients in state hospitals. However, it was soon found that *readmission rates* rose dramatically among those discharged patients who failed to continue taking antipsychotic medication after discharge. Pasamanick, Scarpitti, and Dinitz (1967) provided a dramatic demonstration of the *effectiveness of drug therapy alone in maintaining schizophrenic patients in the community.* Decompensating schizophrenic patients were assigned randomly to one of three groups as follows: home on drugs (40 percent), home on placebo or inert medication (30 percent), and hospital care (control group, 30 percent). More than 77 percent of the first group (home on drugs) but only about 34 percent of the patients taking placebos remained in the community throughout their participation in the project. Even after initial hospitalization averaging 83 days, the third group (hospital controls) failed more often at the termination of treatment than did the home-care patients. Various related findings pointed to long-term drug therapy in the community as the preferred treatment for many schizophrenic patients who would otherwise have been admitted routinely to state hospitals.

In another major study, Philip May (1968) compared five treatments for schizophrenic inpatients: ataraxic (antipsychotic) drugs alone; individual psychotherapy alone; a combination of psychotherapy and ataraxic drugs; electroshock; and milieu therapy without specific treatments. The results showed clearly and convincingly that either drug therapy or a combination of drugs with psychotherapy was the most effective form of treatment for most hospitalized schizophrenic patients. Milieu therapy alone was the least effective treatment for most hospitalized schizophrenic patients.

to be ineffective. Electroshock therapy was intermediate in effectiveness between the two drug treatments and the two nondrug treatments. The results of a five-year follow-up on these 228 patients are now being reported. Patients in the original milieu therapy or psychotherapy alone groups required more days in hospital after the initial discharge, whether rated successes or failures during their experimental treatment, and in spite of the fact that follow-up care was not experimentally controlled and therefore was optimized for all patients.

In spite of the demonstrated effectiveness of outpatient medication, many patients fail to take psychotherapeutic drugs in recommended doses over a prolonged period of time. Sometimes the accidental omission of a few doses leads to rapid decompensation, with disruption of marginal relationships with employers, fellow employees, or family members, and readmission to hospital. The adverse consequences of *repeated relapses may be preventable by administration of long-acting injectable fluphenazine enanthate* or *fluphenazine decanoate.* Denham and Adamson (1971) reported that they were able to maintain 96 of 103 patients on continuous medication for a period of 12 to 40 months. During the follow-up period there was a significant reduction in psychiatric readmission rates from a previous total of 191 to a total of 50 during identical periods of time.

Brown and his associates (1972) noted an *interaction between medication and family relationships* on the course of schizophrenic disorders. In their carefully controlled study, relapse was strongly associated with expression of emotion by key relatives, particularly dissatisfaction and criticism of the patient. Those patients living with highly critical relatives (and therefore the most vulnerable to relapse) were also most susceptible to protective effects from maintenance drug therapy.

In a review of 24 controlled studies on the use of maintenance antipsychotic drugs, Davis (1975) noted that 65 percent of patients receiving a placebo relapsed, in contrast with 30 percent of those receiving maintenance antipsychotics. However, the possibility of a severe *postschizophrenic depressive syndrome* should not be overlooked, particularly in view of a North American tendency to overdiagnose schizophrenia while underdiagnosing mood disorders. McGlashen and Carpenter (1976) rated the frequency of postpsychotic depressive syndrome as high as 50 percent; such patients merit appropriate psychotherapeutic intervention as well as realistic modification of their drug treatment.

PARANOID DISORDERS

Theoretical Descriptive Continuum of Paranoid Psychoses

Paranoid psychotic disorders are characterized by the presence of one or more *delusions,* usually of persecution or grandeur. Hallucinations are usually absent, and any disorders of thinking, mood, or behavior are attributable to the basic delusional beliefs. Delusions appear relatively logical and well systematized, and there may be little evidence of regression in social behavior and no deterioration of personality over a period of years.

There is a theoretical descriptive continuum, extending from *true paranoia* at one extreme, to *paranoid schizophrenia* at the other extreme, with other *paranoid disorders* or *paraphrenias* occupying intermediate positions.

PARANOIA. Paranoia is derived from Greek roots meaning beside (or beyond or near) one's mind (or intellect or reason). In ancient times it was applied to any form of insanity, but was gradually restricted to mental disorders characterized by delusional thinking. Kahlbaum (1863) defined paranoia as a well-systematized delusional state of gradual development, little influenced by life experience, and without hallucinations or other disturbances in thinking. Many years later, however, Kolle (1931) undertook a long-term study of 66 patients with an initial diagnosis of paranoia (including 19 patients described by Kraepelin). Ninety percent of these patients had first become psychotic after the age of 35 years, and a number of family histories were positive for schizophrenia. Many of the patients themselves appeared to have

developed primary symptoms of schizophrenia by the time of the follow-up study. The diagnosis is now extremely rare, and is used mainly as a theoretical construct.

OTHER PARANOID DISORDERS. Other paranoid disorders, or paraphrenias, consist of delusional systems that are less logical than those of true paranoia, but are not associated with the disturbances of thinking and affect that characterize schizophrenia. However, many of these disorders develop during the involutional age range, in persons with a positive family history for schizophrenias (and *not* for mood or affective disorders). A long-term follow-up study of 78 patients diagnosed as paraphrenic by Kraepelin revealed that more than half of them had subsequently developed typical signs of schizophrenia. Hence, there is a strong tendency to regard paranoid disorders as late-onset forms of paranoid schizophrenia; however, late onset is *not* an essential component of such syndromes.

PARANOID PERSONALITY. Paranoid personality characteristics are usually present long before the development of established delusions. These characteristics include mistrust, hypersensitivity, unwarranted suspiciousness, jealousy, envy, inability to accept criticism, and a tendency to *project* unacceptable motives onto others. Ascribing evil motives to others often leads to a self-fulfilling prophecy, whereby the negative expectations are communicated nonverbally, thus inviting rejection and abuse. The role of jealousy as a basis for delusions of infidelity is further illustrated by the following quotation from *Othello:* "Trifles light as air are to the jealous confirmations strong as proofs of holy writ."

PARANOID MISINTERPRETATION OF REALITY. Paranoid misinterpretation of reality involves three defense mechanisms discussed in Chapter 1: repression, denial (of unacceptable motivation in oneself), and projection of evil intentions onto others. The reader is referred back to the initial chapter for discussion of Freud's interpretation of paranoid psychoses as being based on latent homosexuality, as well as repression, denial, and projection. His analysis was derived from the autobiography of Schreber, a paranoid psychotic who reported the fantasy of being female during sexual intercourse.

Social isolation appears to be the common denominator for the development of many paranoid psychoses, including: (1) those following the onset of deafness; (2) those occurring in aliens following migration (with lingual and cultural isolation, compounded by horizontal and vertical displacement, loss of status, etc.); (3) those occurring during the involutional or senile age ranges, often associated with death or loss of spouse and friends, including former fellow employees (through retirement).

Kay and Roth (1961) undertook a clinical follow-up and genetic study of 99 patients aged 60 years and over with "late paraphrenia," who had been admitted to either of two mental hospitals (one in England, the other in Sweden). Both groups showed similar characteristics, which included a *predominance of females over males* (in a ratio of about 7 : 1), and an excess of unmarried patients among both sexes. In contrast to comparable patients with mood disorders, significantly more paranoid patients were *living alone* at the time they became psychotic and many more of the paranoid patients were socially isolated. This social isolation resulted from a variety of factors including deafness, personality abnormalities, and relatively few surviving relatives. It was partly a consequence of self-segregation but also partly a contributing causal factor.

FOLIE À DEUX. Folie à deux is a relatively rare disorder in which two closely related persons, usually in the same family, share the same delusions. It has been referred to by a variety of other terms, the best known of which is probably *the psychosis of association.* Among 109 pairs recorded in the literature by 1942, Gralnick reported that 40 consisted of two sisters, 26 pairs of husband and wife, 24 of mother and child, 11 of 2 brothers, 6 of brother and sister, and 2 of father and child.

The prevailing mood of paranoid patients may be one of extreme apprehension, of misery, or of rage and hostility. This prevailing mood will often determine the direction taken by irrational behavior. The latter may consist of social withdrawal to the life of a recluse; flight to escape from imagined persecutors; suicide; or various forms of counterattack. These may involve repeated litigation, assault, or sometimes homicide. The well-known M'Naghten test for criminal responsibility was developed in relation to a paranoid patient who had committed homicide.

TREATMENT. Treatment follows the same principles applied in the treatment of schizophrenic disorders. The main differences are related to age at onset, duration of delusions prior to treatment, and the reality situation to which the patient must adapt. This usually involves a combination of psychosocial therapies with antipsychotic medication. This approach has resulted in an improved prognosis for patients with paranoid disorders, provided long-term maintenance therapy is undertaken.

REVIEW QUESTIONS

156. The most frequent type of hallucination experienced by schizophrenics is:
    (A) visual
    (B) tactile (haptic)
    (C) olfactory
    (D) gustatory
    (E) auditory

157. Bleuler's primary symptoms of schizophrenias include each of the following except:
    (A) association disturbance
    (B) autism
    (C) ambivalence
    (D) affective disturbance
    (E) acting out

158. The prognosis in schizophrenias is *less* favorable:
    (A) when there is emotional blunting
    (B) in women than in men
    (C) when there is a rapid onset of psychosis
    (D) when anxiety is prominent
    (E) for patients of higher intelligence

159. Which of the following is most characteristically disturbed in schizophrenias?

(A) thinking
(B) interpersonal relations
(C) perception
(D) volition
(E) impulse control

160. During which age range is the hospital *first admission rate* for schizophrenia the highest?
    (A) 15 to 24 years
    (B) 25 to 34 years
    (C) 35 to 44 years
    (D) 45 to 54 years
    (E) 55 years and older

Directions: For questions 161 through 168, *match* the description or statement with the subtype of schizophrenia for which it is most true. Each of the subtypes might be used once, more than once, or not at all as a correct answer.

    (A) simple schizophrenia
    (B) hebephrenic schizophrenia
    (C) paranoid schizophrenia
    (D) schizo-affective schizophrenia
    (E) catatonic schizophrenia

161. Lability and inappropriateness of affect is most commonly seen in which subtype?

162. Which is the most frequently diagnosed subtype (in the United States) among schizophrenics recently admitted to the hospital?

163. Delusions and hallucinations are *least* prominent in which subtype?

164. Which subtype of schizophrenia is most likely to be difficult to distinguish from manic-depressive psychosis?

165. Phases of excitement or stupor, echopraxia, and negativism are likely to be observed in which subtype?

166. Insidious loss of interests, progressive social withdrawal, and deterioration of school or occupational performance are the most common early signs of which subtype?

167. The highest risk of suicide is associated with which subtype?

168. Poorly structured or silly behavior, with grimacing, mannerisms, and bizarre clothing and grooming are commonly seen in which subtype?

Summary of Directions

A	B	C	D	E
1, 2, 3 only	1, 3 only	2, 4 only	4 only	All are correct

169. The *empirical lifetime risk* of schizophrenia is currently estimated as:
    (1) 1% for the entire population
    (2) 40% to 65% among the offspring of two schizophrenic parents
    (3) 10% to 15% among siblings of schizophrenic patients
    (4) 10% to 15% if only one parent is schizophrenic

170. Examples of paranoid characteristics include:
    (1) grandiosity
    (2) litigiousness
    (3) mistrust
    (4) assaultiveness

171. The prognosis for recovery following an acute schizophrenic episode is *more favorable* if:
    (1) there are clear precipitating factors that can be modified
    (2) the patient is married
    (3) the symptoms are distressing to the patient
    (4) the premorbid personality type was schizoid

172. Process schizophrenias are *more likely* than reactive schizophrenias to be associated with:
    (1) family history of schizophrenia
    (2) simple, hebephrenic, and catatonic diagnostic subtypes
    (3) onset during adolescence
    (4) low socioeconomic status

173. Symptoms that strongly favor a diagnosis of schizophrenia rather than any other mental disorder include:
    (1) sudden and pronounced deterioration of social habits
    (2) neologisms
    (3) paranoid delusions
    (4) mutism and waxy flexibility

174. Good principles to follow in the treatment

of nonschizophrenic paranoid patients include:

(1) avoidance of medications unless the patient requests them

(2) confrontation of the patient about the irrational nature of his delusions

(3) outpatient treatment rather than involuntary hospitalization if voluntary admission to hospital is refused

(4) scrupulous honesty on the part of the therapist

175. Patients with a diagnosis of paranoid state usually differ from patients with a diagnosis of paranoid schizophrenia on the basis of:

(1) absence of long-term regression and personality deterioration

(2) later age of onset of psychosis

(3) the logical, systematized nature of the delusions

(4) relatively lower levels of anxiety and depression

SELECTED REFERENCES

1. Ayd, F.J., Jr. (1975). The depot fluphenazines: A reappraisal after 10 years' clinical experience. *American Journal of Psychiatry,* vol. 132, pages 491–500.

2. Bateson, G., Jackson, D.D., Haley, J., and Weakland, J.H. (1956). Toward a theory of schizophrenia. *Behavioral Science,* vol. 1, pages 256–264.

3. Brown, G.W., Birley, J.L.T., and Wing, J.K. (1972). Influences of family life on the course of schizophrenic disorders: A replication. *British Journal of Psychiatry,* vol. 121, pages 241–258.

4. Cohen, S.M., Allen, M.G., Pollin, W., and Hrubec, Z. (1972). Relationship of schizoaffective psychosis to manic depressive psychosis and schizophrenia. *Archives of General Psychiatry,* vol. 26, pages 539–545.

5. Davis, J.M. (1975). Overview: Maintenance therapy in psychiatry. I. Schizophrenia. *American Journal of Psychiatry,* vol. 132, pages 1237–1245.

6. Denham, J., and Adamson, L. (1971). The contribution of fluphenazine enanthate and decanoate in the prevention of re-admission of schizophrenic patients. *Acta Psychiatrica Scandinavica,* vol. 47, pages 420–430.

7. Fleck, S., Lidz, T., and Cornelison, A. (1963). Comparison of parent-child relationships of male and female schizophrenic patients. *Archives of General Psychiatry,* vol. 8, pages 1–7.

8. Glick, I.D., Hargreaves, W.A., Drues, J., Showstack, J.A. (1976). Short versus long hospitalization: A prospective controlled study. IV. One-year followup results for schizophrenic patients. *American Journal of Psychiatry,* vol. 133, pages 509–514.

9. Gottesman, I.I., and Shields, J. (1966). Schizophrenia in twins: 16 years' consecutive admissions to a psychiatric clinic. *British Journal of Psychiatry,* vol. 112, pages 809–818.

10. Gralnick, A. (1942). Folie à deux: The psychosis of association. *Psychiatric Quarterly,* vol. 16, pages 230–260.

11. Gregory, I. (1960). Genetic factors in schizophrenia. *American Journal of Psychiatry,* vol. 116, pages 961–972.

12. Haley, J. (1969). The art of being schizophrenic. In *The Power Tactics of Jesus Christ and Other Essays.* New York: Grossman.

13. Harlow, H.F. (1962). The heterosexual affectional system in monkeys. *American Psychologist,* vol. 17, pages 1–9.

14. Heston, L.L. (1966). Psychiatric disorders in foster home reared children of schizophrenic mothers. *British Journal of Psychiatry,* vol. 112, pages 819–825.

15. Hollingshead, A.B., and Redlich, F.C. (1959). *Social Class and Mental Illness.* New York: John Wiley and Sons. Chapter 8.

16. Inouye, E. (1961). Similarity and dissimilarity of schizophrenia in twins. In *World Congress of Psychiatry,* vol. 1, pages 524–530. Montreal, Canada: McGill University Press.

17. Kay, D.W., and Roth, M. (1961). Environmental and hereditary factors in the schizo-

phrenias of old age ("late paraphrenia") and their bearing on the general problem of causation in schizophrenia. *Journal of Mental Science,* vol. 107, pages 649–686.

18. Kety, S.S. (1974). From rationalization to reason. *American Journal of Psychiatry,* vol. 131, pages 957–963.

19. Laing, R.D. (1967). *The Politics of Experience.* New York: Ballantine Books. Chapter 5.

20. Lidz, T., and Fleck, S. (1960). Schizophrenia, human integration and the role of the family. In *The Etiology of Schizophrenia,* edited by D. D. Jackson. New York: Basic Books. Chapter 11.

21. Matthyse, S., and Kety, S.S. [Eds.] (1975). *Symposium on Catecholamines and Their Enzymes in the Neuropathology of Schizophrenia.* New York: Pergamon Press.

22. May, P.R.A. (1968). *Treatment of Schizophrenia.* New York: Science House.

23. May, P.R.A., Tuma, A.H., Yale, C., Potepan, P., and Dixon, W.J. (1976). Schizophrenia – A followup study of results of treatment. II. Hospital stay over two to five years. *Archives of General Psychiatry,* vol. 33, pages 481–486.

24. McGlashan, T.H., and Carpenter, W.T., Jr. (1976). An investigation of the postpsychotic depressive syndrome. *American Journal of Psychiatry,* vol. 133, pages 14–19.

25. Pasamanick, B., Scarpitti, F.R., and Dinitz, S. (1967). *Schizophrenics in the Community.* New York: Appleton-Century-Crofts.

26. Rosenthal, D. (1959). Some factors associated with concordance and discordance with respect to schizophrenia in monozygotic twins. *Journal of Nervous and Mental Disease,* vol. 129, pages 1–10.

27. Rosenthal, D., and Kety, S.S. [Eds.] (1968). *The Transmission of Schizophrenia. Journal of Psychiatric Research,* vol. 6, suppl. 1. New York: Pergamon Press.

14. Mood Disorders (Affective Disorders)

Ah, could my anguish but be measured and my calamity laid with it in the scales, they would now outweigh the sands of the sea!
The Book of Job

*And if I laugh at any mortal thing,
'Tis that I may not weep.*
George Noel Gordon, Lord Byron

OVERVIEW OF MOOD DISORDERS

Mood disorders, or *affective disorders,* have been defined as any mental disorders in which a disturbance of mood (affect) is predominant. Unfortunately, this simple definition conceals several uncertainties and disagreements that need some elaboration.

In the first place, these affective disorders refer only to extreme depression or elation, and not to either of the other primary moods (i.e., fear or anger).

In the second place, the disturbances in mood may so dominate the syndrome that they are regarded as basic, whereas accompanying disturbances in thinking or behavior are regarded as accessory to the prevailing mood disorder. Beck (1967) argued strongly that representing depression as an affective disorder is as misleading as it would be to designate scarlet fever as a disorder of the skin or as a primary febrile disorder. There are many aspects to depression other than the mood deviation, and Beck recognized five components: (1) a specific alteration in mood (sadness, loneliness, apathy); (2) a negative self-concept (with self-reproach and self-blame); (3) regressive and self-punitive wishes (desires to escape, hide, or die); (4) vegetative changes (anorexia, insomnia, and loss of libido); and (5) change in activity level (retardation or agitation).

A third major difficulty in our initial definition concerns the breadth or narrowness of the category. When defined broadly, disorders of mood have included depressive neuroses (neurotic depressive reactions) and psychotic depressive reactions, as well as the affective psychoses, or major mood disorders. Defined more narrowly, the latter disorders include only involutional melancholia and manic-depressive illness. Manic-depressive illness has recently been recategorized as *unipolar* if it involves deviations of mood in only one direction (i.e., repeated episodes of mania or depression, but *not* both), or *bipolar* when it involves both manic and depressive episodes in the same person (formerly called the circular type).

Reactive vs Endogenous Mood Disorders

It appears likely that at least some forms of mood disorder involve varying interactions between biological predisposition and psychosocial precipitating factors. The latter precipitating factors are obvious in reactive or exogenous disorders — depressive neuroses and psychotic depressive reactions. Sometimes they appear to be absent in the major affective disorders (involutional melancholia and manic-depressive illnesses), so that the latter are regarded as endogenous. However, even manic episodes may sometimes develop immediately following severe psychosocial stress, such as loss of health with impending death. The relative contributions of biological and psychosocial factors to the development of mood disorders do *not* currently constitute a firm basis for their classification. However, the essential characteristics of the tradional categories may now be summarized.

GRIEF. Normal grief has three characteristics: (1) It is a response to a real external loss that is consciously recognized. (2) It is appropriate in degree or severity. (3) It is within the normal limits of duration for the type of loss sustained. The most severe grief reactions are usually those associated with the death of a dearly loved person. Lindemann (1944) made a systematic study of this reaction in an adult population and reported the following as symptoms of normal grief: sensations of somatic distress; preoccupation with the image of the deceased; guilt feelings involving real or imagined negligence regarding the deceased; feelings of hostility toward physicians and others, charging them with not properly caring for the deceased prior to death; and a change in patterns of conduct, such as restlessness and inability to organize normal activities or to carry on customary social pleasantries. He further stated that normal acute grief lasts four to eight weeks, but most authors and clinicians recognize that normal grief and sorrow may be prolonged up to a year or two after a severe loss. It should also be noted that the symptoms may be more intense and intrusive several months after the loss than immediately following the event, as the defensive maneuver of denial loses effectiveness and the full impact of the loss is recognized.

Grief and other depressive reactions of varying intensity and duration are quite commonly encountered among patients (and their relatives) on general medical, surgical, and pediatric wards of hospitals. In addition to impending separation from loved ones by death, significant losses encountered among this group include loss of productive capacity and financial security, ability to engage in previously valued activities, and ability to remain self-sustaining. Proper psychological management in these patients has a major impact on prognosis, and must take into account the previous personality characteristics of the individuals involved and the unconscious significance of the loss in addition to its external nature.

DEPRESSIVE NEUROSIS. Depressive neurosis, or neurotic depressive reaction, has been distinguished on the following bases: (1) It is a response to a precipitating event or situation that may be either an external loss or an internal conflict. (2) It is usually excessively severe in degree relative to the precipitating circumstances but does not involve gross impairment of reality testing nor functional inadequacy so excessive as to be labeled psychotic. (3) It is likely to be of disproportionately long duration. (4) There may be a long history of neurotic personality characteristics and symptoms, which usually include anxiety, apprehensiveness, emotional lability, and previous episodes of depression.

PSYCHOTIC DEPRESSIVE REACTION. This has long been considered a controversial label, defined on the basis of: (1) precipitating events or circumstances similar to those in a neurotic depressive reaction (i.e., external loss or internal conflict); (2) impairment of reality testing or functional adequacy that is severe enough to be considered psychotic rather than neurotic; and (3) the absence of a previous history of severe depression or marked cyclothymic mood swings. The last requirement is meant to exclude recurrent unipolar or bipolar affective disorders, but sometimes the first episode may be not recognized as such and therefore mislabeled.

INVOLUTIONAL MELANCHOLIA. This is another category over which there has been considerable controversy throughout the present century. It has traditionally been defined on the basis of the following: (1) Onset is during the involutional age range (roughly 40 to 55 or 60 years) in women, and after the age of 55 or 60 years in men. These ages have corresponded with the maximum frequencies of successful suicide in the corresponding sex. (2) Significant exogenous stress or adverse life experiences are minimal or absent. This is a highly debatable criterion, since aging is often accompanied by cumulative experiences of loss (e.g., of personal health, interpersonal relationships, or economic security). (3) The depression is severe in degree, with psychotic impairment of reality testing and functional adequacy. Untreated patients were likely to be severely agitated and grossly delusional, expressing delusions of extreme sinfulness, nihilism (e.g., "I have no bowels"), bizarre somatic changes, and sometimes persecution. Auditory hallucinations, usually of reproachful or accusing voices that may suggest suicide or threaten retribution, may also be experienced. (4) Without treatment, the duration is often prolonged for many years in the absence of death from suicide or other complications. (5) The previous personality is usually described as obsessive-compulsive, with perfectionistic striving and meticulous attention to detail and cleanliness. (6) The family history is usually negative for relatives with recurrent episodes of unipolar or bipolar mood disorders, and often has an increased incidence of schizophrenic or paranoid disorders.

MANIC-DEPRESSIVE PSYCHOSIS. Manic-depressive psychosis (unipolar or bipolar) has been distinguished on the following bases: (1) absence of consistent external precipitating stress; (2) severe deviations in mood (mania or depression or both), with psychotic impairment of reality testing and social function; (3) a strong tendency to remission and recurrence; (4) a history of cyclothymic personality characteristics with alternation between (a) cheerful, energetic, and extraverted behavior, and (b) discouragement, inertia, and social withdrawal; (5) a frequent family history of major mood disorders with mania, depression, or suicide. The contrast between manic excitement and the despair of melancholy has been recognized since antiquity. It is nearly 2,000 years since Aretaeus noted the occurrence of both extremes in the same individual, and it is more than 100 years since Falret described such mood alternations as *la folie circulaire* or *la folie à double forme*. Kraepelin (1899) proposed the term *manic-depressive psychosis* and later reported a large series of patients in which the relative frequency of various forms was as follows: recurrent depressive episodes only, 49 percent; recurrent manic episodes only, 17 percent; and circular or combined, 34 percent. In a longer-term follow-up study in the United States, Rennie (1942) reported as follows: depression only, 67 percent; manic only, 9 percent; and combined, 24 percent. The strong tendency toward recurrence is also illustrated by Rennie's series of 208 cases that were followed for more than 30 years. Only 21 percent of these patients had a single episode, whereas 79 percent had at least two, 63 percent had at least three, and 45 percent had four or more episodes. The duration of each successive episode remains about the same (formerly an average of three to six months), but the symptom-free interval tends to decrease following each successive attack, particularly in circular or bipolar disorders.

Manic and Hypomanic Disorders

HYPOMANIA. Manic episodes are usually preceded by a prodromal phase known as hypomania, which may last from a few hours to many weeks. The classic triad of hypomanic symptoms is: (1) elated but unstable mood; (2) pressure of speech; and (3) increased motor activity. These symptoms are usually accompanied by reduced attention to physical needs (sleeping and eating), which may go unnoticed for a long period since the patient is unlikely to complain about them. Other changes that are quite characteristic include carelessness or flamboyance in appearance, a gay and animated attitude, loss of social inhibitions (sometimes resembling mild alcohol intoxication), and reckless, impulsive, and sometimes dangerous behavior. In the early stages hypomanic patients are viewed as outgoing, friendly, genial, witty, and good-natured. As the disorder progresses they become sarcastic, irritable, vulgar, aggressive, impatient, and intolerant.

MANIA. The hypomanic state may subside as abruptly or as gradually as it arose or it may progress to full-blown mania, in which case spontaneous speech increases in speed and volume until the patient may become hoarse. He is constantly stimulated by both new thoughts arising internally and by the external environment. It is therefore usually possible to hold his attention long enough to obtain brief answers or attempts at appropriate answers to questions. Thought disorder becomes apparent in the form of flight of ideas and tangentiality, which in severe cases may progress to clang associations and even incoherence. The content of speech tends to reflect a mood of unwarranted optimism, and is filled with puns, rhymes, and obscure jokes that the patient finds hilariously funny.

There is little or no impairment of intellectual functions accompanying mild hypomanic symptoms, but increasing carelessness and shortness of attention span results in numerous errors, and impairment of measured intellectual function can become extreme in advanced mania. Memory and orientation may be difficult to assess, but they are only likely to be grossly impaired in the most severe cases of delirious mania.

Perceptual disturbances (illusions and hallucinations) are not characteristic, but were formerly reported in about 30 percent of cases and can be present in advanced manic states. True delusions are also associated only with severe cases, and then will usually involve ideas of grandeur or great wealth, and occasionally of persecution.

The prevailing emotional tone is euphoric, but is likely to be quite labile and unstable. In some cases there may be short-lived episodes of tearfulness and other manifestations of depression. Mania has in fact been interpreted dynamically as a defense against depression, that involves both denial and reaction formation. There may also be considerable hostility directed toward those in the immediate environment, which may take the form of sarcasm, ideas of persecution, and even assaultive behavior. In public, the manic patient may be viewed as severely drunk.

The loss of inhibitions and internal controls results in various manifestations of diminished or absent superego, such as sexual promiscuity or aggressiveness, financial irresponsibility, dangerous automobile driving, threatening or injurious behavior toward others, and other blatantly antisocial behaviors. Judgment and insight are severely impaired.

A manic state can be a life-threatening illness. Some patients die from physical exhaustion or dehydration or from adverse effects on preexisting somatic conditions (e.g., cardiovascular disease). Others die from reckless behavior or accident and a few commit suicide. There is also danger of accidental or deliberate harm to innocent bystanders or to concerned relatives or friends who attempt to intervene. It should not be overlooked that the social consequences can also be severe, since the manic patient may deplete his family's resources, alienate himself from significant persons (family, employers, friends), and suffer harm to personal reputation, credit rating, etc. For these reasons, manic episodes require hospital care in a setting that is prepared to deal with disruptive, aggressive, hyperactive behavior. Because of the likelihood of recurrence, family and friends should be educated about the nature of the illness and alerted to the necessity of seeking assistance whenever clearcut hypomanic symptoms return.

DELIRIOUS MANIA. Delirious mania is the most extreme state, and is fortunately rare. All of the previously mentioned symptoms may be present in extreme form. The patient is totally out of contact, with incoherent speech and extremely agitated behavior. Hallucinations and delusions are common, and urinary and fecal incontinence are not unusual. Since the patient is completely unable to cooperate, the condition may be difficult to distinguish from catatonic excitation or from a severe acute brain syndrome of delirium. Because of its similarity to the latter, and the multitude of physical complications, some authorities consider this condition to be a true organic brain syndrome. Rapid medical intervention (by ECT or high doses of an antipsychotic drug such as haloperidol which has minimal effect on blood pressure) is crucial.

BECK'S DEPRESSION INVENTORY

It is not difficult to make a diagnosis of depression when the patient's chief complaint is dysphoric mood, or when he first receives medical attention following an episode of self-destructive behavior. The physician may suspect depression when the patient comes unwillingly, at the behest of his family who are concerned about irritability or other severe changes in behavior. However, the number and variety of symptoms accompanying depressive disorders is great, and a large proportion of these patients will first consult their primary care physician with some combination of somatic complaints. Among the most common of these are: fatigue, exhaustion, and loss of energy; loss of appetite and weight (or an increase in both); sleep disturbances of all sorts, including both insomnia and hypersomnia; changes in sexual function or behavior; headaches; constipation; loss of interest or enjoyment in previously valued activities; and a recent increase in accident-proneness. The physician should also suspect depression when the patient's symptoms elude explanation on a physiological or anatomical basis; when they fail to respond well to usual treatment methods; when the pattern of symptoms is vague or constantly changing; and when patterns of alcohol or other drug use begin to emerge. The depressed patient often becomes hypersensitive to pain and is preoccupied with trivial problems (although he may not always complain of them).

Many rating scales and check lists have been constructed in attempts to measure various aspects of psychopathology quantitatively. One widely used self-reporting index of depression is scale 2 of the Minnesota Multiphasic Personality Inventory (MMPI), which was reviewed briefly in Chapter 4. The score on this scale is derived from the responses to 60 true-false questions distributed among the 566 items in the entire test. The scale was derived empirically, and it would be difficult for a person to falsify his responses along a single dimension such as depression. Moreover, the test includes three validity scales that permit interpretation of the subject's test-taking attitude (inferences about defensiveness, cooperation, or overstatement of problems).

These advantages account for the widespread use of this standardized instrument in studies of depression and other psychiatric disorders and response to treatment. Factor analysis has identified five separate components of this scale, which were termed hypochondriasis, cycloid tendency, hostility, inferiority, and depression.

A number of tests consisting of adjective check-lists have been developed in order to measure the intensity of depression. However, the major mood disorders also involve cognitive, motivational, and behavioral components. Beck therefore constructed a self-reporting inventory having 21 categories of symptoms and attitudes. Each category consists of a graded series of four self-evaluative statements. Numerical values from 0 to 3 are assigned to each statement, corresponding with the severity of depression or associated impairment. The subject is asked to select the single statement in each category that corresponds most closely with the way he feels at the time. The sum total of all the numbers corresponding with those statements will therefore fall within the range of 0 to 63. A total Depression Inventory score of 25 or more indicates a severe or high level of depression. A score of 14 to 24 indicates a medium level of depression,

and scores from 0 to 13 indicate a relative lack of depression.

Beck's Depression Inventory is clearly subject to voluntary distortion or falsification by the subject if he wishes. However, it has been found to correlate highly with scale 2 of the MMPI and with the Hamilton Depression Scale, which involves a clinical interview and ratings made by the interviewer (correlations approximately + 0.75). It has also been found to correlate more highly than the MMPI with other pretreatment and posttreatment clinical ratings in studies of depressed patients. Its convenience has therefore led to widespread clinical application, by family practitioners as well as psychiatrists. It is reproduced here to demonstrate the various gradations of impairment in each of the 21 categories, and the many different types of symptoms which may accompany depression.

Beck's Depression Inventory

A. 0 I do not feel sad.
   1 I feel sad.
   2 I am sad all the time and I can't snap out of it.
   3 I am so sad or unhappy that I can't stand it.

B. 0 I am not particularly discouraged about the future.
   1 I feel discouraged about the future.
   2 I feel I have nothing to look forward to.
   3 I feel that the future is hopeless and that things cannot improve.

C. 0 I do not feel like a failure.
   1 I feel I have failed more than the average person.
   2 As I look back on my life, all I can see is a lot of failures.
   3 I feel I am a complete failure as a person.

D. 0 I get as much satisfaction out of things as I used to.
   1 I don't enjoy things the way I used to.
   2 I don't get real satisfaction out of anything any more.
   3 I am dissatisfied or bored with everything.

E. 0 I don't feel particularly guilty.
    1 I feel guilty a good part of the time.
    2 I feel quite guilty most of the time.
    3 I feel guilty all of the time.

F. 0 I don't feel I am being punished.
    1 I feel I may be punished.
    2 I expect to be punished.
    3 I feel I am being punished.

G. 0 I don't feel disappointed in myself.
    1 I am disappointed in myself.
    2 I am disgusted with myself.
    3 I hate myself.

H. 0 I don't feel I am any worse than anybody
       else.
    1 I am critical of myself for my weaknesses
       or mistakes.
    2 I blame myself all the time for my faults.
    3 I blame myself for everything bad that
       happens.

I. 0 I don't have any thoughts of killing myself.
    1 I have thoughts of killing myself, but I
       would not carry them out.
    2 I would like to kill myself.
    3 I would kill myself if I had the chance.

J. 0 I don't cry any more than usual.
    1 I cry more now than I used to.
    2 I cry all the time now.
    3 I used to be able to cry, but now I can't cry
       even though I want to.

K. 0 I am no more irritated now than I ever am.
    1 I get annoyed or irritated more easily than
       I used to.
    2 I feel irritated all the time now.
    3 I don't get irritated at all by the things that
       used to irritate me.

L. 0 I have not lost interest in other people.
    1 I am less interested in other people than I
       used to be.
    2 I have lost most of my interest in other
       people.
    3 I have lost all of my interest in other people.

M. 0 I make decisions about as well as I ever could.

    1 I put off making decisions more than I
       used to.
    2 I have greater difficulty in making decisions
       than before.
    3 I can't make decisions at all any more.

N. 0 I don't feel I look any worse than I used to.
    1 I am worried that I am looking old or un-
       attractive.
    2 I feel that there are permanent changes in my
       appearance that make me look unattractive.
    3 I believe that I look ugly.

O. 0 I can work about as well as before.
    1 It takes an extra effort to get started at
       doing something.
    2 I have to push myself very hard to do any-
       thing.
    3 I can't do any work at all.

P. 0 I can sleep as well as usual.
    1 I don't sleep as well as I used to.
    2 I wake up 1–2 hours earlier than usual and
       find it hard to get back to sleep.
    3 I wake up several hours earlier than I used to
       and cannot get back to sleep.

Q. 0 I don't get more tired than usual.
    1 I get tired more easily than I used to.
    2 I get tired from doing almost anything.
    3 I am too tired to do anything.

R. 0 My appetite is no worse than usual.
    1 My appetite is not as good as it used to be.
    2 My appetite is much worse now.
    3 I have no appetite at all any more.

S. 0 I haven't lost much weight, if any, lately.
    1 I have lost more than 5 pounds.
    2 I have lost more than 10 pounds.
    3 I have lost more than 15 pounds.

    I am purposely trying to lose weight by
    eating less. Yes_____ No_____

T. 0 I am no more worried about my health than
       usual.
    1 I am worried about physical problems such
       as aches and pains; or upset stomach; or
       constipation.

2 I am very worried about physical problems
   and it's hard to think of much else.

3 I am so worried about my physical problems that I cannot think about anything
   else.

U. 0 I have not noticed any recent change in my
       interest in sex.

    1 I am less interested in sex than I used to be.

    2 I am much less interested in sex now.

    3 I have lost interest in sex completely.

Reprinted by permission from A. T. Beck, M.D. Copyright 1975, Philadelphia, Pa.

SUICIDE

Suicide has been reported among roughly 5 percent
of patients with a history of one or more hospital-
izations for manic-depressive or other depressive
disorders. This is roughly five times the lifetime
expectation of suicide in the United States, which
averages about 1 percent for both sexes combined.
In this country, suicide accounts for roughly 0.5
percent of all deaths of females and 1.5 percent of
all deaths of males. This sex ratio for successful
suicide (3 males to 1 female) has remained fairly
consistent over a period of many years, as has a
similar tendency for suicide to be relatively more
frequent in old age than in young adult life. (See
Tables 14-1 and 14-2.) Successful suicide has

Table 14-1. Death Rates from Suicide,
by Age, United States, 1974

Age Group (Yrs.)	Suicide Rate per 100,000 Population
5–14	0.5
15–24	10.9
25–34	15.7
35–44	16.8
45–54	19.6
55–64	19.7
65–74	18.8
75–84	20.9
85 and over	17.5
All ages	12.1

Table 14-2. Age-adjusted Death Rates from
Suicide, by Race and Sex, United States, 1974

Race and Sex	Suicide Rate per 100,000 Population
White male	19.0
White female	7.1
White, both sexes	12.8
Nonwhite male	11.7
Nonwhite female	3.3
Nonwhite, both sexes	7.2
Total male	18.2
Total female	6.7
Total, both sexes	12.2

therefore been several times as frequent among
old men as among young women, but there has
been a recent reduction in this ratio. There have
also long been higher rates of successful suicide
among whites than blacks, and among those of
high socioeconomic origin who are in the process
of losing property and status (i.e., downward social
mobility). This finding corresponds with the increased suicide rates associated with economic
adversity in times of high unemployment, as discussed in Chapter 9 (Fig. 9-1).

In a retrospective study of 134 successful
suicides, Robins and his associates (1959) found
60 with manic-depressive depression, 31 with
chronic alcoholism, 5 with chronic brain syndromes, 3 with schizophrenia, and 2 with drug
addiction. Twenty-five were undiagnosed, but
were considered definitely psychiatrically ill, 5
were suffering from terminal medical illnesses, and
only 3 were apparently clinically well. It is a popular misconception that people who speak of committing suicide do not carry out their threats. In
the same study, Robins and his associates found
that at least 68 percent of suicides had communicated suicidal ideas, and 38 percent specifically
stated that they intended to kill themselves. *The
communication of suicidal intent is the best single
predictor of a successful attempt.*

Suicide *attempts* are more frequent among
women, the young, and persons with neuroses or
personality disorders who are more angry and

impulsive than persistently depressed. However, it is essential that suicidal potential be evaluated carefully on an individual and not a statistical basis. It should be remembered that suicide is more frequent *when a patient is recovering* from an episode of psychotic depression than at the time he is most immobilized by his despair and loss of initiative. This finding may be attributed to temporary reversal (with anticipated return to intolerable suffering), to increased opportunities during therapy, and to improvement in energy level and removal of the incapacitating inhibitions associated with the illness before the dysphoric affect is ameliorated. Suicidal risk may be greatest during weekend leaves from hospital and shortly after discharge. Among discharged patients, the risk of suicide is about four times as high in the first six months as in the second six months after discharge.

Homicide is far less likely to be carried out by patients with mood disorders than by those with antisocial personalities or paranoid disorders. However, a person who is suicidally depressed may also extend this death wish to immediate family members for whom the person feels most responsible. A severely depressed woman may kill her dependent infant preparatory to attempting suicide. A severely depressed man may kill his wife and children preparatory to his own attempted suicide. However, homicide involving members of the family is more likely to result from paranoid schizophrenic disorders than from depression.

PSYCHOSOCIAL DETERMINANTS OF MOOD DISORDERS

Karl Abraham (1911) regarded *ambivalence* as the basic characteristic of the depressed patient. In his classic paper on mourning and melancholia, Freud (1917) analyzed the self-reproaches of depressed patients and found them to have meaning if the name of an ambivalently regarded person (i.e., both loved and hated) was substituted for the patient's own name. The patient may say, "I am bad because I am a liar," when he has reason to say, "X is bad because he is a liar," or more specifically, "I am angry with X because he has lied to

me." This *introjection* of the ambivalently regarded person has been considered the opposite of the defense mechanism of projection, and the most characteristic defense observed in depression. However, depression also involves subjugation of the ego by a dominant and punitive (sadistic) superego. This would be expected to develop from an unduly moralistic upbringing, with emphasis on perfectionistic striving through constant criticism.

Abraham concluded that, "In the last resort melancholic depression is derived from disagreeable experiences in the childhood of the patient." However, he viewed these disagreeable experiences as sensitizing the patient, so that repetition of disappointment later in life would lead to the onset of depression. In recent years there have been a number of attempts to establish relationships between adult traumatization and possible childhood deprivation or sensitization.

Bereavement

Bruhn (1962) compared the histories of 91 persons who had attempted suicide with those of 91 nonsuicidal outpatients. Controlled comparisons between members of both groups indicated that the following *precipitating factors* were more frequent among those who had attempted suicide: (1) absence or death of a family member in the preceding year; (2) unemployment of the breadwinner in the family; (3) greater residential mobility; and (4) a greater degree of marital disharmony. The data also provided some confirmation of an increased frequency of parental loss during the childhood of those who had attempted suicide (42 percent versus 25 percent), and an increased sensitization of these orphaned persons to bereavement as adults. The precipitating factor of prolonged absence or death in the family during the preceding year was found among 66 percent of the attempted suicides from broken homes, as contrasted with 22 percent of nonsuicidal psychiatric outpatients from broken homes ($p < 0.0001$) or as contrasted with 42 percent of those attempted suicides who had not come from broken homes ($p < 0.05$).

Parental Death

Beck and his associates administered the Depression Inventory to a group of 297 psychiatric patients and found a significantly higher frequency of orphanhood (before age 16) among the 100 patients scoring highest on the Depression Inventory than among the 100 patients scoring lowest. Although the strength of the initial association was partly attributable to age of the patients (older patients tending to have experienced a higher frequency of orphanhood), statistical analysis indicated that childhood bereavement was probably a significant predisposing factor. Further evidence of relationships between childhood death of parents and adult depression comes from a well-controlled study by Dennehy (1966). In a series of 1,020 consecutive patients (under the age of 60) admitted to psychiatric wards in three hospitals serving areas of London, there were 111 males and 250 females with depressive diagnoses. Among the patients with depressive diagnoses she found an excess of *males* who had lost their *mothers,* and an excess of *females* who had lost their *fathers* before the age of 15 years. While some excess of parental loss was observed before the age of 10 years, it was most marked and statistically significant for depressed patients of both sexes when occurring between the ages of 10 and 15 years.

In a more recent study, Birtchnell (1970) found no overall difference in the frequency of death of a parent during the childhood of depressed as opposed to nondepressed patients. However, he found significant differences between the frequency of both early and recent parent death according to the severity of the depression. The incidence of early parent death and of recent parent death were both significantly higher in the severely depressed group, and in both instances this was found to be due to an excess of deaths of the mothers.

Family Characteristics

Paffenbarger and Asnes (1966) searched the college records obtained years previously from 225 male suicides and double the number of matched controls. Several contrasting features of their *family backgrounds* are indicated in Table 14-3.

Among the suicides, a higher proportion of both mothers and fathers had attended college, and father's occupation was more often professional, than among the controls. More of these male suicides had lost their father by death during childhood, and their parents had more frequently separated, than had those of the controls. Among the data *not* included in this table are other findings to the effect that suicides had more often attended secondary boarding schools; that they had more frequently reported insomnia, social isolation, anxiety, and depression; and that they had more frequently failed to graduate from college than had the control population. Apart from the high frequency of paternal death and parental separation, therefore, the suicides appeared to have come from families of higher socioeconomic status that placed a higher premium on achievement, which they themselves had failed to attain.

SOCIOECONOMIC FACTORS. The latter findings correspond with those in Breed's (1963) sociological study of 103 suicides by white males in New Orleans. Compared with 206 men matched for age, race, and residence, the suicides were disproportionately lower class. However, this finding was directly attributable to their *downward occupational mobility* when compared with controls. Decreasing income characterized more than half of the suicides, but just over 10 percent of the controls.

INTELLIGENCE. Because industrialization of society creates more nonmanual jobs, upward social mobility is more frequent than downward mobility (and becomes the prevailing norm). In our open society, there is a strong positive correlation between *intelligence* and socioeconomic status (roughly + 0.5), and there is pressure on the intelligent for achievement. This is probably the basis for a relatively high frequency of suicide among those of superior intelligence. In their 35-year follow-up study of intellectually superior California school children, Terman and Oden (1959) found that by a median age of 44 years, suicide among the gifted women had already passed the corresponding lifetime

Table 14-3. Family Background Data Obtained from College Records of Male Suicides and Controls

Item	Percent of Suicides	Percent of Controls	P
Parental education			
Father, college	74.7	59.1	< 0.01
Mother, college	42.3	30.6	0.03
Father's occupation			
Professional	56.7	40.0 ⎫	
Managerial	23.2	28.6 ⎬	< 0.01
Other	20.1	31.4 ⎭	
Parents separated	17.0	10.4	0.05
Parental morbidity			
Father, poor health	10.5	6.3	0.08
Mother, poor health	13.6	10.1	0.21
Parental mortality			
Father dead	14.3	6.7	< 0.01
Mother dead	7.2	7.2	0.99
Parents separated or father ill or dead	34.4	21.8	< 0.01

Adapted from Paffenbarger, R.S., Jr., and Asnes, D.P. Chronic disease in former college students. III. Precursors of suicide in early and middle life. *American Journal of Public Health*, 56:1026–1036, 1966.

expectation of suicide in the general population. Similarly, the suicide rate among the gifted men had reached two-thirds of the lifetime expectation of suicide among the corresponding male population, with the years of the highest suicide rates still ahead of them.

Religion

The Hutterites are members of a religious sect living mainly in rural areas of the American and Canadian prairies. Shortly after World War II they became the object of sociological and psychiatric study because it was noted that they were underrepresented in nearby mental hospitals, and presumably had few psychiatric disorders. On closer scrutiny, Eaton and Weil (1955) reported that the Hutterites did, indeed, have far less schizophrenic disorders than nine other cultural groups with whom they were compared. However, they also appeared to have an unduly high frequency of mood disorders. Although this finding might be attributable to differences in hereditary predisposition, the authors pointed to the Hutterites' extreme emphasis on communal cohesiveness. "There is much stress on religion, duty to God and

society, and there is a tendency in their entire thinking to orient members to internalize their aggressive drives. Children and adults alike are taught to look for guilt within themselves rather than in others."

The Learned-Helplessness Model of Depression

Seligman (1975) extensively documented many similarities between symptoms of depression in humans and learned helplessness in experimental animals. The theory of helplessness may be summarized as follows: *The expectation that an outcome is independent of responding* reduces the motivation to control the outcome and interferes with learning that responding does control the outcome. *If the outcome is also traumatic* (as in the inescapable punishment discussed in Chapter 5) it produces *fear* for as long as the subject is uncertain of the uncontrollable nature of the outcome, *and then produces depression.*

Seligman concluded there are six symptoms of learned helplessness, each of which has parallels in depression: (1) reduced initiation of voluntary responses; (2) negative cognitive set (difficulty in learning that responses will produce outcomes);

(3) persistence over time (increased by multiple exposures to uncontrollable shock); (4) reduced aggressive and competitive responses, with lowered dominance status; (5) loss of appetite, weight, and libido; (6) physiological changes, including nor-epinephrine depletion in helpless rats, and cholinergic overactivity in helpless cats.

Biochemical findings in patients with mood disorders are controversial and may be attributable to various factors including the following: genetic predisposition; developmental stress or deprivation (including too little stress); or therapeutic intervention already attempted. However, any of the preceding findings may be relevant to our therapeutic efforts to restore normal activity and function.

BIOLOGICAL DETERMINANTS OF MOOD DISORDERS

Hereditary Predisposition

Depression is so frequent that it has been regarded as the "common cold" of psychiatric disorders. Estimates of frequency (prevalence, incidence, or life-time expectancy) are highly unreliable, due to changing definitions and methods of case-finding, as well as to substantial fluctuations over a period of time.

Suicide, on the other hand, has been regarded as the tip of the depression iceberg, occurring in some small fraction of all depressed persons. Unfortunately, the latter represent a heterogeneous group that includes many persons with schizophrenia, alcoholism, and drug dependence. Moreover, estimates of frequency may be less reliable than is often assumed, due to underreporting in a number of population subgroups.

Many attempts have been made to estimate the lifetime expectancy of *manic-depressive disorders,* but these depend on diagnostic criteria that have differed between the United States and Europe, and that have also changed during the past generation. In European studies, the lifetime expectation of manic-depressive psychosis has usually exceeded that of schizophrenia, and has been within the range of 1 to 2 percent of the population. In the United States, the combined frequency of all major mood disorders (manic-depression and involutional melancholia) has been less than that of schizo-

phrenia (i.e., less than 1 percent) and diminishing since World War II. *There is no reason to believe that this represents anything more than changing fashions in diagnosis.*

In spite of the difficulties just mentioned, relatively reliable estimates have been made of the frequency of major mood disorders (resulting in hospitalization or suicide) among various relatives of persons with established mood disorders. These lifetime expectancies among primary relatives of patients have tended to be *higher* in the case of manic-depressive psychosis than in schizophrenia. In most studies the frequencies have ranged from about 10 percent to more than 20 percent, whether for parents, siblings, or children of a person with manic-depressive disorder.

These data were long considered more compatible with the hypothesis of transmission by a single dominant-autosomal gene (with incomplete penetrance or expressivity) than any other form of monogenic (single gene) transmission. However, Burch (1964) suggested the possibility that predisposition to manic-depressive psychosis required one dominant gene at an X-linked locus, and another dominant gene at an autosomal locus. Mendlewicz and his associates later reported seven extensive pedigrees of families with manic-depressive illness in whom *color blindness* also happened to be present. These two characteristics (manic-depressive illness and color blindness) tended to remain associated throughout the generations studied, suggesting the possibility that both were transmitted on the same chromosome — which was known to be the X chromosome in the case of color blindness.

More recent data suggest that X-chromosome transmission is more likely in the bipolar form of affective disorder than in unipolar disorders. However, Gershon and his associates (1976) raised serious questions concerning association versus linkage, analytic methods, ambiguous pedigrees, and chromosomal map distance incompatibity. A sophisticated statistical analysis of the data was compatible with the hypothesis of X-linkage, although not at the levels of significance required by the method used.

In spite of the conflicting data concerning possible methods of genetic transmission, earlier studies of *manic-depressive twins* have suggested that heredity plays a strong role (estimated between 38 and 100 percent). The results of the relevant twin studies are summarized in Table 14-4.

Neuropharmacology of Mood Disorders

According to the catecholamine hypothesis of mood disorders, *depression* is sometimes associated with a *deficit* of catecholamines, particularly norepinephrine, at central adrenergic receptor sites. *Elation,* or euphoria, by contrast, may be associated with a relative *excess* of such amines. Data supporting this hypothesis were derived from pharmacological studies of antidepressants and other drugs carried out mainly in animals. Monoamine oxidase inhibitors were found to increase brain concentrations of norepinephrine, while tricyclic antidepressants were found to potentiate the physiological effects of norepinephrine. However, the results of short-term, high-dosage studies in animals may be misleading, since clinical antidepressant effects may not become evident for two or three weeks. Hence, more recent investigations have turned to the biochemical effects accompanying long-term administration of these agents in animals and man. Earlier emphasis on norepinephrine depletion has been replaced by more complex hypotheses involving interactions between catecholamines and other brain neurotransmitter systems.

Gershon, Murphy, and their associates reported that platelet monoamine oxidase (MAO) activity is reduced in patients with bipolar mood disorders, and also in first degree relatives of such patients. However, the low platelet MAO activity is present both in relatives who also have mood disorders and in those who show no evidence of illness. This platelet MAO activity is known to be genetically determined, but these studies suggest it may be necessary but not sufficient for the development of bipolar mood disorders. This group of investigators has suggested that reduced platelet MAO activity identifies a genetically determined factor that increases vulnerability to both bipolar mood disorders and schizophrenias, but that other genetic factors determine both which individuals will develop overt psychiatric disorder and what form the disorder will take.

Iatrogenic Depression

Although a clearcut biochemical model for affective disorders remains elusive, one very important result of the search for such a model has been an increased appreciation of the fact that medical

Table 14-4. Estimated Concordance Rates in Monozygotic and Dizygotic Co-twins of Manic-depressive Twins

Investigator	Apparent Zygosity of Twins	Number of Pairs	Estimated Concordance Rate (percent)	Heritability $H = \dfrac{CMZ - CDZ}{100 - CDZ}$
Rosanoff	MZ	23	70	0.64
et al, 1935	DZ	67	16	
Luxenburger, 1942				
(cited by Gedda,	MZ	56	84	0.81
1951)	DZ	83	15	
Kallmann, 1953	MZ	27	100	1.00
	DZ	58	26	
Slater, 1953	MZ	8	57	0.39
	DZ	30	29	
Da Fonseca, 1959	MZ	21	75	0.60
	DZ	39	38	
Cohen et al, 1972	MZ	13	38	0.38
	DZ	27	0	

treatments may cause depression as well as alleviate it. One drug, reserpine, is so notorious for this property that "reserpinized" animals are commonly used in laboratory investigations of potential antidepressant drugs. Large doses (5 to 10 mg or more) were once used in the treatment of schizophrenia, but this treatment is now considered obsolete, partly because of the availability of clearly superior antipsychotics and partly because of the very high incidence of depression as a side effect. However, several studies have reported incidences from 10 to 30 percent of serious depression among persons taking relatively low antihypertensive doses of this drug (less than 1 mg per day) for extended periods of time.

The occurrence of depression, sometimes of psychotic intensity and resulting in suicidal activity, is a well-documented side effect of a number of drugs. The most important classes include: *antipsychotics* (especially chlorpromazine and haloperidol); *antihypertensives* of all types, including reserpine and other *Rauwolfia* derivatives, diuretics (if electrolyte imbalance develops), guanethidine, and alpha-methyldopa; and *progestins* (including oral contraceptives which contain them). The patients most vulnerable to this side effect are those who have a history or predisposition for depression or an existing depression that is aggravated by the drug. However, the physician should keep this possibility in mind and monitor the mental status of all patients taking one of these drugs.

Physicians must also guard against contributing to depression by conveying an attitude of hopelessness (defeat and helplessness), or by inappropriate psychotherapy.

TREATMENT

Some years ago a cartoon appeared in which a patient was lying on an analyst's couch with his head and arm in bandages. The caption read as follows: "I think I was better off when my hostility was latent." The cartoon illustrates one of many difficulties involved in treating patients with mood disorders by means of *psychotherapy*. Helping the patient to become more self-assertive

carries the risk of retaliation by key persons (e.g., spouse or employer) with whom he may be in conflict. In general terms, psychotherapeutic approaches must be selected carefully and applied skillfully or they may be: (1) ineffective; (2) directly damaging (e.g., by reinforcing dependency and disability and providing secondary gain); (3) indirectly damaging, by exposing the patient to adverse consequences of his behavior; or (4) dangerous, by increasing despair and potential for suicide.

Reactive or situational depression often involves conflict with the spouse, and it may be more productive to involve both partners in family therapy. However, relatively mild depression associated with predominantly intrapsychic conflict may require long-term intensive psychotherapy. When the mood disorder is more acute or severe, supportive psychotherapy will usually be more appropriate, and decisions about longer-term psychotherapy should be deferred until later.

Experiments on learned helplessness have suggested that depression results from the belief that any action is futile (since experience has demonstrated that responding does not affect the outcome). Hence, *forced exposure to the fact that responding does produce reinforcement* should be the most effective way of breaking up learned helplessness or depression. Animals subjected to repeated traumatization beyond their control have required a correspondingly long period of forced responses in the absence of trauma before they have initiated any further responses themselves. These findings have been reviewed at length by Seligman (1975) and have major significance for those undertaking appropriate psychotherapeutic intervention in depressed persons.

Antidepressant medications should always be considered for moderate or severe depression, the usual choice being one of the tricyclics. Amitriptyline is often preferred when there is concurrent anxiety or insomnia (and may be given in a single dose at bedtime). In other cases imipramine is considered preferable, particularly for those with retarded endogenous depression, and there are some persons who respond better to one than to the other type of agent. Persons with cardiac disease should probably receive a trial of doxepin in preference to any of the other tricyclics. Monoamine oxidase inhibitors may help some depressed patients that fail to respond to tricyclics, but involve many risks and should not be given without a preceding drug-free interval of one week. Details on antidepressant medication have already been discussed in Chapter 8.

Convulsive therapy was originally introduced in the treatment of schizophrenic disorders, but was soon found to be much more effective for the treatment of severe depression, particularly involutional melancholia and manic-depressive disorders. It is still the most reliably effective treatment for severe unipolar or bipolar depression, where there is no obvious exogenous perpetuating situational stress or prominent associated manifestations (neurotic anxiety, schizophrenic thought disorder, or organic intellectual impairment). Convulsive therapy is often reserved for drug-resistant depressive disorders. The usual course of treatment lasts somewhere between two to four weeks (the number of treatments per week depending on the response, and on such factors as whether electrode placement is bilateral or unilateral). Convulsive therapy is most likely to be the initial treatment of choice if the depression is unusually severe, if there is urgent need for rapid recovery, or when there are complications such as sensitivity to medications.

Maintenance treatment of depression is directed toward preventing relapses, which are most frequent during the first six months or year after a major depressive episode. Frequent and severe recurrences were formerly reduced or partially prevented by maintenance convulsive therapy (from once a week to once a month), or sometimes by means of psychosurgery (particularly bimedial lobotomy). In recent years, placebo-controlled double-blind studies have clearly demonstrated the effectiveness of tricyclic drugs in preventing relapse, including relapse among patients who have received convulsive therapy. This literature was reviewed by Davis (1976).

Manic excitement also responds to convulsive therapy, but less favorably than does severe depression. Manic patients are more likely to require a longer course of treatment and to relapse more frequently within a week or two after its termination. The introduction of the major tranquilizing drugs constituted a major advance in the rapid management of acute manic excitement, but they are less satisfactory than lithium for long-term maintenance therapy. Davis (1976) reviewed a number of studies, establishing "beyond a doubt" the effectiveness of lithium in preventing recurrence of manic episodes. There is also strong evidence that lithium is effective in preventing recurrence of many unipolar depressive episodes and in controlling the target symptoms of mood disorder in patients with schizo-affective psychoses. However, except in the case of bipolar mood disorders, the precise indications for long-term lithium therapy are still subject to continuing investigation and debate.

REVIEW QUESTIONS

176. The manic patient, in contrast to the excited schizophrenic patient:
    (A) is less responsive to environmental stimuli
    (B) never has hallucinations or delusions
    (C) seldom shows incongruity between affect and thought content
    (D) all of the above
    (E) none of the above

177. Paranoid delusions are *incompatible* with a diagnosis of:
    (A) organic brain syndrome
    (B) involutional melancholia
    (C) acute mania
    (D) all of the above
    (E) none of the above

178. Females are reported to outnumber males in which of the following diagnostic categories?
    (A) paranoid state
    (B) involutional melancholia
    (C) manic-depressive illness
    (D) all of the above
    (E) none of the above

179. The premorbid personality of females with a

205

diagnosis of involutional melancholia is most
frequently described as:

(A) introverted
(B) extroverted
(C) schizoid
(D) obsessive-compulsive
(E) inadequate

180. Which of the following is most likely to be a
major psychodynamic factor in a psychotic
depressive reaction?

(A) unrelieved sexual tension
(B) sibling rivalry
(C) hostility toward a loved person
(D) castration anxiety
(E) unresolved Oedipal complex

181. A 36-year-old married man with no history
of psychiatric disturbance has become progressively more elated and excited, with
increasing capacity for work. He is now
humorous and overactive to the point that he
irritates others; his sleep has decreased to
four hours per day without distressing him.
This is most likely a description of:

(A) catatonic excitement
(B) agitated depression
(C) an acute schizophrenic episode
(D) hebephrenia
(E) hypomania

182. Of the following list, the item *least* characteristic of involutional melancholia is:

(A) good response to ECT
(B) high risk of suicide
(C) many somatic complaints and delusions
(D) family history of manic-depressive illness
(E) signs of functional intellectual impair-
ment

Summary of Directions

A	B	C	D	E
1, 2, 3 only	1, 3 only	2, 4 only	4 only	All are correct

---

183. Manic states can be alleviated by:
(1) convulsive therapy
(2) lithium salts

(3) antipsychotic drugs
(4) benzodiazepines

184. Psychodynamic interpretations or descriptions of affective disorders include:

(1) retroflexion of latent hostility in depression
(2) diminished superego influence in mania
(3) subjugation of the ego by a dominant
and punitive superego in depression
(4) manic elation is a defense against depression

185. Symptoms commonly present in acute manic
states include:
(1) flight of ideas
(2) emotional lability
(3) psychomotor agitation
(4) hallucinations

186. As described by Lindemann, a *normal* grief
reaction following bereavement includes:
(1) sensations of somatic distress
(2) preoccupation with the image of the
deceased
(3) guilt feelings in which the bereaved
accuses himself of negligence
(4) acquisition of symptoms similar to
those of the final illness of the deceased

187. In contrast with schizophrenia, the diagnosis
of manic-depressive illness (unipolar and
bipolar affective disorders) is:
(1) relatively more frequent in upper and
middle social classes
(2) relatively more frequent among married
persons
(3) relatively more frequent among persons
whose first psychotic episode occurs during middle age
(4) equally frequent in males and females

188. Convulsive therapy (ECT) is generally ac-
knowledged as superior to drug therapy in
the treatment of:
(1) involutional melancholia
(2) acute mania
(3) psychotic depressive reaction
(4) paranoid state

189. Manifestations of depression include:
(1) poverty of ideation

    (2) irritability

    (3) psychomotor agitation or retardation

    (4) ambivalence

190. Depression in children and adolescents may be manifested by:

    (1) delinquent or antisocial behavior

    (2) drug abuse

    (3) poor school work

    (4) withdrawal

SELECTED REFERENCES

1. Akiskal, H.S., and McKinney, W.T. (1975). Overview of recent research in depression. *Archives of General Psychiatry,* vol. 32, pages 285–305.

2. American Psychiatric Association (1975). The current status of lithium therapy: Report of the APA Task Force. *American Journal of Psychiatry,* vol. 132, pages 997–1001.

3. Beck, A.T. (1967). *Depression: Clinical, Experimental, and Theoretical Aspects.* New York: Hoeber.

4. Birtchnell, J. (1970). Depression in relation to early and recent parent death. *British Journal of Psychiatry,* vol. 116, pages 299–306.

5. Breed, W. (1963). Occupational mobility and suicide among white males. *Sociological Review,* vol. 28, page 183.

6. Bruhn, J.G. (1962). Broken homes among attempted suicides and psychiatric outpatients: A comparative study. *Journal of Mental Science,* vol. 108, pages 772–779.

7. Burch, P.R.J. (1964). Manic-depressive psychosis: Some new aetiological considerations. *British Journal of Psychiatry,* vol. 110, pages 808–817.

8. Cohen, M., Allen, M.G., Pollin, W., and Hrubec, Z. (1972). Relationship of schizo-affective psychosis to manic-depressive psychosis and schizophrenia. *Archives of General Psychiatry,* vol. 26, pages 539–546.

9. Davis, J.M. (1976). Overview: Maintenance therapy in psychiatry. II. Affective disorders. *American Journal of Psychiatry,* vol. 133, pages 1–13.

10. Dennehy, C.M. (1966). Childhood bereavement and psychiatric illness. *British Journal of Psychiatry,* vol. 112, pages 1049–1069.

11. Eaton, J.W., and Weil, R.J. (1955). *Culture and Mental Disorders.* Glencoe, Illinois: The Free Press, Division of Macmillan Co.

12. Farberow, N.L. (1975). *Suicide in Different Cultures.* Baltimore: University Park Press.

13. Freud, S. (1917). Mourning and Melancholia. In *Collected Works.* London: Hogarth Press, pages 243–248.

14. Gershon, E.S., et al (1976). Is there X-linkage in bipolar affective illness? (and three related papers). American Psychiatric Association, *Scientific Proceedings,* pages 124–129.

15. Murphy, D.L. (1976). Neuropharmacology of Depression. In *Drug Treatment of Mental Disorders,* edited by L. L. Simpson. New York: Raven Press. Chapter 8.

16. Paffenbarger, R.S., and Asnes, D.P. (1966). Chronic disease in former college students. III. Precursors of suicide in early and middle life. *American Journal of Public Health,* vol. 56, pages 1026–1036.

17. Paykel, E.S., Myers, J.K., Dienelt, M.N., Klerman, G.L., Lindenthal, J.J., and Pepper, M.P. (1969). Life events and depression. *Archives of General Psychiatry,* vol. 21, pages 753–760.

18. Perlin, S. [Ed.] (1975). *A Handbook for the Study of Suicide.* New York: Oxford University Press.

19. Rennie, T.A.C. (1942). Prognosis in manic-depressive psychoses. *American Journal of Psychiatry,* vol. 98, page 801.

20. Robins, E., Murphy, G.E., Wilkinson, R.H., Gassner, S., and Kayes, J. (1959). Some clinical considerations in the prevention of suicide based on a study of 134 successful suicides. *American Journal of Public Health,* vol. 49, pages 888–899.

21. Schildkraut, J.J., and Klein, D.F. (1975). The classification and treatment of depressive disorders. In *Manual of Psychiatric Therapeutics,* edited by R. I. Shader. Boston: Little, Brown and Co. Chapter 3.

22. Seligman, M.E.P. (1975). *Helplessness.* San Francisco: W. H. Freeman and Co.

23. Shneidman, E.S., and Farberow, N.L. [Eds.] (1957). *Clues to Suicide.* New York: McGraw-Hill.

24. Terman, L.M., and Oden, M.H. (1959). *The Gifted Group at Mid-Life.* Stanford, California: Stanford University Press. Pages 30–32.

25. Zung, W.W.K. (1973). From art to science: The diagnosis and treatment of depression. *Archives of General Psychiatry,* vol. 29, pages 328–337.

15. Anxiety and Hysterical Disorders (Neurotic Disorders)

But first of all let me assert my firm belief that the only thing we have to fear is fear itself — nameless, unreasoning, unjustified terror which paralyzes needed efforts to convert retreat into advance.
Franklin D. Roosevelt, Inaugural Address, 1933

FEAR, ANXIETY, PANIC, PHOBIC, AND RELATED DISORDERS

Fear

Fear is one of the four most basic and universal, or primary, emotions. (The other three are joy, sorrow, and anger.) Normal fear consists of subjective apprehensions and objective physiological changes, both of which are appropriate in degree and duration to a consciously recognized external source of danger. It involves recognition and arousal, with preparation for action to be taken in the immediate future, which may consist of violent muscular activity (i.e., fight or flight). Fear dissipates when such action is taken, leading to escape or avoidance of danger.

The physiological concomitants of fear are the same as those resulting from an injection of epinephrine, or from generalized stimulation of the sympathetic nervous system. There is tachycardia and rapid respiration with hyperventilation, as well as tremor of skeletal muscles, with redistribution of blood from skin and viscera. There is a cold sweat, with clammy palms, pallor, and piloerection. The pupils are dilated, and there may be nausea ("butterflies" in the stomach), vomiting, diarrhea, or frequency of urination.

Anxiety

Anxiety consists of apprehension, tension, and excessive concern over danger that is either minor in degree or largely unrecognized. Anxiety is usually accompanied by signs of increased activity of the sympathetic nervous system, and is described as *free-floating* when there is no conscious recognition of a specific external danger. Anxiety has been regarded as the chief characteristic of all neurotic disorders, with various other symptoms (e.g., phobic, obsessive, compulsive, or hysterical) representing maladaptive defenses against intolerable conscious anxiety.

Neurotic anxiety differs from normal fear, or "signal anxiety," by: (1) being unrelated to a perceived realistic threat, or disproportionate to such threats; (2) resulting from intrapsychic conflict, which must be controlled by repression and other mechanisms; (3) leading to various forms of altered activity and awareness and to inhibitions and other neurotic defenses and symptoms; and (4) not being relieved by amelioration of the objective situation.

Generalized Anxiety Disorder

Generalized anxiety disorder (anxiety neurosis) is characterized by the frequent presence of excessive free-floating anxiety and overconcern, to the extent that these conditions interfere with effectiveness in living, the achievement of desired realistic goals and satisfactions, or emotional comfort. The more specific symptoms associated with other neurotic disorders (e.g., phobias, obsessions, and compulsions) are minimal or absent, although there are usually multiple minor somatic complaints.

According to psychoanalytic theory, neurotic symptoms result from unconscious conflicts involving fantasies of punishment for instinctual wishes and originating in childhood. The typical dangers that lead to fear and sometimes to neurotic conflict may be conscious in early childhood but are unconscious later on, and include: (1) loss of, or separation from, a person on whom the child depends for care and love; (2) loss of love through anger or disapproval expressed by such a person; (3) damage to or loss of the genitals (also known as the *castration complex*); and (4) bad conscience, guilt, or superego anxiety, with disapproval of oneself based on internalized moral standards.

Other concepts of neurosis emphasize the overlearning of escape and avoidance behavior, and overexposure to situations involving ambiguity and unpredictability of outcome. It is characteristic of many neurotic persons that they must constantly strive to avoid even minor disapproval by others. They appear insecure, wanting to be loved by everybody all the time, and unable to say no to additional responsibilities. They conform with institutionalized strivings for upward social mobility, and work long hours (although sometimes ineffectively). They tend to be regarded as reliable, responsible, and conscientious. However, their thoughts and behavior are overly inhibited, and they have difficulty in recognizing or tolerating sexual or hostile impulses in themselves as well as in others. Neurotic women tend to be frigid and unable to enjoy sex, while neurotic men often show some form of sexual dysfunction such as impotence or premature ejaculation. Neurotic persons try not to express anger or hostility directly, but may hurt or frustrate others unintentionally as a consequence of their behavior. In part, this results from their high expectations for achievement and postponement of pleasure by members of their family, employees, or other associates.

Panic Disorder

Panic disorder consists of discrete episodes of fearfulness (i.e., panic attacks) that occur at least half a dozen times in as many weeks, against a background of milder anxiety and nervousness. The panic attacks themselves are characterized by several of the following symptoms: dyspnea; palpitations; chest pain or discomfort; choking or smothering sensation; dizziness, vertigo, or feelings of unreality; paresthesias (tingling); sweating; faintness; trembling or shaking; and fear of dying during the attack.

Phobic Disorders

Phobic disorders are characterized by intense fear of an external object or situation that the person consciously recognizes as harmless. However, the irrational fear is persistent, and the person tends to avoid the object, activity, or situation that arouses fear. In the past a great many words were coined from Greek roots for specific phobias, but there has been a tendency to abandon these and recognize three major groups of phobia: (1) *agoraphobia*

consists of fear of the street or open places, and hence of leaving one's home (usually associated with other phobias that may involve crowds, heights, or closed spaces); (2) *social phobias* concern situations that involve interaction with other people (as in public speaking or attending school); (3) *simple phobias* are specific phobias involving neither of the preceding characteristics (e.g., fear of animals).

Psychoanalytic therapy of persons with phobic disorders led to the belief that the fear originates internally (as a fear of punishment for forbidden sexual or aggressive impulses), and that ego defenses operate so that the inner danger seems to become an outer one (which can then be *avoided*). The characteristic defense employed in this process of externalization is the mechanism of *displacement*.

Obsessive-compulsive Disorder

Obsessive-compulsive disorder is characterized by the persistent intrusion of unwanted thoughts, urges, or actions that the person is unable to stop. *Obsessive* thoughts often involve the mechanism of *isolation* of affect, by means of which aggressive and other unacceptable ideas (e.g., of attacking someone) can occur without the corresponding emotion. *Compulsive* behavior is usually recognized by the individual as foreign to his personality (i.e., *ego-alien*) and is accompanied by a desire to resist. However, failure to carry out the compulsive action or ritual may result in intolerable anxiety. Compulsive rituals may represent both the symbolic expression of a forbidden impulse, and atonement for this impulse through the defense mechanism of *undoing* (e.g., by repeated hand-washing). Obsessive-compulsive personality characteristics include excessive cleanliness, orderliness, perfectionistic striving, and meticulous attention to detail.

Hypochondriacal Disorder

Hypochondriacal disorder (somatic preoccupation) is characterized by preoccupation with bodily functions and with *fears* of presumed diseases of various organs. These fears are not delusional in intensity, but persist in spite of reassurance concerning normal findings on physical examination and laboratory investigations. This disorder should be distinguished from hysteria, but there is a strong correlation (coefficient roughly + 0.7) between the scores on scale 1 (hypochondriasis) and scale 3 (hysteria) of the MMPI. Persons with a somatic preoccupation disorder are apt to consult many physicians, to have repeated admissions to hospital, and to be vulnerable to *polysurgery*.

HYSTERICAL DISORDERS (CONVERSION AND DISSOCIATIVE)

Conversion Disorders

Conversion disorders are characterized by involuntary psychogenic loss or disturbances of bodily functions that are mediated by cranial nerves or the *voluntary* skeletal nervous system. This contrasts with *psychophysiological disorders* (sometimes known as *psychosomatic disorders*) that are mediated mainly through the *involuntary* muscular and autonomic nervous system.

The major forms of conversion disorders include the following: (1) *altered sensation,* such as anesthesia or paresthesia, partial or complete blindness, or deafness; (2) *ataxia or paralysis,* including inability to stand or walk (astasia-abasia) and loss of voice, with inability to whisper (aphonia); (3) *involuntary movements* or dyskinesias, and pseudo-epileptic seizures; and (4) *pain,* which may affect any part of the body (e.g., abdominal cramps, headache, chest pains, etc.) and if incorrectly diagnosed may lead to unnecessary surgery. The mechanism by which the pain is produced is poorly understood, but this is now considered the most common form of conversion hysteria.

The onset of conversion symptoms is often sudden and dramatic. The presenting symptoms appear neurological, but careful examination and tests are likely to show obvious discrepancies between the dysfunction and known anatomical distribution of motor and sensory nerves (e.g., anesthesia with a "glove" or "stocking" distribution). There may be gross disability over which the patient shows no apparent anxiety or concern,

to which Charcot referred as *la belle indifférence* (beautiful indifference).

The somatic disability results both in *primary gain* (relief from emotional conflict and freedom from anxiety) and *secondary gain,* consisting of such external benefits as release from unpleasant responsibility, increased personal attention, and financial rewards.

Dissociative Disorders

Dissociative disorders are hysterical neuroses in which there are alterations in the person's state of consciousness or in his sense of identity. The most frequent form consists of an episode of *amnesia* during which there is total loss of memory, either for the entire previous life (including his identity) or for a circumscribed period of time (usually including a traumatic incident or experience). Unlike the diffuse amnesia associated with organic mental disorders, hysterical amnesia usually has an abrupt onset following emotional stress rather than some biological insult to the brain.

Another form of dissociative disorder is the hysterical *fugue,* in which amnesia is combined with physical flight, usually from a situation that has become intolerable. Loss of memory and identity may be total and lasting, and the person may move to a new locality and establish a new life. A similar loss of identity occurs in *sleepwalking* (somnambulism), and in *multiple personality.* The latter is the rarest and most spectacular form of dissociative disorder. One of the best documented cases was described in *The Three Faces of Eve* by Thigpen and Cleckley (1957). The first identity (Eve White) was neurotic and unduly inhibited. The second identity to appear (Eve Black) misbehaved in ways that would have been unacceptable to Eve White (and made the former's life more difficult). The third identity (Jane) appeared during therapy, and the patient was enabled to effect a compromise between conflicting drives that had previously been dissociated.

Briquet's Hysteria

In Briquet's hysteria there is a dramatic, vague, or complicated medical history, beginning before the age of 25 years. In most instances, patients believe they have been sickly a good part of their life. Often they have a definite history of conversion disorder or of dissociative symptoms. Otherwise, the main symptoms involve complaints of bodily pain in the absence of organic somatic disease. Abdominal pain or vomiting spells are the most frequent. Other common complaints include back pain, joint pain, pain in the extremities, and frequent headaches. Women with this disorder are likely to complain of dysmenorrhea or excessive menstrual bleeding. There is often a history of pain or lack of pleasure during intercourse if the person has an opportunity for an active sex life. The somatic complaints are apt to lead the person to consult many doctors, to be admitted to hospitals repeatedly, and to be vulnerable to polysurgery.

Hysterical Personality

Hysterical personality characteristics include histrionic (theatrical) tendencies toward self-dramatization, together with dependency and seductiveness, of which the patient may not be aware. The lack of awareness is attributable to excessive use of the defense mechanism of *denial,* which the hysteric applies to anything felt to be unpleasant, including sexual or aggressive feelings, childhood or recent conflict, and the extent or consequences of disability. This naive defensive attitude is revealed by certain psychological tests, including the validity scales of the MMPI (as discussed in Chap. 4). It is also evident in the following responses to an Incomplete Sentence Blank that were given by a young hysterical woman who had been married a few months previously, but who was currently separated from her husband.

Marriage . . . has brought me more happiness than I ever dreamed possible.
Most women . . . should strive to remember to be feminine, though capable and not overly feminine.
My body . . . satisfies me the way it is. I won't let it be defiled. I know I must not be ashamed of it.
Most bosses . . . aren't nearly as nice as mine. He is the best in the world, I'm sure.

A husband . . . must be prepared to stand by and understand through thick and thin — as mine is doing now. His love for his wife must take second place only to his love for God.
I like . . . to like people and to be liked by them. Perhaps love would be a better word. I like to be in the wild free outdoors and to run uninhibitedly.
My mother . . . is one of the dearest, most precious persons in the whole world. I'd do almost anything to make her happy.
If I were in charge . . . of the world, I'd arrange things so that everyone loved everyone else all of the time.
My father . . . has always and still does refuse to let me grow up. At least he won't admit to himself that I have.
Most men . . . are wonderful, fascinating creatures who never forget that women are female.
This place . . . is wonderful. It is more like a hotel than a hospital and does everything possible to prevent us from thinking we're really very, very sick.
My job . . . is perfect. Though the work gets boring, the people are wonderful beyond words.
It is easy for me to . . . love many people and animals and friends all at the same time.
My health . . . is good and bothers me only when I think something is psychosomatically wrong again.
Nothing cheers me up as much as . . . my husband or a good talk with God.
I'm the sort of person who . . . is so full of love it just bursts out and sometimes in the wrong ways.
I am ashamed when I think of . . . my past relations with a man named X — also hurt and regretful.
Things look hopeless when . . . I'm all depressed, excited, angry, and don't know why. Really, I don't think things have ever looked really hopeless!
I need . . . help to understand myself and loads of love.
Most of the time I am . . . a very pleasant, likeable (I think and hope) person.
If I saw a fire truck . . . I'd like to follow it and always hope no one was hurt and that it wasn't too bad.
Everywhere . . . around me I find people who love me and want to help me now when it is so important.
If I were the boss, I . . . would arrange for everyone to love everyone else.
I really think my place in life . . . is and will be wonderful and satisfying.
Some people don't like me because . . . I don't know of anyone who dislikes me.

BIOLOGICAL AND PSYCHOSOCIAL DETERMINANTS

Biological Factors

The only consistent physiological findings in neurotic disorders are those of *increased autonomic nervous system activity*. The relative preponderance of epinephrine activity versus norepinephrine activity may be estimated by measuring the hypotensive effect of an injection of Mecholyl. Anger tends to be associated with norepinephrine secretion, and relatively minor hypotensive effects from Mecholyl, whereas fear is associated with epinephrine secretion and marked hypotensive effects from Mecholyl. It has been proposed that the tendency to react to danger or stress with fear rather than anger may be based on individual variations in hypothalamic sympathetic excitability. However, this type of mediating mechanism would not provide evidence on the relative importance of hereditary predisposition versus avoidance learning through early experience.

The *frequency* of neurotic disorders is extremely difficult to estimate, as noted in Chapter 9. Estimates based on patients being treated at a given time represent only the tip of the iceberg, depending on such factors as: (1) severity of disability; (2) public awareness, demand, and ability to pay for services; (3) professional availability; and (4) use of diagnostic terminology. For many years these factors have combined to result in a much higher frequency of neuroses being treated in females than in males (ratios range from 3:2 to more than 2:1) and among those of higher socioeconomic status (largely because they remain in treatment longer). Moreover, there are no firm cutoff points to determine the presence or absence of neurosis, since neurotic traits and symptoms appear to vary quantitatively along continuous distributions (such as those represented by individual scales of the MMPI).

FAMILY AND TWIN STUDIES. Former attempts to estimate the *lifetime frequency* of neurotic disorders among the parents and siblings of neurotic patients suggest some degree of specificity within families. One such study reported anxiety disorders among roughly 20 percent of the parents and 10 percent of the siblings of patients with anxiety disorders. There were corresponding frequencies of hysterical disorders among the parents and siblings of patients with hysterical disorders, with substantially lower frequencies (but still the corresponding diagnosis) among the relatives of patients with obsessive-compulsive disorders. These findings of familial concentration and specificity still fail to provide indications of possible hereditary factors, and the information obtainable from twin studies is very limited.

Slater (1953) provided data concerning 52 pairs of twins, one of each having been diagnosed as "psychopathic or neurotic." In this relatively small and mixed group, he recorded an age-corrected frequency of similar abnormality among 26 percent of their siblings and 32 percent of their parents. The *concordance rates* for their co-twins were only 2 of 8 pairs diagnosed as monozygotic and 8 of 43 pairs diagnosed as dizygotic. Computing Holzinger's index of heritability from these data suggests that the overall contribution of heredity in this sample accounted for roughly 10 percent of the total variation. However, the small numbers involved and the mixed diagnostic grouping make the results unconvincing. In a later study, Gottesman (1962) administered the MMPI to 34 pairs of monozygotic and 34 pairs of same-sexed dizygotic adolescent twins. Several of the clinical scales had appreciable indices of heritability in this study, including an index of 33 percent on scale 7 (psychasthenia, corresponding with a variety of neurotic manifestations, including anxiety, phobias, and obsessive-compulsive traits).

Psychosocial Factors

The importance of psychosocial factors in the development of neurotic disorders is supported by a variety of evidence including: (1) the history of interpersonal relationships prevailing during childhood; (2) the frequent exacerbation of neurotic symptoms in response to situational stress and interpersonal difficulties of adult life; (3) remission in response to diminished environmental stress, and relatively favorable response to psychotherapies. Psychoanalytic theory and therapy, as well as learning theory and behavior therapies, have their maximum applicability in neurotic disorders. These concepts have been discussed in detail in Chapters 1, 5, and 6, and it is only necessary to review certain aspects briefly in the present chapter.

In their conformity to social ideals and expectations, persons with neurotic disorders tend to make excessive use of the unconscious ego defense mechanisms of *repression, sublimation,* and *displacement* of affect. In those with anxiety disorders, such defenses have proved inadequate, and unconscious conflict is associated with conscious anxiety. Hysterical patients rely heavily on the mechanism of *denial,* and conscious anxiety is largely prevented by the maladaptive defenses of *conversion* or *dissociation.* The development of phobic disorders involves *displacement* of fear associated with the danger of punishment for forbidden sexual and hostile impulses. Obsessive thinking involves *isolation* of affect, and compulsive behavior consists of both symbolic *acting out* and *undoing* or atonement for unacceptable fantasies. Reactive depression is often associated with neurotic conflict, loss, or frustration, *introjection* or retroflexed rage, and guilt with need for punishment.

There are many individual differences in developmental dynamics and adult personality characteristics in various neurotic disorders, but there are certain *common denominators in their early experiences.* They have become conforming, inhibited, and anxious to please others because this type of behavior has been expected and demanded of them. Parents and other significant adults have strongly emphasized and reinforced "good" behavior, while attempting to extinguish or actively punishing all signs of "bad" impulses and behavior.

The superego is developed partly through the *internalization* and automatization of the repeated instructions and prohibitions of childhood, and partly through *identification* with the ideals and example of those in authority. Typically, parents of a neurotic patient have fostered the development of an unusually *harsh and rigid superego,* so

that the patient feels as guilty over perceiving unacceptable impulses as most persons would feel if they had acted on such impulses. Although antisocial impulses are universal, the neurotic attempts to avoid guilt by repressing them from consciousness and adopting various other defenses.

Since *mother* is the primary agent of socialization during the preschool years, it has generally been assumed that her personality and behavior are more likely than those of *father* to have both positive and negative effects on the development of the child. However, there is a strong tendency for persons to marry others of equivalent emotional maturity, and therefore for psychiatric disorders in the mother to be associated with various forms of psychiatric disorder in the father. In recent years there has also been an increasing tendency to recognize the direct effects of father's behavior on the child from an early age, as well as the indirect effects on the child of father's behavior toward mother.

One or both parents of neurotic persons are likely to be *overprotective.* They are overconcerned not only with good behavior and moral development, but also with attempting to protect the child against physical illnesses, and they will caution him excessively against common physical or social dangers. It may soon appear to the child that the physical environment and interpersonal relationships are dangerous, and should therefore be feared. Verbal reassurance about the absence of danger is easily contradicted by nonverbal communication, or by the example of an apprehensive parent who is forever expressing concern over trivialities. Overprotection also implies overcontrol and possessive domination of the child. If he is never given the responsibility for making decisions and learning from his own mistakes, he then becomes overdependent on the parent, and may remain so in adult life.

Along with the parents' concern that the child be a credit to them goes undue *emphasis on achievement.* This often leads to attempts to elicit behavior that is normally expected at a later stage of development, as in premature attempts at toilet training that have been reported in patients with obsessive-compulsive disorders. Such parents are usually also intolerant of dirt and disorder, and establish the child's compulsive cleanliness, meticulous attention to detail, and perfectionistic strivings.

The parents are often undemonstrative of affection toward each other and the children. They also tend to inhibit all expression of anger by the child, through either harsh retribution or guilt-provoking moralization. Greenfield (1959) reported that patients with neurotic and schizophrenic disorders had suffered less *direct* discipline (such as scolding, spanking, and isolation) than *indirect* discipline, such as being made to feel that one is not as good as other children, being made to feel that one had hurt his parents, being made to feel that one had fallen short of expectations, and being denied any demonstration of affection. These techniques of indirect discipline, combined with frequent criticism or nagging, give the neurotic person a lasting sense of guilt and inadequacy.

Some parents indulge in violent temper outbursts, which are particularly frightening to the child because of their *unpredictability.* Seligman (1975) summarized extensive experimental evidence about the consequences of such circumstances. When traumatic events are predictable (through some advance signal or warning) the absence of a traumatic event is also predictable (by the absence of the predictive signal or warning). When traumatic events are unpredictable, however, safety is also unpredictable. According to the *safety-signal hypothesis,* people and animals remain in a state of constant anxiety or chronic fear following traumatic events, except in the presence of a stimulus that reliably predicts safety.

The worst bridges may be those we never cross, and *uncertainty* may be more anxiety-provoking than unpleasant experiences that cannot be avoided. The child who develops a neurotic disorder has often been warned of dangers that remain vague and undefined, notably in the area of sexual behavior. The child's simple questions about where babies come from or how they start to develop may be met with embarrassment and evasion or, alternatively, with detailed explanation far beyond

the child's current interest or ability to understand. There is a lack of easy communication of such simple sexual information, so that it often remains shrouded in mystery and danger or disgust. Any breach of modesty with a neighbor child may result in further play with that child being forbidden. In spite of sex education in the schools, and liberalization of sexual mores, it is not surprising that the neurotic's relationships with members of the opposite sex should be marred by conflict and sometimes frigidity or impotence. It was the latter observation that led to Freud's dictum that with a normal sex life no neurosis was possible. However, this was to some extent related to the prevailing culture (nineteenth-century Vienna), and nowadays repressed aggression or hostility may be relatively more significant than repressed sexual impulses.

SOCIOECONOMIC FACTORS. The frequency and form of neurotic disorders vary considerably in different cultures, social classes, and over a period of time. Hollingshead and Redlich (1958) found hysterical disorders virtually absent in social classes I, II, and III, but present in limited numbers in classes IV and V of the New Haven, Connecticut, population. The prevalence of obsessive-compulsive disorders, neurotic depressive disorders, and "character neuroses" (in patients receiving treatment) were all *positively* correlated with socioeconomic status (i.e., more frequent at upper than at lower levels) (see Chap. 9). They simplified their observations to the following statement: "The Class V neurotic behaves badly, the Class IV neurotic aches physically, the Class III patient defends fearfully, and the Class I-II patient is dissatisfied with himself." However, it should be recognized that these generalizations may involve local ethnic or cultural factors as well as prevailing vagaries of psychiatric diagnosis.

TREATMENT OF NEUROTIC DISORDERS

Neurotic disorders are usually considered to be less severe than psychotic disorders because they do not involve gross distortion or misinterpretation of external reality, or gross personality disorganization. However, their course is often chronic or intermittent, with a strong tendency toward episodes of severe exacerbation that are at least temporarily incapacitating. Neurotic disorders are sometimes more disabling than isolated or recurrent psychotic disorders. In addition to causing subjective distress, they may also lead to great inconvenience or hardship among close relatives, particularly the spouse or offspring, who may themselves be greatly handicapped through long interaction with a severely neurotic parent.

All forms of psychotherapy have been employed in the treatment of neurotic disorders. The choice of therapy depends on a variety of factors including severity and duration of the disorder, as well as the person's age, intelligence, marital status, socioeconomic status, other aspects of his reality situation, and the experience and preference of the therapist.

Supportive therapies and environmental manipulation (with or without tranquilizing medication) are likely to be at least temporarily helpful in patients with relatively mild disorders, and may be most appropriate for middle-aged or elderly patients with strong precipitating factors. However, the tendency to recurrence, and the possible severity of disability, should lead to consideration of *long-term intensive individual psychotherapy,* particularly for younger patients. Those with hysterical and phobic disorders tend to respond more favorably to analytically oriented insight therapy than do those with obsessive-compulsive disorders. However, all forms of neurotic disorder with anxiety as a prominent component tend to respond more favorably than those associated with reactive depression or those with underlying personality disorders involving diminished impulse control and antisocial behavior.

In recent years, *systematic desensitization* (with the associated techniques of relaxation and reciprocal inhibition) has often been regarded as the treatment of choice in simple phobic disorders. This approach has also been applied to more diffuse anxiety disorders, and techniques of behavior modification have been applied to other forms of neurotic disorder. However, the application of learning theory to other forms of psychotherapy may be a more significant development than simplistic attempts to apply these principles exclusively. Since neurotic conflicts originate in childhood relationships and find expression in current interpersonal relationships, group or family therapies are frequently indicated, either alone or in combination with individual psychotherapies.

Minor tranquilizing drugs are effective antianxiety agents, and have been reviewed in Chapter 8. Three major problems associated with their use in treating neurotic disorders should be kept in mind: (1) Mild anxiety acts as a stimulus to learning and problem-solving, so that removal of all neurotic symptoms may reduce motivation for lasting relief through psychotherapy; (2) learning or unlearning that takes place under the effects of tranquilizing medication will probably be reversed (i.e., eliminated) as soon as that medication is discontinued; (3) the minor tranquilizing drugs have a strong potential for misuse by physicians and abuse by patients. The patient with a neurotic disorder may not use the drug to obtain a high, but the relief from anxiety may involve psychological habituation and tolerance for increased dosage, with the development of physical dependence and a withdrawal or abstinence syndrome.

The *benzodiazepines* are the most effective and widely prescribed antianxiety agents. Shader and Greenblatt (1975) pointed out that they are not associated with clinically important enzyme induction, that they have a relatively low addiction risk at therapeutic dosages, and that they rarely cause serious outcomes in deliberate or accidental overdosages. Side effects include drowsiness and ataxia, and all drugs in this group are likely to act synergistically with other CNS depressants (which increases the prospect of fatality in the event of concurrent overdosage with alcohol or other sedative drugs).

As of 1976, diazepam (Valium) was the most frequently prescribed drug in the United States, with 75 percent of such prescriptions written by nonpsychiatrists. Chlordiazepoxide (Librium) is also widely used, but has roughly half the therapeutic potency of diazepam (i.e., requires about twice the dose) and is eliminated roughly twice as quickly (i.e., is shorter acting and must be given roughly twice as frequently). Neither drug is well absorbed intramuscularly, but both drugs may be carefully given intravenously in the event that extreme panic prevents initial dosage by mouth.

Many other drugs have been tried in the treatment of neurotic disorders, and tricyclics such as amitriptyline may be indicated *where anxiety is combined with significant depression.* Electroshock therapy may produce temporary relief of depression in patients with neurotic disorders, but should usually be avoided because: (1) depression is apt to recur when it represents a reaction to loss or frustration that remains unchanged; (2) convulsive therapy may accentuate symptoms of anxiety and apprehension, and lasting relief requires more intensive efforts directed toward treatment of the neurotic disorder.

Short-acting barbiturates and propanediols such as meprobamate have been used in the treatment of anxiety, but they have a high potential for abuse and dependency, as well as a significant risk of fatal overdosage. Beta-adrenergic blocking agents such as DL-propranolol (Inderal) reduce many of the somatic symptoms associated with anxiety, but may cause or exacerbate symptoms of depression, and are not currently approved by the Food and Drug Administration for treatment of anxiety states.

Major tranquilizing drugs (antipsychotic agents) have often been prescribed in the treatment of anxiety or other neurotic disorders. However, their use may also be complicated by accentuation of depression, and they have many undesirable side effects even when given in relatively low doses. They are also believed to be less effective in the treatment of neurotic disorders than are the benzodiazepines.

There are many reports that imipramine has a specific therapeutic effect against certain panic disorders, even though the patient is not clinically depressed. These reports emphasize that a relatively low dosage may be adequate, and that dosages in the usual antidepressant range may produce toxic effects in nondepressed patients. However, the Food and Drug Administration currently classifies this as an experimental use of imipramine.

REVIEW QUESTIONS

191. *Neurotic illnesses* are best defined as those psychiatric disorders in which:
    (A) reality testing is relatively unimpaired
    (B) the chief complaint is inability to achieve one's innate potential
    (C) early childhood experiences are the determining factors
    (D) anxiety is the chief characteristic
    (E) defense mechanisms can no longer exclude painful memories from awareness

192. The two psychiatric disorders generally believed to be less frequently diagnosed in the United States since World War II than previously are general paralysis and:
    (A) hysterical paralyses and anesthesias
    (B) obsessive-compulsive neuroses
    (C) neurotic depressions
    (D) phobic disorders
    (E) neuroses of all types

193. Each of the following may result from conversion hysteria except:
    (A) epileptiform seizures
    (B) blindness
    (C) extensor plantar response
    (D) astasia-abasia
    (E) abdominal pain

194. The *primary gain* of a neurotic illness refers to:
    (A) relief from internal conflict by symptom formation
    (B) external benefits derived from illness, such as increased attention
    (C) masochistic punishment derived from the symptoms
    (D) all of the above
    (E) none of the above

195. Gross motor hysteria:
    (A) is increasing in frequency in urban western society
    (B) is best treated by reinforcement of dependency needs

(C) is usually learned by identification rather than reinforcement

(D) all of the above

(E) none of the above

196. In a phobic disorder, the fear is:
    (A) always associated with specific objects or situations
    (B) avoidable
    (C) consciously recognized as irrational
    (D) displaced from its true object
    (E) all of the above

197. In which form of neurotic disorder is the patient *least* likely to complain of feeling anxious?
    (A) conversion hysteria
    (B) phobic disorder
    (C) obsessive-compulsive disorder
    (D) hypochondriacal disorder
    (E) neurotic depression

198. A 46-year-old man, previously well adjusted, has developed early morning insomnia, increasing anergia, and the obsession that God has given him cancer as punishment for his failures. Despite repeated medical examinations and assurances that he does not have cancer, he maintains his belief that he does. The correct diagnosis is:
    (A) neurotic depression
    (B) hypochondriacal disorder
    (C) obsessive-compulsive disorder
    (D) Briquet's hysteria
    (E) psychotic depression

Summary of Directions

A	B	C	D	E
1, 2, 3 only	1, 3 only	2, 4 only	4 only	All are correct

---

199. Examples of secondary gain include:
    (1) release from unpleasant responsibility
    (2) increased personal attention
    (3) financial compensation
    (4) relief from emotional conflict

200. Examples of dissociative disorders include:
    (1) multiple personalities
    (2) fugue
    (3) functional amnesia
    (4) compensation neurosis

201. A 30-year-old man consulted his physician because of several hour-long episodes of severe chest pains during the past month. Thorough physical examination revealed no somatic disorder but during an interview the patient stated that heart disease must run in his family, since his father had died unexpectedly of a myocardial infarction three months previously. In response to questioning, he stated that he felt little grief following his father's death, and he described his father as difficult to like, harsh, and emotionally distant. This situation appears to represent:
    (1) hypochondriacal preoccupation
    (2) a pathological grief reaction
    (3) Ganser's syndrome
    (4) conversion hysteria

202. Neurotic symptoms:
    (1) are produced by defense mechanisms
    (2) may be seen in functional psychoses
    (3) are manifestations of anxiety or fear
    (4) may be seen in organic brain syndromes

203. Characteristics of anxiety neurosis include:
    (1) excessive free-floating anxiety and over-concern
    (2) episodes of panic
    (3) multiple somatic complaints
    (4) infrequent appearance of symptoms related to other neuroses

204. The following may be observed as part of a hysterical conversion disorder:
    (1) dystonias and dyskinesias
    (2) a lump in the throat
    (3) bruises and tissue atrophy
    (4) pain

205. Defense mechanisms prominent in obsessive-compulsive disorders include:
    (1) intellectualization
    (2) isolation
    (3) undoing
    (4) repression

SELECTED REFERENCES

1. Eisenstein, V.W. (1956). *Neurotic Interaction in Marriage.* New York: Basic Books.

2. Fenichel, O. (1945). *The Psychoanalytic Theory of Neurosis.* New York: W.W. Norton and Co.

3. Freud, S. (1920). *A General Introduction to Psychoanalysis.* (Reprinted 1953) New York: Perma Books, No. M-5001.

4. Greenfield, N.S. (1959). The relationship between recalled forms of childhood discipline and psychopathology. *Journal of Consulting Psychology,* vol. 23, pages 139–142.

5. Hollender, M.H. (1965). Perfectionism. *Comprehensive Psychiatry,* vol. 6, pages 94–103.

6. Hollingshead, A.B., and Redlich, F.C. (1958). *Social Class and Mental Illness.* New York: John Wiley and Sons.

7. Horney, K. (1937). *The Neurotic Personality of Our Time.* New York: W.W. Norton and Co.

8. Leveton, A.F. (1962). Reproach: The art of shamesmanship. *British Journal of Medical Psychology,* vol. 35, pages 101–111.

9. May, R. (1950). *The Meaning of Anxiety.* New York: The Ronald Press Co.

10. Seligman, M.E.P. (1975). *Helplessness.* San Francisco: W. H. Freeman and Co. Chapter 6.

11. Shader, R.I., and Greenblatt, D.J. (1975). The psychopharmacological treatment of anxiety states. In *Manual of Psychiatric Therapeutics,* edited by R. I. Shader. Boston: Little, Brown and Co. Chapter 2.

12. Sullivan, H.S. (1953). *The Interpersonal Theory of Psychiatry.* New York: W.W. Norton and Co.

13. Thigpen, C.H., and Cleckley, H.M. (1957). *The Three Faces of Eve.* (Reprinted 1961) New York: Popular Library.

16. Personality Disorders: Antisocial and Other

The only way to get rid of a temptation is to yield to it.
Oscar Wilde, The Picture of Dorian Gray

OVERVIEW OF PERSONALITY DISORDERS

Personality is a term derived from the Latin word *persona* for the mask worn on the stage by an actor in ancient Rome. The term is used in psychiatry to refer to a person's deeply ingrained patterns of behavior, especially as they affect interpersonal relationships and social skills. These patterns are assumed to evolve from a combination of innate and learned tendencies, and to be modified by life stresses and neurological changes.

Personality types are descriptive labels referring to frequently encountered constellations, or "syndromes," of personality characteristics. Depending on the context, such labels may emphasize adaptive capacity (e.g., rigid), social temperament (i.e., introverted or extraverted), behavior characteristics associated with the stages of psychosexual development (e.g., oral, anal), or characteristic patterns of defense mechanisms (e.g., hysterical, obsessive-compulsive). Such labels are used to describe habitual tendencies, and therefore are not always pejorative or suggestive of pathology.

Personality disorders are defined as deeply ingrained *maladaptive* patterns of behavior that tend to persist throughout a person's lifetime and are often recognizable by the time of adolescence. The disorder leads to behavior that limits the person's use of his potential assets and often provokes retaliation on the part of others that is not intended consciously or deliberately. Personality disorders differ qualitatively from neuroses by the relative absence of long-term anxiety or subjective distress, and from psychoses by the relatively unimpaired capacity for reality testing.

There are three major groups of personality disorders, as follows: (1) *prepsychotic,* involving patterns associated with vulnerability to paranoid, schizophrenic, or mood (affective) psychoses; (2) *neurotic,* involving traits associated with vulnerability to symptoms of obsessive-compulsive or hysterical disorders; and (3) *antisocial* characteristics, involving extractive and manipulative behavior for short-term personal gains, without appropriate consideration for other members of society. A summary of characteristics or traits associated with each of the personality disorders given diagnostic labels by the American Psychiatric Association's *Diagnostic and Statistical Manual* follows.

Paranoid personality involves deep-seated mistrust of other persons, with a strong tendency to use the defense of *projection,* and to ascribe evil motives to others. Other paranoid traits include hypersensitivity, unwarranted suspiciousness, jealousy, and unrealistic ambition or feelings of self-importance. There is often a history of social isolation either by choice or by accident (e.g., deafness, cultural and lingual displacement, or death of spouse and peers). Paranoid attitudes and behavior result in alienation of others with resultant rejection and ostracism, which thus becomes a self-fulfilling prophecy.

Schizoid personality traits include shyness, seclusiveness, and avoidance of interpersonal relationships. Avoidance may be based on fear, as in some children with "school phobia" involving fear of peers or teachers. However, long-established social isolation (i.e., *asocial* as opposed to *antisocial* behavior) may be based on life-long habit. The social introversion scale of the MMPI is the one with the highest index of heritability, but lack of social participation may also be reinforced by unsocial parents, who provide an example or model to be emulated. Other characteristics associated with lack of social participation are passivity, dependency, and increased fantasy or daydreaming.

Cyclothymic (affective) personality characteristics are those associated with vulnerability to major mood (bipolar) disorder. At times persons with this disorder appear exceptionally energetic and socially extraverted, warm, optimistic, and enthusiastic. At other times there may be great reduction in energy level and social participation, accompanied by doubts, fears, and pessimism. These changes are not readily attributable to environmental events, and there has been an increasing tendency to regard this form of personality disorder as indicative of the major mood disorder to which such persons are vulnerable. The term *depressive personality* is sometimes used to refer to persons who lack the frequent mood swings and who consistently show only the depressive features of cyclothymic personality.

Obsessive-compulsive (anankastic) personality traits are those associated with conflict over autonomy in the toilet-training or anal phase of personality development. There is undue rigidity, inhibition, and perfectionistic striving, with excessive cleanliness and meticulous attention to detail.

Hysterical (histrionic) personality traits involve emotional lability and self-dramatization. The latter is always attention-seeking and often unconsciously seductive. The person is usually dependent on others, and obtains secondary gains from disability when it develops.

Antisocial personality characteristics involve uninhibited acting out of selfish impulses that bring the person into repeated conflict with society. (The term *acting out* refers to behaviors that express unconscious conflicts or feelings, so that the individual remains unaware of his true motives.) Such persons may be referred to as *sociopaths* or *psychopaths,* although these terms are no longer included in the standard nomenclature. However, not every person who habitually violates the norms and rules of society should be considered sociopathic. The term *dyssocial behavior* applies to individuals who manifest disregard for the usual social codes and who often come into conflict with them as a result of having lived all their lives in an abnormal moral environment. Unlike true sociopaths, they may be capable of strong loyalties to their own moral code or to members of their own cultural subgroup, and they typically do not show significant personality deviation other than that implied by adherence to such loyalties.

The history of a true sociopath usually indicates a lack of effective social controls during childhood, with inadequate development of conscience. There is a low level of achievement in school and employment. Behavior toward others is extractive and manipulative, and there is likely to be a history of persistent and poorly motivated lying, stealing, vandalism, and unusually early or aggressive sexual behavior. There is often extreme promiscuity, leading to frequent divorces and marital separations, and sometimes experimentation with a wide variety of deviant sexual behaviors. Often there is abuse of alcohol or other drugs, as well as tendencies to repeated automobile accidents, traffic violations, and arrests for both public disorder and criminal offenses. Typical antisocial personality characteristics are contrasted with typical neurotic personality characteristics in Table 16-1.

Explosive (epileptoid) personality is a relatively rare diagnosis applied to persons who exhibit gross outbursts of rage or of verbal or physical aggressiveness, which are strikingly different from the person's usual behavior, and for which he may be regretful and repentant.

Asthenic personality is characterized by easy fatigability, consistently low energy level, lack of enthusiasm, marked incapacity for enjoyment, and oversensitivity to physical or emotional stress.

Passive-aggressive personality is characterized by both passivity and aggressiveness, although the latter is usually expressed passively, as by obstructionism, pouting, procrastination, intentional inefficiency, or stubbornness. This behavior often reflects hostility of which the individual is aware, but which he feels he dare not express openly.

Inadequate personality is characterized by ineffectual responses to emotional, social, intellectual, and physical demands. Although the person seems neither physically nor mentally deficient, he manifests inadaptability, ineptness, poor judgment, social instability, and lack of physical and emotional stamina.

BIOLOGICAL DETERMINANTS OF ANTISOCIAL BEHAVIOR

Extreme difficulty in modifying long-standing patterns of antisocial behavior has sometimes been used to support a belief that they are based on

Table 16-1. Typical Antisocial vs Neurotic Personality Characteristics

Antisocial Personality	*Neurotic Personality*
Psychopathic or sociopathic personality; instinct-ridden character; character or behavior disorders	Symptomatic, situational, or character neuroses
Predominantly male (approx. 3:1)	Predominantly female (approx. 3:2)
First psychiatric contact prior to age of 40 years	First psychiatric contact at any age
Concentration in lower socioeconomic classes and areas	Equal distribution of new cases in all classes, but concentration of treated cases in upper classes
Defective or absent superego	Rigid superego
Minimal or no regrets, guilt, or depression over serious past antisocial behavior	Frequent regrets, guilt, and depression over minor or imagined past mistakes or misdeeds
Uninhibited acting out of hedonistic impulses, with inability to postpone immediate gratification for future reward. Reckless antisocial behavior	Excessive inhibition of present impulses (particularly sexual or aggressive) in anticipation of long-range advantage. Conformity with standards of civilized society
Amoral, unreliable, irresponsible. Pathological liar, cheat, swindler, thief. May be promiscuous, violent, or addicted to alcohol or drugs. Indifferent to religion	Moral, reliable, responsible, but lacks self-confidence and may be indecisive. Devout or conflicted over religion
Absence of long-range plans or efforts, and freedom from worry or anxiety; confident and carefree	Ambitious plans and striving for goals in remote future, and intangible ideals with much doubt, fear, anxiety, and apprehension
Does not care what other people think of him, so long as this does not frustrate his immediate goals	Strives to attain and retain affection of others. Insecure and sensitive to criticism. Frequent feelings of inadequacy and worthlessness
Incapable of true affection for others, but uses superficial charm and plausibility to manipulate others	Capable of deep affection, but latent (unconscious) hostility often interferes with ability to maintain warm relationships
Transient enjoyment of uninhibited sexual behavior with wide variety of partners	Sexual impulses or behavior appear dangerous or disgusting, with resulting frigidity or impotence
Hostility may be expressed directly and violently if this does not interfere with goals of the moment	Aggressive impulses not permitted direct expression, but may be displaced onto others, or achieved by indirect expression
Frequent electroencephalographic abnormalities and tendency to mesomorphic body build	Autonomic lability and tendency to ectomorphic body build (except in hysteria)
Frequent history of similar disorder in parents and siblings. Parental deprivation, discord (often illegitimacy or desertion by parents), deceit, and lack of supervision, poor example or controls (occasionally overindulgence); association with delinquent peers or siblings; truancy, job instability, and nomadism; record of conflict with the police or military authorities and often jail sentences	Frequent history of similar disorder in parents and siblings; parental deprivation, discord, domination, and demands; restricted relationships with siblings and peers; high achievement in school and occupation with continued social conformity

hereditary or constitutional psychopathic inferiority. This post hoc reasoning is no more valid than claiming a hereditary basis for the structural damage resulting from severe vitamin deficiency, on the grounds that the damage was not reversed by belated massive doses of the vitamin, deficiency of which had indeed caused the damage. However, some tentative evidence has been provided concerning possible contributions of hereditary or somatic factors in the development of antisocial personality.

Shields and Slater (1961) combined the results reported in five studies of adult *twins,* at least one of whom was involved in criminal behavior. The concordance rate among monozygotic co-twins was 68 percent, and among same-sexed dizygotic co-twins was 35 percent. Holzinger's index of heritability computed from these rates is 0.51, suggesting that hereditary and environmental factors were about equally important in the development of criminal behavior among these samples. In a comparable study of twins with persistent juvenile delinquency, Rosanoff and his associates reported concordance rates of 85 percent in monozygotic pairs and 75 percent in same-sexed dizygotic pairs, resulting in a Holzinger index of heritability of 0.40 for this series. However, all these twin studies were conducted prior to World War II, and therefore prior to the availability of modern serological techniques for the determination of zygosity.

O'Neal and her associates (1962) supplied interesting data concerning *parental deviance* and the genesis of antisocial personality. In a follow-up study of over 500 children seen in a child guidance clinic about 30 years previously, they identified 84 males who were diagnosed sociopathic (antisocial) as adults, and they compared the characteristics of their parents with those of the parents of 166 males with other psychiatric disorders and also with 75 males showing no gross psychopathology. Only 13 percent of the antisocial males had *mothers* with a probable diagnosis of antisocial personality, as compared with 9 percent of males with other psychiatric disorders, and 4 percent of males without psychopathology. However, 51 per-

cent of the antisocial males had *fathers* with a probable diagnosis of antisocial personality, as compared with 33 percent of the males with other psychiatric disorders, and 19 percent of the males without obvious psychopathology.

These figures do not conform with any simple mechanism of heritance, and do not indicate whether antisocial males inherit or learn their antisocial behavior from their parents. However, they do suggest a much stronger contribution by father than by mother. This tendency may be mediated in part by *physique,* or *body build.* In their detailed analysis of physique (somatotype) among 500 matched pairs of persistently delinquent and nondelinquent boys, Glueck and Glueck (1956) reported a strong statistical association between delinquency and mesomorphic or athletic body build. Far more delinquents than nondelinquents were predominantly mesomorphic (60 percent versus 30 percent), whereas fewer were predominantly ectomorphic (14 percent versus 39 percent).

Lykken (1957) undertook a study of anxiety in persons with antisocial personality. He divided 49 persons diagnosed as psychopaths into two groups, according to whether they met criteria listed by Cleckley for "primary" sociopathy, and compared them with 15 control subjects on a battery of tests related to anxiety reactivity and anxiety conditionability. In comparison with control subjects, the primary sociopaths showed significantly less anxiety by questionnaire, less galvanic skin response reactivity to a conditioned stimulus associated with electroshock, and less avoidance of punished responses on a test of avoidance learning than the controls. The remaining, or "neurotic," sociopaths scored significantly higher on two psychological tests for levels of anxiety. Subsequent studies have discriminated between subgroups of persons with antisocial personalities on the basis of their physiological responses to intramuscular injections of epinephrine, and the subsequent rate at which physiological parameters returned to a resting level. Normalization of physiological response has been accomplished experimentally by means of imipramine, but the long-term effects of this drug on antisocial behavior are not yet adequately documented.

PSYCHOSOCIAL DETERMINANTS OF ANTISOCIAL BEHAVIOR

Levy (1951) pointed to two contrasting patterns in the development of delinquency: parental rejection and other forms of deprivation, and parental indulgence, permitting the child uncontrolled expression of his aggressions and desires. Sometimes the child is exposed to both of these apparently contradictory patterns, but it is not difficult to interpret overindulgence as either a manifestation of rejection (by a parent who doesn't care enough to control the child), or as a reaction formation against feelings of guilt (that would arise if the parent consciously recognized his hostility and rejection). Moreover, the child may be exposed to inconsistent rewards and punishments, indulgence, and rejection, whether he or she lives with both parents continually, or one or both parents are absent from the home, or he or she is moved from one home or institution to another.

There is an unduly high frequency of both *parental death* and *separation* during the childhoods of those who develop antisocial personality characteristics. Among their extensive comparisons between 500 matched pairs of persistently delinquent and nondelinquent boys, Glueck and Glueck (1950) recorded detailed data concerning various forms of family disruption and parental loss. Sixty percent of the delinquents, as compared with 34 percent of the nondelinquents, came from homes that had been broken by separation, divorce, death, or prolonged absence of a parent, by the time of the boy's inclusion in the research project at a mean age of roughly 14½ years. The first breach in family life had occurred before the age of 5 years in 170 delinquents, as compared with 80 nondelinquents. Significantly larger numbers of delinquents than nondelinquents had been deprived of one or both parents for each of five categories of deprivation: sporadic separation of parents, permanent separation or divorce, death, absence from the home for at least a year on account of criminality or illness, and abandonment at birth.

Bowlby (1951) reviewed data from many countries concerning the high frequency of broken homes and admission to institutions during the childhood of persons with delinquency and other behavior disorders. He contended that loss of *mother* during early childhood was more damaging than loss of father. However, many studies show that loss of *father* is both more frequent and more statistically significant in the case of *male* delinquents. In the study mentioned previously, Glueck and Glueck noted that 41.2 percent of their *male* delinquents (as compared with 24.8 percent of the nondelinquent controls) were no longer living with their own *father*; whereas only 15.6 percent of these male delinquents (as compared with 7.2 percent of the nondelinquents) were no longer living with their own *mother*.

In a subsequent study involving a large sample of Minnesota school children, Gregory (1965) analyzed frequencies of delinquency during high school years among those with various kinds of parental loss recorded previously (at the time they were in the ninth grade). Delinquency *in boys* was found to be much more frequent than average among those who had lost their *father* by parental separation or divorce, and somewhat more frequent than average among those who had lost their father by death, as well as among boys who had experienced other forms of parental loss during childhood (Table 16-2). These findings were not restricted to any socioeconomic group. Delinquency *in girls* was most frequent among those whose parents had separated or divorced, those who had lost their *mother* by death, those who were living with their father only, and those who were not living with either parent. These findings suggest that the identification model provided and the control normally exercised by the *parent of the same sex* are more crucial in preventing delinquency during adolescence than any aspect of the relationship with the parent of the opposite sex.

However, the majority of persistent delinquents and adults with antisocial personality have grown up in homes where both parents were present throughout most of their childhood. Studies on

Table 16-2. Frequencies of Subsequent Delinquency among a Statewide Sample of Minnesota Boys, According to Persons with Whom Boy was Living During Ninth Grade

Person with whom boy was living during ninth grade	Number of boys	Percentage subsequently rated as delinquent	Statistical significance of deviation from average
Both parents	4,682	22.9	
Father only	78	24.4	
Mother only (father dead)	159	31.4	P < 0.025
Mother only (divorced or separated)	164	40.2	P < 0.0005
One parent and step-parent	115	28.7	
Neither parent	94	34.0	P < 0.025
Total	5,292	24.1	

Adapted from Gregory, I. Anterospective data following childhood loss of a parent. I. Delinquency and high school dropout. *Archives of General Psychiatry,* 13:99–109, 1965.

the *quality of parental relationships* existing within these homes indicate that various hidden factors may contribute to the development of *superego lacunae* (holes or blind spots in the superego) of children with severe antisocial attitudes and behavior. Johnson and Szurek (1952) emphasized the subtle conscious and unconscious ways in which parental behavior directs the development of the child's superego, and pointed out that the child internalizes not only the positive, socially consistent attitudes of the parents, but also the frequently unexpressed, ambivalent, antisocial feelings. They maintained that antisocial acting out in a child is unconsciously fostered and sanctioned by the parents, who *vicariously achieve gratification* of their own poorly integrated forbidden impulses through the child's acting out. In addition, one or both parents unconsciously experience gratification for their own hostile and destructive wishes toward the child, who is repeatedly harmed by his own behavior.

Thus, the *predominant patterns of childhood experiences* which precede sociopathy in adulthood involve various combinations of parental absence, rejection, and indifference; inconsistent rewards and limits; parents' conflict with each other and

also with society at large; deceit; and the example or covert approval of antisocial behavior. Often there are no incentives or rewards for good behavior at home or at school, and the values of the peer group tend to be accepted uncritically.

Achievement in school, therefore, tends to be lower than native ability would suggest, although there may be some success in athletic and other extracurricular pursuits. In a high proportion of cases there is a history of temper tantrums in childhood, repeated difficulty with teachers, resentment of discipline, or open rebellion and truancy. Often such children are expelled or otherwise leave school prematurely, and have to be satisfied with jobs below their native capability. There are frequent changes of occupation and residence and moves to other localities, often resulting from situational difficulties of their own making. They tend to spend money freely when they have it, and they are usually in financial difficulties. They are apt to accumulate a long record of conflict with police or military authorities, interspersed with jail sentences followed by repeated offenses of the same nature, so that it appears they are unable to learn from the unpleasant consequences of past mistakes.

Socioeconomic Factors

It has long been recognized that high rates of delinquency are found among boys who live in underprivileged areas of large cities. Shaw and McKay (1942) undertook a detailed ecological analysis of such rates within the city of Chicago for three 6-year periods, commencing in 1900 and ending in 1933. In the first of their three series, the four areas with the highest rates were all immediately adjacent to the Loop; other areas with high rates were in the stockyards district and in south Chicago. The areas with low rates, on the other hand, were located for the most part near the city's periphery. The correlation coefficient for delinquency rates in the early and later series (in 113 geographical areas) was found to be + 0.70. This coefficient was much lower than it would otherwise have been, due to radical changes in only six of the areas studied. Most of the areas with high rates in the early series also corresponded with those ranking highest in the two later series. Their principal conclusion was that sociological delinquency was a subcultural tradition in the areas of the city inhabited by the lower socioeconomic classes. The rates of delinquency in these areas did not tend to change much in spite of marked changes in the ethnic origin of the persons living in these areas.

Many subsequent statistical studies tended to confirm the popular impression that gang delinquency is primarily a working-class phenomenon. Thus Lander (1954) reported that in Baltimore the correlation between the juvenile delinquency rate and overcrowding was + 0.73. The correlation between the juvenile delinquency rate and substandard housing conditions was + 0.69. On the basis of similar correlations a number of persons have argued that bad housing has a direct causal effect on the delinquency rate and that removal of slums would lead to removal of social ills, but Lander rejected this interpretation as insufficient. He reported that the correlation between delinquency and median years of schooling for the adult population was − 0.51 and that the correlation between delinquency and median rentals was − 0.53, but more sophisticated analysis indicated

that these variables were not fundamentally related to the prediction or understanding of juvenile delinquency. He concluded that adequate explanations of the differential delinquency rates must involve consideration of the direct motivation of behavior, and he invoked the concept of *anomie:* "When the group norms are no longer binding or valid in an area or for a population sub-group insofar is individual behavior likely to lead to deviant behavior. Delinquency is a function of the stability and acceptance of the group norms with legal sanctions and the consequent effectiveness of the social controls in securing and forming juvenile behavior."

Cohen (1955) attempted to account for the delinquent subculture on the basis of the valid observation that birds of a feather flock together. Lower-class children tend to be reared in surroundings that are quite different from the middle-class standards of schools they must attend. Status frustration and loss of self-esteem leads such children to draw together in small groups or gangs. The delinquent subculture thus rewards those who attack or assault the middle-class status system. However, not all boys from a high delinquency area rebel against the standards of the larger society.

Scarpitti and his associates (1960) pointed to the long-term stability of "good" boys living in poor areas. They concluded that once a favorable self-image has been internalized by preadolescents with respect to friends, parents, schools, and the law, there is every reason to believe that it is as difficult to alter as a delinquent self-image.

Prediction of Delinquency

Hathaway and Monachesi (1963) reported on delinquency occurring over a period of several years, among a sample of more than 11,000 adolescents, for whom psychological tests and social background information had been obtained when they were in the ninth grade. High points on three of the scales of the Minnesota Multiphasic Personality Inventory were associated with subsequent low rates of delinquency, whereas high points on three other scales were associated with subsequent high rates of delinquency. The three *suppressor* scales were 2, 5, and 0 (depression, femininity, and social introversion), whereas the three *excitor* scales were 4, 8, and 9 (psychopathic deviate, schizoid, and hypomanic). In this sample, the rates of delinquency showed a relatively limited association with intelligence and with parental socioeconomic status. However, those children from broken families had much higher rates of delinquency (as discussed previously), as did those who dropped out of school before graduating.

Using subsamples of these data, Wirt and Briggs (1959) analyzed environmental factors related to delinquency among those with MMPI scores characterized by extremes of low and high vulnerability to delinquency. Those from both groups who remained nondelinquent came from a background with a high index of family sufficiency and family occupational-educational achievement. Members of both groups who became delinquent came from backgrounds with a low index of family sufficiency and occupational-educational achievement, together with low achievement by the child and a high frequency of conflict with parents. In a subsequent study, Briggs, Wirt, and Johnson (1961) showed that interaction between the MMPI profile obtained during the ninth grade and frequency of family disruption would identify subgroups of the population having very high vulnerability to subsequent delinquent behavior. If the highest two MMPI scales were among the three excitor scales (4, 8, and 9) and there was a history of three or more family disruptions by the ninth grade, the frequency of severe delinquency in the next few years was about 80 percent in this particular study.

Identification of sub-groups with high vulnerability may permit effective intervention before overt delinquent behavior occurs. However, a major problem in the use of such predictive data is the occurrence of "false positives," subjects incorrectly labeled as predelinquent and thereby subjected to unnecessary (or perhaps even adverse) intervention. In a 1975 Puerto Rican study, Ferracuti, Dinitz, and Acosta de Brenes were able to achieve correct retrospective classification of all 202 subjects by means of a stepwise discriminant

function analysis. Each of 101 delinquent boys (ages 11 to 17 and living in the slums of San Juan) was paired with a nondelinquent boy matched for age (within 6 months), area of residence, socioeconomic level, family income, and, for most pairs, class in school. All subjects were very carefully screened to ensure that no boys were incorrectly placed in either group (e.g., on the basis of avoiding police contact). Dependent variables included medical history and laboratory tests (78 items), psychological test and psychiatric interview items (70 items), characteristics of the subject's home and family (48 items), subject's school record and behaviors (52 items), and electroencephalographic tests (19 items). Each of the groups of items except the last provided statistically significant discrimination (i.e., correct labeling of most subjects as delinquents or nondelinquents), but some subjects remained incorrectly classified in each case. However, the combined pool of items provided error-free classification by means of a prediction equation involving only 13 items (2 items from the medical group, 3 from the psychiatric, 3 from the school records, and 5 from the family histories). These results underscore the value of *multidisciplinary* approaches to the prediction of vulnerability to delinquency and to its remediation.

COURSE AND TREATMENT

Psychiatric statistics show a much higher frequency of antisocial personality disorders among young adults than among middle-aged or older members of the population. This has often led to the conclusion that such persons tend to mature and behave more responsibly with advancing age. This belief may find some support in the substantial reduction in rates of automobile accidents (and corresponding insurance premiums) among male drivers after the age of 25 years. However, it should not be overlooked that reckless antisocial behavior may result in removal from society in a number of ways, including: (1) an increased rate of deaths and permanent disability from automobile and other accidents; (2) increased vulnerability to being killed or injured by other antisocial persons, police, or their own victims; (3) a tendency for some antisocial personalities to become incapacitated by chronic alcoholism and drug dependence; (4) prolonged or repeated imprisonment for felonies. Rates of diagnosable sociopathy as high as 40 percent have been reported in some studies of penitentiary populations.

Not only does the nature and frequency of antisocial behavior vary according to socioeconomic status, but so does *society's response to similar behavior* by members of different socioeconomic or cultural groups. This has been well documented by a number of authors including Hollingshead and Redlich (1958). Antisocial behavior is more likely to be viewed as evidence of illness at upper socioeconomic levels, and antisocial persons in those classes are more likely to be involved in individual psychotherapy than are members of lower socioeconomic groups. However, in recent years there has been a strong tendency to emphasize *group therapies* as being more effective than individual therapy in modifying antisocial behavior. The delinquent is much more likely to accept the judgment of peers, than that of representatives of authority, to the effect that certain antisocial attitudes and behavior are "just plain stupid" (i.e., have obvious negative consequences). Unfortunately, long-term studies of offenders subjected to compulsory group therapy (as a condition for probation or parole) do not show a convincing reduction in rates of recidivism. This may suggest that for some persons, compulsory therapy results only in their learning another role, namely, that of the false penitent who is able to "con" the parole board or probation officer.

There have also been a number of innovative attempts at behavior modification, including the use of aversive conditioning techniques. However, these techniques may well constitute "cruel and unusual punishment," and offenders have been increasingly vocal in asserting their right to freedom from treatment. From a practical viewpoint, they may indeed be better off when treated as "bad" than when treated as "mad." This is because the punishment for an offense is more likely to be associated with a definite and shorter period of incarceration than is therapy for long-standing personality disorder. There are many aspects of the criminal justice system that are currently under review. Among reforms that are under consideration or implementation in certain areas are the following: (1) elimination of indeterminate sentences for some offenses; (2) reduction in inconsistency of sentencing from one locality or court to another; and (3) increasing emphasis on rehabilitation and restitution.

In the Puerto Rican study of delinquency referred to previously, Ferracuti and his associates concluded that one of the critical areas for intervention appears to be the school. When family socialization fails, the child has a second (although lesser) chance of being socialized if his peer group or school structure can assume this task. Compulsory school attendance should therefore be accompanied by efforts toward extracurricular involvement, as contrasted with the process of stigmatization and rejection that fosters high school dropouts and delinquents.

REVIEW QUESTIONS

206. Characteristics of the hysterical personality include each of the following *except:*
    (A) easy fatigability
    (B) emotional instability
    (C) attention seeking behavior
    (D) dependency
    (E) seductiveness

207. Characteristics of the schizoid personality include each of the following *except:*
    (A) avoidance of close relationships with others
    (B) inability to express aggression
    (C) dependency
    (D) multiple personality
    (E) shy, obedient childhood

208. Characteristics of the cyclothymic personality include each of the following *except:*
    (A) personal warmth
    (B) avoidance of competition
    (C) alternating moods
    (D) enthusiasm
    (E) pessimism

209. The mechanism of projection is most closely associated with:
    (A) paranoid personality
    (B) hysterical personality
    (C) passive-aggressive personality
    (D) schizoid personality
    (E) obsessive-compulsive personality

Directions for questions 210 to 212: For each of the numbered items which follow, answer *A* if true of antisocial personality but *not* of dyssocial behavior, or *B* if true of dyssocial behavior but *not* of antisocial personality, or *C* if true of *both* antisocial personality and dyssocial behavior, or *D* if true of *neither* antisocial nor dyssocial behavior.
    (A) antisocial personality
    (B) dyssocial behavior
    (C) both
    (D) neither

210. Repeated behaviors which endanger public order or safety, or which are either illegal or viewed as deviant by society.
211. Superego is absent or defective.
212. Incapable of strong loyalties.

Summary of Directions

A	B	C	D	E
1, 2, 3 only	1, 3 only	2, 4 only	4 only	All are correct

213. Personality disorders as a group are characterized by:
    (1) persistent high levels of anxiety
    (2) relatively unimpaired reality testing
    (3) usually high degree of motivation for treatment
    (4) persistent (life-long) behavior patterns
214. Johnson and Szurek described some antisocial persons as characterized by:
    (1) relatively stable childhood family situation
    (2) superego lacunae
    (3) acting out by the child of the parents' forbidden impulses
    (4) parents obtaining vicarious satisfaction from the child's self-defeating acts

215. Countertransference problems are prone to arise in the treatment of patients with personality disorders because such persons:
    (1) by their actions invite others to displace anger onto them
    (2) are often viewed as bad rather than sick
    (3) have insatiable needs for nurturance, but tend to pick out persons least able to meet these needs
    (4) don't care how other people feel about them

SELECTED REFERENCES

1. Andry, R. (1960). *Delinquency and Parental Pathology.* London: Methuen.
2. Bowlby, J. (1951). *Maternal Care and Mental Health.* Geneva: World Health Organization (Monograph Series No. 2).
3. Briggs, P.F., Wirt, R.D., and Johnson, R. (1961). An application of prediction tables to the study of delinquency. *Journal of Consulting Psychology,* vol. 25, pages 46–50.
4. Cleckley, H. (1976). *The Mask of Sanity: An Attempt to Clarify Some Issues About the So-called Psychopathic Personality* (5th ed.). St. Louis: C. V. Mosby Co.
5. Cohen, A.K. (1955). *Delinquent Boys: The Culture of the Gang.* Glencoe, Illinois: The Free Press, Division of Macmillan Co.
6. Ferracuti, F., Dinitz, S., and Acosta de Brenes, E. (1975). *Delinquents and Non-Delinquents in the Puerto Rican Slum Culture.* Columbus, Ohio: Ohio State University Press.
7. Glueck, S., and Glueck, E. (1950). *Unraveling Juvenile Delinquency.* Cambridge, Mass.: Commonwealth Fund and Harvard University Press.
8. Glueck, S., and Glueck, E. (1956). *Physique and Delinquency.* New York: Harper & Row.
9. Gregory, I. (1965). Anterospective data following childhood loss of a parent. I. Delinquency and high school dropout. *Archives of General Psychiatry,* vol. 13, pages 99–109.
10. Hathaway, S.R., and Monachesi, E.D. (1963). *Adolescent Personality and Behavior: MMPI Patterns of Normal, Delinquent, Dropout, and*

Other Outcomes. Minneapolis: University of Minnesota Press.

11. Hollingshead, A.B., and Redlich, F.C. (1958). *Social Class and Mental Illness.* New York: John Wiley and Sons.

12. Johnson, A.M., and Szurek, S.A. (1952). The genesis of antisocial acting out in children and adults. *Psychoanalytic Quarterly,* vol. 21, page 323.

13. Lander, B. (1954). *Towards an Understanding of Juvenile Delinquency.* New York: Columbia University Press. Pages 77–90.

14. Levy, D.M. (1951). Psychopathic behavior in infants and children: A critical survey of the existing concepts. *American Journal of Orthopsychiatry,* vol. 21, pages 250–254.

15. Lykken, D.T. (1957). A study of anxiety in the sociopathic personality. *Journal of Abnormal and Social Psychology,* vol. 55, pages 6–10.

16. O'Neal, P., Robins, L.N., King, L.J., and Schaefer, J. (1962). Parental deviance and the genesis of sociopathic personality. *American Journal of Psychiatry,* vol. 118, pages 1114–1123.

17. Scarpitti, F.R., Murray, E., Dinitz, S., and Reckless, W.C. (1960). The "good" boy in a high delinquency area: 4 years later. *American Sociological Review,* vol. 25, pages 555–558.

18. Shaw, C.R., and McKay, H.D. (1942). *Juvenile Delinquency and Urban Areas.* Chicago: University of Chicago Press. Pages 60–68.

19. Shield, J., and Slater, E. (1961). Heredity and Psychological Abnormality. In *Handbook of Abnormal Psychology,* edited by H.J. Eysenck. New York: Basic Books. Pages 298–343.

20. Wirt, R.D., and Briggs, P.F. (1959). Personality and Environmental Factors in the Development of Delinquency. American Psychological Association, *Psychological Monographs* No. 485, vol. 73, no. 15.

17. Psychosomatic Factors in Physical Disorders (Psychophysiological Disorders)

The sorrow which has no vent in tears may make other organs weep.
Henry Maudsley

AFFECT-EQUIVALENTS, BIOLOGICAL STRESS, AND SPECIFICITY OF TARGET-ORGAN

Psychosomatic disorders are those disorders of bodily function or structure that develop at least in part because of emotional factors. In other words, the pathology of somatic tissues is at least partly attributable to psychological determinants; i.e., to psychogenic factors. By contrast, *somatopsychic disorders* consist of emotional manifestations that are determined by or secondary to physical or somatic pathology. However, this distinction has often been overlooked, and the term psychosomatic has been used to include both of the preceding interactions between the mind and body.

Earlier in the present century, psychoanalysts used the term *organ neurosis* to distinguish psychosomatic disorders from the disturbances in bodily function due to conversion hysteria. At first it was thought that the somatic pathology might be symbolic of unconscious conflict (as had previously been established in the case of conversion symptoms). This led to the interpretation of psychosomatic disorders through a superficial *organ language,* some of which is a matter of everyday usage. Thus, nausea and vomiting are associated with disgust in such phrases as, "You make me sick to my stomach." Similar expressions may be related to bowel and bladder functions that are relatively voluntary. However, many persons came to the conclusion that there was no symbolic relationship between unconscious conflict and physiological functions that were involuntary and automatic. The bodily manifestations of

psychosomatic disorders are therefore *distinguished from those of conversion hysteria* by the following: (1) involvement of organs and viscera innervated by the autonomic nervous system and hence not under full voluntary control or perception; (2) failure of the symptoms to alleviate anxiety; (3) physiological rather than symbolic origin of symptoms; (4) structural changes often produced, sometimes life-threatening.

Affect-Equivalents

It is only a few decades since physiologists first studied the somatic concomitants of fear, hunger, pain, and rage. Direct observation of changes in the gastric mucosa were reported by Wolf and Wolff. When their subject became angry, his stomach lining was red, and there was an increase in both rhythmic contractions and secretion of acid. When the same man was depressed or frightened, his stomach was pale, and there was a decrease in its movements and acid secretion.

Ax (1953) reported that a number of physiological responses differentiated reliably between fear and anger in humans. Further studies have suggested that the response to fear resembles that following an injection of epinephrine, whereas the response to anger resembles that following a combined injection of both epinephrine and norepinephrine. Central sympathetic reactivity appears to be increased during anger and decreased during depression. These and similar findings led to psychosomatic disorders being regarded as *somatic equivalents of chronic dysphoric affect* (fear, anger, or depression).

This concept is explicit in the definition of **psychophysiological autonomic and visceral disorders** as representing the visceral expression of affect, which may thereby be largely prevented from becoming conscious. Psychophysiological disorders involve a single organ system, usually innervated by the autonomic nervous system. The bodily changes are those that normally accompany certain emotional states, but the changes are more intense and sustained. However, the person may not be consciously aware of the emotional state that is usually associated with such bodily changes. Often they appear to result from chronic stress that is likely to involve more than one of the basic dysphoric affects. It is therefore appropriate to consider briefly some of the known biological consequences of various forms of stress.

Biological Stress

Walter Cannon (1926) used the term *homeostasis* to describe physiological processes of regulation that maintain constancy in the internal environment. He also applied the term *stress* to those external and internal conditions that affect the regulators of homeostasis, and that thereby tend to disturb the constant state of the fluid matrix. Among these stresses he included cold, oxygen deficiency, loss of blood, and low blood sugar.

Hans Selye and his associates found that many animals responded in a stereotyped manner to a large variety of different stresses, including infection, intoxication, trauma, nervous strain, heat, cold, muscle fatigue, and x-rays. Each of these agents had some specific effects, but the common denominator of the stereotyped response involved a reaction to stress itself. The first signs of this stress response were enlargement of the adrenal cortex (with microscopic evidence of hyperactivity), involution of the thymus and lymph gland system (with accompanying changes in blood count), and ulcers of stomach and intestines, often accompanied by other signs of damage or "shock." In view of the involutional or degenerative changes of most organs of the body, it was striking that the adrenal cortex should *increase* in size and activity. This nonspecific defense mechanism was therefore termed an *alarm reaction.*

Further studies showed that the alarm reaction was merely the first stage of a much more prolonged *general adaptation syndrome,* evolving in three distinct stages: (1) the *alarm reaction* (with an initial phase of *shock,* followed by a phase of *countershock*); (2) the stage of *resistance* (involving successful adaptation to the specific stress or agent); and (3) the stage of *exhaustion,* following prolonged exposure to the stressor (to which resistance had

developed, but could no longer be maintained).

Nonspecific changes in bodily function and structure may occur in any of the three stages, with tissue degeneration such as that producing ulcers of the stomach and intestines being most marked in the initial phase of the alarm reaction, and again in the final stage of exhaustion. It is well established that these changes in bodily function and structure may follow prolonged emotional stress, but it remains uncertain what determines the vulnerability of a specific *target-organ* or organ system.

Specificity of Target-Organ

Except in some disorders with a major voluntary component (e.g., ingestion or elimination), a symbolic basis for unconscious conflict has been discounted. Moreover, most psychosomatic disorders do not appear to be consistently associated with the prolonged experience of a single dysphoric affect. It is even often difficult to establish that such affects were antecedent rather than subsequent to the development of severe somatic symptoms and disturbed relationships with family members and others.

The search for specific causal relationships has therefore included long-standing personality characteristics of the patient, predisposing and precipitating interpersonal relationships, and predisposing constitution or heredity. *The development of some psychosomatic disorders appears to require interaction between several of these factors,* which may be summarized as follows: (1) precipitating stress or conflict; (2) the prevailing dysphoric affect-equivalent; (3) personality characteristics of the patient; (4) interpersonal relationships of childhood; (5) hereditary and constitutional factors.

PEPTIC ULCER

The term *peptic ulcer* is applied to both gastric and duodenal ulcers, but there is a marked difference in their pattern of distribution and probable causation. Gastric ulcer is associated with either normal or abnormal gastric secretion, and is equally frequent in males and in females. Duodenal ulcers are associated with a marked *increase* in gastric secretion, and are currently about four times as frequent in males as in females. They are infrequent in rural areas and in underdeveloped countries, but frequent among administrative and professional persons in industrial countries. They appear to be precipitated or made worse by stressful life circumstances, and improve when the latter are diminished.

What constitutes stressful experience is not always obvious, as illustrated by some experiments on the production of ulcers in monkeys. The first such studies were reported by Brady (1958), who subjected pairs of yoked monkeys to experimental shock during alternating periods of six hours at a time. During the experimental periods, *both* monkeys received a mild electric shock on the foot every 20 seconds, unless *one* of them (the experimental monkey) pressed a nearby bar at least once within each 20-second interval. In his series of studies, several of the experimental monkeys (those that pressed the bar) died or were found at autopsy to have developed ulcers, whereas none of the yoked control monkeys did so. The results were mistakenly assumed to demonstrate that "executive" behavior, involving vigilance and avoidance action, was more stressful than passive inescapable punishment.

Unfortunately, this outcome appears to have been produced by an experimental design in which the first four monkeys to learn avoidance behavior became executives, whereas the slower monkeys to learn were assigned to the yoked group. In a subsequent study, Weiss (1968) assigned rats randomly to executive, helpless, or no-shock conditions, and found that the helpless animals receiving shock developed the most ulcers. This is consistent with the view that helplessness usually produces more stress than does control. Moreover, when no control or escape is allowed, ulceration occurs with unpredictable rather than with predictable shock. Seligman (1975) interpreted these findings in terms of the safety-signal hypothesis of anxiety. The fact that more ulcers occur when shock is uncontrollable reflects the fact that shock is also unpredictable, and unpredictable shock produces more ulcers than predictable shock.

INTERACTION BETWEEN PREDISPOSITION AND PRECIPITATING STRESS. A study of human subjects suggests that neither predisposition nor precipitating stress alone is ordinarily sufficient to produce duodenal ulcers, but that both are necessary. Weiner and his associates (1957) obtained measurements of serum pepsinogen for each of 2,073 Army inductees. From this total sample they selected 63 men with values in the upper 15 percent and 57 men with values in the lower 9 percent of the blood pepsinogen distribution. Each of these subjects was given a battery of psychological tests and a radiological examination of the upper gastrointestinal tract before being sent to basic training. One hundred and seven subjects were reexamined between the eighth and sixteenth weeks of basic training, and nine were found with either healed or active duodenal ulcers. All these men were in the upper 15 percent of the blood pepsinogen distribution, and independent evaluation of the psychological data revealed that these men showed evidence of major unresolved and persistent conflicts about dependency and oral gratification. The authors concluded that neither a high rate of gastric secretion nor a specific psychodynamic constellation is independently responsible for the development of peptic ulcer, but that together they constitute the essential determinants in the precipitation of ulcers on exposure to social situations noxious to the specific individual.

There is an increased frequency of duodenal ulcers among the close relatives of persons with this disorder (11 percent of brothers in one large study, as compared with a base rate of 5.5 percent among the control group). It has also been found that persons with type O blood are about 40 percent more likely to suffer from ulcers than those with other blood types in the ABO system, but this association is far too small to account for the increased frequency of duodenal ulcers in siblings. It therefore appears that both major genes and multiple minor genes may contribute to the genetic component in peptic ulcers.

The sex ratio for peptic ulcer has been changing throughout the present century. Before 1900 peptic ulcer was more frequent in women, and there has been considerable speculation about possible sociocultural determinants of this change. Perhaps nineteenth century men were better able to express both their aggressive and their dependent impulses, whereas women of the same era were more blocked from expressing aggressive and independent impulses. An alternative hypothesis would suggest that stresses associated with modern industrialization have hitherto had their maximum impact on males rather than on females. In any event, *the established data on peptic ulcers provide convincing evidence for the interaction of multiple factors in etiology.*

OTHER PSYCHOPHYSIOLOGICAL DISORDERS

Other Gastrointestinal Disorders
Nausea and vomiting, as well as constipation and diarrhea, are under varying degrees of voluntary modification or partial control. This permits a greater degree of emphasis on symbolic interpretation of symptoms in terms of unconscious conflict than is the case with most other psychophysiological disorders. Persistent constipation and diarrhea may follow conflict over autonomy and control of bowel function during the anal phase of development. This is likely to be associated with obsessive-compulsive, or anankastic, personality traits. Similar personality traits are also associated with *ulcerative colitis,* although this disorder is generally regarded as somatopsychic, with vulnerability determined by strong hereditary or constitutional predisposition.

Obesity
Obesity is the end result of a disturbance in energy balance that involves greater calorie intake than utilization. Dietary intake and exercise are both under voluntary control, and obese persons are often aware of voluntary overeating when they are emotionally upset. However, there are several other significant contributory factors. Obesity is *inversely* related to socioeconomic status, with overweight being about three times more frequent at the lower than at the upper socioeconomic levels. Overweight is also roughly twice as frequent

at age 50 as it is at age 20. In addition, there is probably a larger hereditary component than is generally recognized. Twin studies show much higher correlations for height and weight among monozygotic pairs than among same-sexed dizygotic pairs, so that heritability for both has been estimated as close to 80 percent. In any event, it appears that there are multiple patterns and pathways to obesity.

Anorexia Nervosa
The term *anorexia nervosa* describes a diverse group of conditions with the common denominator of psychogenic malnutrition due to reduced calorie intake. Ninety percent of patients are female, and many are disturbed adolescents who may have a history of obesity. This obesity may have symbolic sexual significance that the patient rejects by rigid diets and sometimes self-induced vomiting. As the condition progresses there is usually amenorrhea, but patients often retain their usual energy despite considerable cachexia, at least until weight drops to critical levels. Severe forms of anorexia nervosa are associated with other symptoms of neurosis or psychosis, particularly depression or schizophrenia. If untreated, there is a 40 percent mortality, so that prompt and energetic intervention is indicated. Further details about this disorder will be included in Chapter 19.

Cardiovascular Disorders
In a large scale epidemiological study, Paffenbarger and his associates (1966) searched for precursors of mortality from *coronary heart disease.* This study involved over 45,000 former students of the University of Pennsylvania and Harvard University and examined relationships between physical, social, and psychological data recorded during college years (1921 to 1950) with later health status as measured by self-administered questionnaires, physical examinations, and death certificates. Observations on coronary heart disease were limited to the first 590 male former students known to have died from this cause, who were contrasted with 1,180 randomly chosen classmates

of the same sex and equivalent age who were known to be still alive. Analyses of college case-taking and other records on these subjects identified nine precursors of fatal coronary heart disease: heavy cigarette smoking, high level of blood pressure, increased body weight, shortness of body height, early parental death, absence of siblings, nonparticipation in varsity athletics, high emotional index, and scarlet fever in childhood.

Other studies have emphasized a more limited group of factors as those associated with increased risk of coronary heart attacks, namely: family history, diabetes, smoking habits, high blood pressure, and high level of blood lipids. In addition, Jenkins and his associates (1971) described what they called a *type-A behavior pattern* characterized by enhanced aggressiveness, ambitiousness, competitive drive, and a chronic sense of time urgency. Men who fell into this behavior pattern were found to be roughly twice as vulnerable to coronary heart attacks as men in the same age group with a more relaxed personality. Once again, the data point to significant interaction between biological and psychosocial determinants of such disorders.

Respiratory Disorders

Bronchospasm in asthma may be brought about by specific allergens or by conditioned stimuli that have previously been presented simultaneously with the allergic substance. Thus an artificial flower may precipitate an asthmatic attack in a person who is allergic to the pollen of that type of flower. This type of learning is a form of classical conditioning (i.e., stimulus substitution), and it is possible that attacks may also be precipitated by unrecognized conditioned stimuli. They are often accompanied by fear and apprehension, which has sometimes been held responsible for the development of the attack (particularly fear of loss of mother). However, both fear and dependency may be secondary consequences of the disorder rather than basic causes. There are no personality patterns consistently associated with asthma, and other psychodynamic interpretations are even more speculative.

Hyperthyroidism

Hyperthyroidism results in autonomic overactivity, tachycardia, tremor, anxiety, and apprehensiveness. It is therefore a differential diagnosis that should always be considered in anxiety and panic disorders. There is also a widespread, but unproved, belief that hyperthyroidism may result from severe emotional trauma in persons with specific hereditary predisposition. However, it is more likely that significant emotional stress would need to occur repeatedly over a period of time, as in most other forms of psychiatric or psychosomatic disorder.

Skin Disorders

Itching, tickling, and pain are all transmitted by the same sensory nerve fibers, and they differ from one another only in the frequency of nerve impulses. The subjective perception of itching, or *pruritus,* will be increased when there is hyperarousal and anxiety, and decreased when there is relaxation and somnolence. Excessive sweating, or *hyperhidrosis,* is also associated with hyperarousal and fear or anger. Prolonged emotional stress with undue sweating may lead to irritation and aggravation of other skin conditions.

Rosacea involves increased vascularity over the blush area of the face and upper part of the body. Subjects are apt to be emotionally labile, and the rash may be associated with unreasonably strong feelings of guilt or shame. *Urticaria* is also frequently associated with emotional stress and either overt irritability or undue compliance associated with repressed hostility.

Atopic dermatitis, or *neurodermatitis,* usually involves excessive itching and lesions that are largely factitious, or the result of scratching by the person affected. Psychodynamic interpretations usually involve overdependency on parents, and unreasonable feelings of rejection or loss of love.

Rheumatoid Arthritis

This disorder is more frequent among women than among men, and also tends to be familial. The etiology is otherwise unknown, but repressed rage has been considered a significant contributory factor. However, it should not be overlooked that the disorder is severely incapacitating, and that disability itself may provoke various combinations of emotional denial, anger, depression, and dependency.

Migraine Headaches

Migraine headaches involve unilateral vascular spasm that is recurrent and usually associated with anorexia. Sometimes there is nausea and vomiting, and the attack may be preceded by visual amblyopia, or other disturbances of sensory or motor function. There is often a positive history in other members of the same family, strongly suggesting predisposition. The most frequent psychological predisposition involves repression of hostility, and associated vulnerability to anxiety or depression. Attacks are often precipitated or aggravated by emotional stress, but are best treated by medication. The most effective treatment of the headache consists of a combination of ergotamine tartrate and caffeine. Other drugs may be necessary to control nausea and vomiting. Prevention of further attacks may be accomplished by means of methysergide maleate.

TREATMENT

Much of the emphasis in treatment of these disorders is necessarily somatic rather than psychological. Severe bodily disease requires medical and sometimes surgical treatment. Hemorrhage from peptic ulcers may necessitate transfusion, and perforation may require prompt surgical intervention. Ulcers that cannot be controlled by an adequate period of medical and psychosocial treatment may lead to severe complications, the prevention of which may also involve surgery. Symptomatic medical treatment of other disorders may require a variety of therapeutic efforts such as the use of specific drugs or diets, or topical application of medication.

Psychosocial therapies have been widely employed in conjunction with medical treatment, and in attempts to diminish vulnerability during quiescent phases of the disorder. However, physicians and surgeons are sometimes reluctant to recognize the significance of psychological factors, and may refer patients for psychiatric treatment only as a last resort, when somatic disease has been firmly established for many years and has proved resistant to all their efforts at treatment. Even in a much shorter period of time, extensive somatic investigations and treatment may convince the patient of the exclusive importance of organic factors, and render him extremely reluctant to accept the significance of the emotional factors in development or in treatment. Unfortunately, some psychiatrists have compounded the problem by unduly optimistic pronouncements about the outcome of therapy when they became involved in treatment that was doomed to failure by the severity of the somatic disease.

In appropriate circumstances, much may be accomplished through supportive psychotherapy and environmental manipulation and, sometimes, through more ambitious efforts at personality reconstruction. However, insight therapy may be accompanied by temporary increases in anxiety or depression, with regression and exacerbation of somatic pathology. Some patients are also vulnerable to the development of overt schizophrenic or paranoid psychoses. Any of these developments may require administration of tranquilizing or antidepressant medication. Occasionally, depression may be so severe that electroconvulsive treatment may be indicated. In any event, the application of both psychotherapies and somatic therapies conforms with principles already outlined in Chapters 6 and 8.

REVIEW QUESTIONS

216. Hyperventilation syndrome (psychophysiological respiratory disorder) is most frequently a sign of:
    (A) fatigue
    (B) petit mal epilepsy
    (C) opiate withdrawal
    (D) anxiety
    (E) consciously suppressed anger

217. In this country, obesity is due to an endocrine disorder or other strictly physical abnormality in approximately what proportion of cases?
    (A)   5%

(B) 25%
(C) 50%
(D) 75%
(E) 95%

218. The psychological complication of cardiac disease most likely to be produced iatrogenically is:
(A) compulsive exercising
(B) persistent overconcern and invalidism
(C) hysterical neurosis, conversion type
(D) neurasthenia
(E) decreased libido and impotence

219. The psychiatric treatment of choice for peptic ulcer patients is usually:
(A) behavior therapy
(B) group therapy
(C) supportive psychotherapy
(D) psychoanalysis
(E) antianxiety medication

220. Rheumatoid arthritis patients:
(A) commonly experience depression shortly after the onset of the rheumatoid arthritis
(B) can neither experience nor express emotions easily, and usually deny or repress anger
(C) experience a temporary remission during pregnancy
(D) all of the above
(E) none of the above

221. The most important reason that premature ejaculation is considered a psychophysiological genito-urinary disorder rather than a hysterical conversion disorder is:
(A) conspicuous absence of secondary gain
(B) lack of association with anxiety
(C) absence of la belle indifférence
(D) other neurotic symptoms are usually absent
(E) autonomic nervous system involvement

Summary of Directions

A	B	C	D	E
1, 2, 3 only	1, 3 only	2, 4 only	4 only	All are correct

222. At the present time in the United States, conditions diagnosed more frequently in the upper socioeconomic classes than the lower include:
(1) obesity
(2) obsessive-compulsive neurosis
(3) antisocial personality
(4) peptic ulcer

223. The typical patient with a duodenal ulcer:
(1) probably has a repressed conflict over suicide
(2) has markedly increased gastric acid secretions
(3) is an alcoholic
(4) experiences remissions and exacerbations related to life changes

224. Migraine headaches are:
(1) familial
(2) often accompanied by nausea and visual disturbances
(3) related to inability to express anger
(4) usually bilateral

225. Psychophysiological disorders have classically been distinguished from hysterical conversion disorders on the basis of:
(1) lack of symbolic origin
(2) autonomic nervous system innervation of affected tissue
(3) frequent production of structural changes in tissue
(4) notable absence of secondary gain

SELECTED REFERENCES

1. Ax, A.F. (1953). Physiological differentiation between fear and anger in humans. *Psychosomatic Medicine,* vol. 15, pages 432–442.
2. Bliss, E.L., and Branch, C.H. (1960). *Anorexia Nervosa.* New York: Hoeber Medical Division, Harper & Row.
3. Block, J., Jennings, H., Harvey, E., and Simpson, E. (1964). Interaction between allergic potential and psychopathology in childhood asthma. *Psychosomatic Medicine,* vol. 26, page 307.
4. Brady, J.V. (1958). Ulcers in "executive" monkeys. *Scientific American,* vol. 199, pages 95–100.

5. Gellhorn, E. (1960). Recent contributions to the physiology of the emotions. In L.J. West and M. Greenblatt (Eds.), *Explorations in the Physiology of the Emotions.* Washington, D.C.: American Psychiatric Association. Psychiatric Research Reports No. 12, pages 209–223.

6. Hanley, W.B. (1964). Hereditary aspects of duodenal ulceration: Serum pepsinogen level in relation to ABO blood groups and salivary ABH secretor status. *British Medical Journal,* vol. 1, pages 936–940.

7. Jenkins, C.D., Zyzanski, S.J., and Rosenman, R.H. (1971). Progress toward validation of a computer-scored test for the type A coronary-prone behavior pattern. *Psychosomatic Medicine,* vol. 33, page 193.

8. Mendelson, M. (1966). Psychological aspects of obesity. *International Journal of Psychiatry,* vol. 2, pages 599–612.

9. Paffenbarger, R.S., Wolf, P.A., Notkin, J., and Thorne, M.C. (1966). Chronic disease in former college students. I. Early precursors of fatal coronary heart disease. *American Journal of Epidemiology,* vol. 83, pages 314–328.

10. Seligman, M.E.P. (1975). *Helplessness.* San Francisco: W.H. Freeman and Co. Pages 116–121.

11. Selye, H. (1946). General adaptation syndrome and diseases of adaptation. *Journal of Clinical Endocrinology,* vol. 6, pages 117–230.

12. Vandenberg, S.G., Clark, P.J., and Samuels, I. (1965). Psychophysiological reactions of twins: Hereditary factors in galvanic skin resistance, heartbeat, and breathing. *Eugenics Quarterly,* vol. 12, pages 7–10.

13. Weiner, H., Thaler, M., Reiser, M.G., and Mirsky, I.A. (1957). Etiology of duodenal ulcer. I. Relation of specific psychological characteristics to rate of gastric secretion (serum pepsinogen). *Psychosomatic medicine,* vol. 19, pages 1–10.

14. Weiss, J.M., Krieckhaus, E.E., and Conte, R. (1968). Effects of fear conditioning on subsequent avoidance behavior. *Journal of Comparative and Physiological Psychology,* vol. 65, pages 413–421.

15. Weiss, J.M., Stone, E.A., and Harrell, N. (1970). Coping behavior and brain norepinephrine in rats. *Journal of Comparative and Physiological Psychology,* vol. 72, pages 153–160.

16. Wolf, S., and Wolff, H.G. (1947). *Human Gastric Function: An Experimental Study of a Man and His Stomach.* New York: Oxford University Press.

18. Sexual Response, Dysfunction, and Deviation

MALCOLM GARDNER, PH.D., IAN GREGORY, M.D., AND WALTER KNOPP, M.D.

. . . and then I asked him with
*   my eyes to ask again yes*
and then he asked me would I yes . . .
and first I put my arms around him yes
and drew him down to me so he could feel my
*   breasts all perfume yes*
and his heart was going like mad
and yes I said yes I will Yes.
James Joyce, <u>Ulysses</u>

The second half of this century has seen a most profound increase in sexual awareness and knowledge, influenced by a number of factors. All forms of media both discuss and display human sexuality with openness and directness. Movements such as women's liberation have received widespread attention and influence. There has been a marked increase in sex research, stimulated notably by the sociological studies of Kinsey and his associates, and the physiological research of Masters and Johnson. The application of research findings by Masters and Johnson to a carefully structured treatment concept and format provided the primary impetus to the new sex therapy, and to the proliferation of sex therapists, ranging from the most capable practitioners to outright quacks. Human sexuality is now included in the curricula of almost all medical schools, and in recent textbooks and professional journals. Educators and practitioners are offered a wealth of audiovisual aids, varying markedly in quality, purpose, and appropriateness.

One of the effects on the public has been that physicians in their individual daily practices are increasingly expected to deal with sex-related problems. The role they assume in the management or treatment of specific sexual problems is a matter of personal preference and preparation, but being able to recognize and understand the problem is a necessity.

The understanding of human sexuality requires some background in psychiatry and the behavioral sciences. Theoretical viewpoints, human psychosexual development, the effect of psychiatric disorders, and the variety of psychotherapeutic approaches are considered in other chapters. This chapter is concerned with the physiology of sexual response, normal and deviant sexual behavior, and the treatment of sexual dysfunction.

HUMAN SEXUAL RESPONSE

Human sexual response has been divided by Masters and Johnson into four separate but progressive phases. Beginning at the onset of effective stimulation, the *excitement phase* varies in duration from minutes to hours. This is followed by a short ½- to 3-minute *plateau phase* of intense sexual tension culminating in a 3- to 15-second *orgasmic phase.* Following orgasm, there is a 10- to 15-minute *resolution phase,* by the end of which the individual is returned to the unstimulated state. If desired orgasm is not achieved, the resolution phase may be extended up to a full day.

The sexual response cycle of *the normal male typically follows the above pattern,* with the indicated variations in duration but little variation of intensity. But the response cycle of the normal female varies in intensity as well as in duration, both from one individual to another and within an individual from one sexual experience to another, producing *an almost infinite variety of female sexual response cycles.* The female response patterns normally may range from very rapid to very extended patterns with varying intensity. She may have multiple orgasms without leaving the high sexual tension of the plateau stage, minor orgasms while at plateau, or move from plateau to resolution with no apparent orgasm — all with subjective and physiological sexual satisfaction. The female may reach full orgasm with minimal, even nonvaginal or nonpelvic stimulation, or she may require intensive stimulation, including the use of vibrators and direct, manual clitoral stimulation along with coital connection.

In both sexes two basic physiological phenomena accompanying increasing response to sexual stimulation have been identified: marked *vaso-congestion,* followed by a generalized *increase in muscle tension.* As tension mounts to the orgasmic phase, pronounced vascular responses occur. At orgasm, pulse may be as high as 180 beats per minute, blood pressure may increase as much as 80 mm Hg systolic and 40 mm Hg diastolic, and respiration rate may exceed 40 breaths per minute. In both sexes, as sexual tension mounts to high levels, accompanied by increased vasocongestion, there is varying but significant increase in the size of sexual parts, including the female breasts, labia, clitoris, and vagina, and the male penis and testes. Inconsistent, although common, is a skin rash similar to measles in varying body patterns at plateau or orgasm, as well as sweating that is unrelated to exercise immediately following orgasm in the resolution phase.

Details about sexual anatomy and physiological responses for each sex in each of the four response cycle phases are available from a number of sources. Here we will be concerned with those aspects of human sexuality that most commonly contribute to distortions and misconceptions, and to unsatisfying and distracting sexual behavior. Knowledge of general reproductive anatomy is assumed.

Female Sexual Response

Although the two sexes do respond alike in many respects, there are a number of ways in which they do not. The most significant *initial response of the female* to effective stimulation is vaginal secretion, which normally occurs within 5 to 10 seconds. This is the counterpart to the male erection, which occurs normally in the same time span. Although equally significant and occurring at the same time as the male erection, the female secretion is not as apparent, since it is entirely internal. Lubrication of the outer labia by vaginal secretions is usually dependent on manual manipulation or penile thrusting. The production of vaginal secretion occurs primarily in the excitement phase and usually diminishes or ceases at higher levels of excitement.

The clitoral glans, although erect and prominent in the excitement stage, will almost inevitably retract into the clitoral hood at the plateau stage. This response has caused undue distraction and frustration for the male who has been instructed (often by a professional authority) to maintain contact with the clitoris, and in turn it has often caused undue discomfort, distraction, and accusations of loss of interest for the female. At high levels of sexual tension, clitoral stimulation is sufficiently maintained by displacement accomplished in spontaneous sexual activity.

Similarly, the nipple of the female breast may be erect in the excitement phase but *appear* to lose its erection at plateau because an increase in breast size of as much as one-fourth over normal enlarges the areola and causes it to impinge on the nipple, thereby masking the erection.

The female vagina is a potential rather than a real space because it accommodates naturally to the size of the object inserted. The sensations experienced during coitus, including the rhythmical contractions of the orgasm, occur only in the outer one-third of the vagina, the area generally designated the *orgasmic platform.* As orgasm approaches, the inner two-thirds of the vagina expand, producing a *tenting* effect, and elevate along with the uterus to elongate the vaginal cavity. At the moment of orgasm, unlike the male, the female has a tendency to increase pelvic thrusting. It may also be noted that the female orgasm differs in no way that depends on the point of stimulation. There is no evidence for making any distinction between clitoral and vaginal orgasm. In both sexes, the orgasm achieved by self-stimulation is usually more intense physiologically than that achieved in coitus.

Male Sexual Response

The most obvious *initial response of the normal male* to effective stimulation is penile erection, which usually occurs in the same 5 to 10 seconds in which female vaginal secretion is produced. In contrast to the female, the male cannot accomplish successful coital connection without first obtaining a sufficient erection. Once he has achieved erection, it will normally wax and wane if the excitement phase is sufficiently prolonged, which can be done voluntarily. At full erection the size of the penis does not vary significantly from one male to another, despite apparent differences in the flaccid state.

As excitement increases in the male, the scrotal sac tightens and lifts, resulting in partial elevation of the testes, and at plateau the size of the testes increases as much as 50 percent. Also at plateau, prior to orgasm, two or three drops of mucoid fluid that contain viable sperm are secreted from the penis (a response worthy of consideration in timing penile withdrawal as a contraceptive measure).

The male orgasm is in two distinct stages. At the point of *ejaculatory inevitability,* an irreversible, all-systems-go signal is triggered by contractions of the testes, prostate gland, and seminal vessels as they collect the sperm and seminal fluid and expel them into the entrance of the urethra. This is followed immediately by the *ejaculatory stage,* in which contractions of the urethra and muscles of the penis eject the seminal fluid through the urethral canal and out of the penis. At orgasm the male, unlike the female, has a tendency to freeze his thrusting activity, holding the penis in deep penetration. Immediately following orgasm, again unlike the female, the male undergoes at the resolution phase a *refractory period,* which cannot be prevented. During this period he generally loses up to 50 percent of his erection, although this may not occur if the erection has been present for a long time. But effective restimulation to higher levels of sexual tension is impossible until the refractory period is complete. Even then, the male's ability to respond to restimulation is much lower than that of the female.

Variations in Sexual Response

Normal variations in the physiology of sexual response occur during the aging process. Assuming physical health, active sexual life in later years is more likely in individuals who have been active in earlier years, who have an available partner, and who live in a social environment accepting of their sexuality. With advancing years, the vasocongestive patterns in the female are diminished and the elasticity and secretory capacities of the vagina decrease. The male takes longer to reach erection, which may not be complete even though sufficient for coital connection, and the expulsive force of his ejaculation diminishes. In both sexes all phases of the response cycle are prolonged. But these changes do not diminish the subjective experience and enjoyment of sexual activity.

Other normal variations in the sexual response cycle occur in the pregnant female, largely due to the massive pelvic vasocongestion already present, and in the multiparous female as compared with her nulliparous counterpart, as a result of the sequelae to reproduction and obstetric procedures.

Variations produced by disease and injury, medical and surgical procedures, drugs, deviant behavior, and psychological factors accompanying these will be considered later.

There is considerable variation in the terminology used to describe human sexual dysfunction, as well as in the definition and organization of the terms. The classification devised by Masters and Johnson is currently the one most widely used and is presented here, although some of the other terms used will be indicated.

MALE SEXUAL FUNCTION DISORDERS

Premature Ejaculation

Premature ejaculation is diagnosed when the penis cannot be contained in the vagina without orgasm occurring, for a period of time sufficient to satisfy the partner, in at least 50 percent of the coital connections. Others have defined premature ejaculation in terms of time in the vagina before orgasm, ranging from 30 to 60 seconds. In practice, many therapists prefer to view this dysfunction in terms of the satisfaction of the male and his partner, with little or no emphasis on the percentage factor or time. Some routinely offer exercises to extend male ejaculatory control to all males. This dysfunction has also been termed *premature orgasm,* defined more broadly than just in terms of partner satisfaction, including the quality of the orgasm as a primary factor.

Paramount in the etiology of premature ejaculation appears to be the nature of first coital experiences. Initial coital experiences that reward speed, with little or no other performance demand placed on the male, tend to foster premature ejaculation. This includes initial experiences with prostitutes, and in settings such as back seats in lovers' lanes or drive-ins, by-the-hour motels, and other "quickie" situations. Premature ejaculation may develop with partners who experience pain with intercourse, submit but are uninterested, or fear the family may become aware of the sexual activity, and in similar situations in which "get it over with" is either stated or implied. Factors that have *not* proved evident in the etiology are masturbatory practices, environmental background, religion, and parental patterns.

Ejaculatory Incompetence

Ejaculatory incompetence is diagnosed when an individual cannot ejaculate intravaginally. He rarely has difficulty achieving or maintaining an erection or ejaculating extravaginally. (Other terms frequently used for this dysfunction are *retarded ejaculation* and *inhibited orgasm*.)

There are generally multiple etiological factors involved in this dysfunction. It is possible for it to be created by one specific traumatic episode of a physical nature, but the etiology is usually psychological. The more common etiological factors are attitudes and inhibitions produced by religious orthodoxy, fear of causing pregnancy, or lack of interest in or physical orientation to the particular female involved.

Impotence

Impotence is an inability to achieve or maintain an erection sufficient to accomplish coital connection. If the male has *never* been able to accomplish coital connection in even a single instance, the condition is termed *primary impotence*. More common is *secondary impotence*, in which there has been at least one instance of successful coitus. Frequently there has been continued successful coitus, even for years, before the episode of failure. In some of these the impotence may be consistent, in others

it may be episodic, and in some males it may exist only in relation to coitus with specific partners. This dysfunction may also be termed *inhibited sexual excitement.*

Both primary and secondary impotence usually derive from multiple etiological factors. Most common in the etiology of primary impotence are parental influences, religious orthodoxy, homosexual involvement, negative experiences with prostitutes, and physiological causes. The same factors contribute to secondary impotence, as well as to premature ejaculation, as also do alcoholic episodes and inept or negative input from professional authority.

Dyspareunia

Dyspareunia, difficult or painful coitus, is much more common in the female than in the male. Although the etiology may be psychological, there are numerous physical sources, especially in the female. These will be discussed later.

FEMALE SEXUAL FUNCTION DISORDERS

Orgasmic Dysfunction

Orgasmic dysfunction denotes the inability of the female to attain orgasmic release. As in male impotence, the female may *never* have attained orgasm in response to any stimuli from any source. This condition is termed *primary orgasmic dysfunction,* and is a much more severe exclusion than that of primary impotence in the male. If the female has experienced at least one instance of orgasmic expression from any stimuli or source, it is termed *situational orgasmic dysfunction.* Masters and Johnson further arbitrarily catagorize the situational orgasmic dysfunction as masturbatory, coital, or random. The female who does reach orgasm by coitus but cannot do so with stimulation by a partner of either sex or with self-stimulation exhibits *masturbatory orgasmic inadequacy.* The reverse of this, the inability to reach orgasm in coital connection while able to do so by other techniques, is termed *coital orgasmic inadequacy.* Some women have had an orgasm at least once during both manipulative and coital activity, but are rarely orgastic and surprised when it happens. This situation is termed *random orgasmic inadequacy.* Some orgasmic dysfunctions may also be referred to as *inhibited sexual orgasm.*

As with male impotence, female orgasmic dysfunction derives from multiple etiological factors. Religious orthodoxy, the social position of the female, different standards of sexual morality for men and for women, and especially the concept that it is the woman's duty to satisfy the male, are all prominent. Also significant are early family patterns and identifications, antagonistic behavioral patterns toward males, the male partner's failure to meet expectations as a provider, or the male being a substitute for someone preferred. Impotence or premature ejaculation by a male partner may lead to either primary or situational orgasmic dysfunction. Homosexual practices or tendencies may be a strong factor in situational orgasmic dysfunction. Random orgasmic inadequacy may result from a low sexual tension in some women, although this is rare. Masturbatory or coital orgasmic inadequacy generally occurs from guilt over masturbatory experimentation and instillation of the "don't touch" syndrome.

Vaginismus

Vaginismus is a classic example of a psychosomatic disorder, involving all components of the pelvic musculature investing the perineum and outer one-third of the vagina. These muscle groups contract spastically as a completely involuntary reflex stimulated by imagined, anticipated, or real attempts at vaginal penetration. The female may be totally unaware of these contractions, and the condition may vary in intensity. Direct pelvic examination is essential to a secure diagnosis of vaginismus.

Multiple factors are usually present in the etiology of vaginismus. It is commonly associated with male sexual dysfunction (especially primary impotence), religious orthodoxy, prior homosexual identification, and prior specific sexual trauma, including insensitively performed pelvic examinations. It may also be associated with dyspareunia, sometimes persisting even after the dyspareunia is relieved.

Dyspareunia

Dyspareunia, as noted earlier, is much more common in the female than in the male. There are numerous medical and surgical causes of dyspareunia in the female, some of which will be considered in the next section. However, in both sexes, with physical causes ruled out, the etiology can be purely psychological. The excuses that can be generated by a sexually dysfunctioning partner to avoid sexual activity are legion. A determined, aggressive partner can overpower or circumvent even the most clever and original excuses, but if coitus causes pain, he or she becomes powerless if there is any residual caring. A grimace, grunt, moan, or spastic reaction on entry usually suffices, but if all else fails a scream or tears will certainly win the day. Dyspareunia will therefore often result in other dysfunctions in the mate.

Other Disorders

Other functional disorders that may be unrelated to the classifications described by Masters and Johnson are frequently presented. Complaints of lack of interest or inhibited sexual desire, routine, boredom, "just something missing," disappointment, diminished response, conflicts in desired frequency, conflicts in desired practices, and similar problems must also be considered dysfunctions.

DYSFUNCTIONS SECONDARY TO OTHER CONDITIONS

Other dysfunctions are secondary to medical illness, physical injury, drug abuse, psychiatric disorder (especially depression), or undesirable complications of treatment for the primary illness. These dysfunctions must be considered in the proper context.

Some dysfunctions may be induced by organic alterations in sexual response *specific* to the illness or treatment. Thus peripheral neuropathy in diabetes or uremia may lead to neurogenic impotence in men. In such cases the specific medical or surgical (prosthetic) treatment of the primary disease has highest priority. In addition, pre- and post-treatment counseling and referral to an appropriate self-help organization is of great importance. The latter assists the patient in finding satisfactory alternatives to old, familiar life patterns or sexual techniques and a new balance with the partner and within the environment. For example, Cole presented an integrated approach to sexuality in the spinal cord–injured patient.

In other cases the dysfunction is precipitated by nonspecific stressful influences or discomfort resulting from the primary medical or surgical illness. A typical example is a postcoronary male patient who fears that sexual arousal or coitus may be dangerous, and whose wife does not dare to even suggest sexual activity for fear she may cause her husband's death. Sexual tensions may lead to irritability, resentment, marital discord, impotence, orgasmic dysfunction, and even separation. None of these is amenable to specific medical or surgical treatment. Reassurance, factual education, and helping the partners to feel comfortable with the resumption of their customary sexual routines as early as possible can obviate emotional crippling and marital tragedy. If this counseling does not suffice, the patient and his wife should be referred to an experienced sex therapist.

Following are some examples of dysfunctions and their more common organic causes:

Ejaculatory incompetence may be associated with lumbar sympathectomy, syringomyelia, parkinsonism, treatment with thioridazine or adrenergic blocking agents, and methaqualone abuse in large doses.

Impotence may be the result of any debilitating illness, diabetes mellitus, severe cardiac or respiratory disease, uremia, myxedema, thyrotoxicosis, pituitary diseases, Addison's disease, high-dosage estrogen treatment, lower spinal cord lesions, hypothalamic and temporal lobe lesions, perineal prostatectomy, abuse of alcohol or other drugs, use of major tranquilizers or antidepressants, or vaginal infection in the partner.

Loss of libido may occur with any severe illness, heroin addiction, depression, hysteria, and following colostomy, ileostomy, hysterectomy, or mastectomy.

Orgasmic dysfunction may be caused by methaqualone in large doses, any debilitating disease, alcohol abuse, physical exhaustion, depression, colostomy, ileostomy, mastectomy, and hysterectomy.

Retrograde ejaculation (dry ejaculation) may be found in patients treated with thioridazine, and after radical prostatectomy.

Vaginismus frequently accompanies local infections of the genital tract and leads to dyspareunia. The latter may also be caused by endometriosis, atrophic senile changes, obstetrical or gynecological scars, arthritis, or imperforated hymen.

Castration (removal of testes or ovaries) and sterilization (vasectomy, hysterectomy, or tubal ligation) may or may not lead to sexual dysfunction, depending on the premorbid personality. Colostomy and ileostomy may be followed by various forms of dysfunction in both sexes due to the physical implications, which are esthetically offensive to some patients. Procedures involving closing of the vagina result in disorders of arousal and orgasmic response unless female patients and their partners are properly warned ahead of time and later helped to find a new and acceptable sexual adjustment.

TREATMENT OF SEXUAL FUNCTION DISORDERS

Sexual dysfunction was long considered a manifestation of serious psychopathology responsive only to psychoanalytic therapeutic intervention. For the most part the object choice and situation disorders described later do manifest deep emotional disturbance and require intensive therapy utilizing the traditional approaches. The sexual function disorders, however, may have their etiology in more immediate and simpler problems, and may occur in people with no other apparent psychological symptoms.

The "new" sex therapies that focus primarily on the sexual function disorders are based on the research and subsequent treatment programs of William Masters and Virginia Johnson. There still remains some confusion between the research program of Masters and Johnson and their treatment program. The research program involved the observation of human subjects in a variety of sexual experiences. In their treatment program, the prescribed sexual exercises are always practiced by the couple in private. Although most reputable sex therapy centers modify and vary the Masters and Johnson program for a variety of practical reasons, they still employ the basic exercises, rationale, theoretical framework, and much of the format of the Masters and Johnson program. For this reason, understanding the new sex therapy approaches must start with an understanding of the Masters and Johnson program on which they are largely based.

Masters and Johnson Therapy Program

Basic to the therapy program of Masters and Johnson is the concept of *the marital unit as the patient*. They maintain that there is no such thing as an uninvolved partner or a "sick half" in sexual dysfunction. The program and its exercises are demanding on both partners, frequently one more than the other, so that complete and willing cooperation is essential to the treatment success. For these reasons Masters and Johnson accept for treatment only persons in an established relationship of sufficient duration who have mutual vulnerability and affection. Their observations have convinced them that "sociocultural deprivation and ignorance rather than psychiatric or medical illness is the basis of most sexual dysfunction." The treatment program is strongly influenced also by the observation that sexual dysfunction is intensified and sustained by the demand to perform and the fear of not performing. They employ a short-term behavior-oriented approach, focusing on corrective or necessary sexual information, constant support and reassurance, improvement of communication, removal of demand to perform, and prescribed exercises appropriate to the specific dysfunction and to the particular couple. The values, needs, and preferences of each individual are thoroughly respected in determining the exercises and course of therapy. Since sex is a natural function, removal of the demand to perform and replacement with emphasis on the relationship, communication, and response to the giving and receiving of pleasurable stimuli lead to a natural response. It is a gradu-

ated, building-to-a-goal model in which exercises are *added to* rather than *substituted for* those previously assigned until the desired goal is achieved. It is not until this goal is attained that the couple is free to alter the pattern in its own way. While recognizing that it is not always practical or possible, Masters and Johnson employ a heterosexual pair of therapists, preferably one from a biological and one from a behavioral discipline. They recommend this combination of therapists where possible because it provides distinct advantages over the single therapist or a team from the same discipline.

Couples entering this program are isolated from all other activities, responsibilities, and contacts for a two-week period, and are seen by the therapy team every day. Regardless of the presenting problem, the first four days of the program are basically the same. The first day consists of a brief intake interview in which the program and its demands on the couple are explained. From the point of entry into the program the couple is instructed to engage in no sexual activity until and as instructed by the therapists. The remainder of the first day consists of an extensive psychosexual and social history of each individual taken by the therapist of the same sex, and completed on the second day by the therapist of the opposite sex. On the third day the medical history, physical examination, and laboratory evaluation are all completed. At this point the basic format for all the remaining therapy sessions is begun with round table sessions, in which the therapy team meets with the couple to discuss, clarify, and understand their specific problem. The couple is instructed in the initial phase of *sensate focus,* a series of exercises designed to increase sensory awareness to self and partner, and promote more effective sexual communication. Each partner in turn is the passive recipient of the other's "pleasuring" with the genitals and breasts excluded in the initial exercise. The therapeutic intervention on the fourth day and in the sessions thereafter begins with a discussion of the couple's success or failure in following the specific instructions of the previous day's therapy session. Reassurance, further explanation of the exercises, additional information about sexual anatomy and functioning, and dealing with the variety of reactions to the exercises that may occur in individual cases may all be a part of this portion of the session. The couple is then instructed to continue with the sensate focus as prescribed, adding to it the inclusion of the genitals and breasts, along with additional responsibility for communicating to the partner the desired response and how to produce it. After the fourth day the program and exercises vary as a function of the specific couple and the dysfunction involved, influenced by factors such as the etiology of the disorder, the degree of psychopathology in the individuals and in the marriage, and the day-to-day progress made toward the desired goal.

PREMATURE EJACULATION. The treatment of premature ejaculation focuses exercises on repeatedly stimulating the male to the point of or near ejaculatory inevitability and then either forcibly preventing ejaculation or ceasing stimulation just before ejaculatory inevitability occurs. The repeated forcible prevention of ejaculation, despite a state of inevitability, is accomplished by firm pressure with the thumb on the frenulum and the first and second fingers on either side of the coronal ridge opposite it. This is referred to as the *squeeze technique.* The repeated withdrawal of stimuli just short of inevitability is commonly referred to as the *stop and go technique.* The almost universal success of the squeeze technique, its simplicity, and the ease with which it can be taught has resulted in many sex therapists offering the exercise to all dysfunctional couples as an option to delay ejaculation, even if this has not been a presenting complaint. Whether or not it is introduced into the treatment program, and at what point, varies with the individual couple and the approach of the particular therapist.

EJACULATORY INCOMPETENCE OR RETARDED EJACULATION. This is approached in almost the opposite manner as premature ejaculation. In almost all of these cases ejaculation can be accomplished by effective stimulation outside of the vagina, the block being to intravaginal ejaculation only. A single intra-

vaginal ejaculation is usually sufficient to break the block, so the treatment program and exercises are aimed toward this goal. The female is instructed in the exercises to stimulate the male manually to high tension levels so that he achieves comfortable orgasm in her presence and to her stimulus. Then from the kneeling superior position she continues this process in ever closer proximity to vaginal entry. Eventually, at the point of ejaculatory inevitability, she is able to insert the penis quickly into the vagina without interrupting ejaculation and the block is broken.

MALE IMPOTENCE AND FEMALE ORGASMIC DYSFUNCTIONS. It must be stressed that it is impossible to will or demand a sexual response. The therapists strive to remove any demand or expectation for performance throughout the entire exercise sequence. Sensate focus exercises are employed until sufficient response (erection or vaginal secretion) is firmly established. At a time considered appropriate by the therapists, the female is directed to assume the kneeling superior coital position where she is "in command," and from where intravaginal containment is started. Initially only containment is experienced, with no thrusting or only that minor thrusting necessary to maintain the level of excitement reached. As thrusting is increased and response mounts, the therapists may direct the couple to a lateral coital position in which both partners have equal freedom of movement. Relieved of the demand to perform and free to respond without threat, nature takes its course and orgasm occurs spontaneously. If one of the partners has no difficulty with sexual arousal and orgasm, the therapists must consider this in their instructions and provide for the tensions produced in this partner.

VAGINISMUS. This condition can be firmly diagnosed only by direct physical examination, and the treatment program should actually begin in this setting. With the partner present, involuntary vaginal spasms are demonstrated and explained to both partners. This setting also offers the best opportunity to explain the use of graduated Hegar dilators, and to obtain the cooperation and understanding of the male partner. Thereafter the exercises are carried out in the privacy of the couple's home. With the female in command, through both verbal and manual control, increasingly larger dilators are inserted into the vagina, always within the limits of comfort. The female is encouraged to maintain the dilators intravaginally for several hours. When these exercises are performed in the presence of the partner and with his cooperation and understanding, treatment is almost invariably successful and the penis can be comfortably and pleasurably contained within three to five days.

DYSPAREUNIA. The treatment of dyspareunia, like that of vaginismus, must begin with physical examination. As has been indicated earlier, there are multiple physical and medical origins of dyspareunia, and when these exist the treatment is the appropriate medical or surgical procedure. Obviously, dyspareunia commonly produces vaginismus, which may persist after the cause of the dyspareunia is removed. In this instance the treatment is that described above for vaginismus. When no physical cause of the dyspareunia is found the problem may be the lack of sexual excitement (and therefore lack of vaginal secretion) or it may be a maneuver to escape an undesired or a feared situation. These situations may require psychotherapy aimed at improving the couple's relationship, or utilization of exercises designed to enhance sexual communication and response in a nondemanding environment, or both.

OTHER SEXUAL FUNCTION COMPLAINTS. The treatment of other sexual function disorders such as lowered libido, boredom, and differences in desired practices or frequency, assuming physical origin is ruled out in a couple with sufficient mutual caring, varies with the complaint and the dynamics of the couple involved. Although Masters and Johnson do not specifically address themselves to these problems in the description of their program, the appropriate approach and exercises in their theoretical framework are readily discerned. The levels of sensate focus, with minor variations and additions, perhaps

in conjunction with the squeeze technique, are commonly employed. In some cases psychotherapy aimed at the marital relationship may be necessary preceding or in conjunction with sex therapy exercises. Problems arising from spinal cord lesions, mental retardation, blindness, and radical pelvic surgery require special techniques.

TREATMENT SUCCESS RATES. Reports of incidence and treatment success rates for various dysfunctions are difficult to assess. There is still considerable variation in the nomenclature of sexual function disorders, the definitions employed, the criteria for successful outcome of treatment, the basis for selection of patients for treatment, and the type of follow-up of these patients. It is also impossible to determine how many of these problems are treated, and with what results, under other primary diagnoses and by other treatment modalities. The statistics reported by Masters and Johnson have been those most commonly substantiated by other recognized clinics. Taking into account the treatment reversals identified in patient follow-up, they report an overall treatment success (combining all dysfunctions) of about 80 percent. They report success in all cases of vaginismus, and in 97 percent of cases of premature ejaculation. They have been least successful with primary and secondary impotence, reporting success rates of 59 percent for primary impotence and 69 percent for secondary impotence. Situational orgasmic dysfunction (75 percent), primary orgasmic dysfunction (82 percent), and ejaculatory incompetence (82 percent) also approached their overall success rate. By far the most common presenting complaints were secondary impotence (213 cases), primary orgasmic dysfunction (193 cases), premature ejaculation (186 cases), and situational orgasmic dysfunction (149 cases). Much less common were primary impotence (32 cases), vaginismus (29 cases), and ejaculatory incompetence (17 cases).

Whether in strict adherence to the Masters and Johnson programs or in any of its modifications and variations, *sex therapy is not a cookbook application of programmed exercises.* The therapy or round table sessions are crucial. The application, timing, sequence, pacing, repetition, elimination, variation, and modification of the exercises are determined by the therapist's understanding of and sensitivity to the individual personalities and dynamics of the couple involved, as well as the dysfunction presented. A couple may bring to their relationship the same or different dysfunctions (sometimes the source of their attraction to each other), or a dysfunctional partner may produce a corresponding dysfunction in the mate. It is quite common, for example, for a female with vaginismus to produce premature ejaculation or secondary impotence in her mate. A male with premature ejaculation or impotence may cause his mate to develop a situational orgasmic dysfunction. An impotent male and an unresponsive female may "solve" their problems by selecting each other as partners, only to become unhappy with their solution. Such situations may require varied treatment approaches.

Most sex therapy clinics cannot rigidly follow the Masters and Johnson program for a variety of reasons. Most couples cannot afford, for financial or other practical reasons, to remove themselves from all responsibilities and isolate themselves in a motel or hotel for two weeks. Dual therapists and daily sessions create problems in manpower and cost for many clinics as well as for the population that they serve. Private practitioners often either are unable or do not care to enter into a dual-sex co-therapy relationship. Some patients have no mate, or a mate who refuses to join in the treatment. Programs such as that of Kaplan and her associates at Cornell University and of Annon and Pion and associates at The University of Hawaii are typical of the approach of most clinics and private practitioners. In these programs couples are treated by both individual therapists and dual-sex teams. The exercises and approaches have been modified and applied to individuals without a mate. Group psychotherapy, relaxation therapy, and other approaches have been employed. Homosexual couples are accepted in some programs and by some therapists, and at least one successful application of the new sex therapy approach to a

heterosexual pedophile has been reported. The two-week format has been adapted to weekends, once-a-week clinic visits, and combinations of these. Additional exercises are employed, such as close examination of partners' genitals and their response; the discovery, use, and exercise of the pubococcygeal muscles; self-stimulation exercises; and fantasy exercises — to name only a few. Fingers have been used instead of Hegar dilators in vaginismus exercises. Audiovisual aids to sex therapy treatment are being developed and are in increasing use as an adjunct to the treatment.

The PLISSIT model of therapy, developed by Annon, has influenced many clinics and clinicians, and serves as an example of the levels at which sex therapy may be employed. The acronym is formed from the initials of the four levels of approach to sexual disorders, from the simplest to the most complex. Some people need only to know that they are normal, so that reassurance and permission (P) from authority for their behavior is all that is necessary. In other people limited information (LI) directly relevant to the specific concerns of the couple is necessary in conjunction with permission. These two levels do not require the patient to take active steps to alter his or her behavior. In more complex problems specific suggestions (SS), designed to alter behavior to a desired goal, are necessary and are made in the brief therapy framework. The treatment program of Masters and Johnson described earlier is basically at this level. Though these approaches are successful with many sexual problems, some require a highly individualized approach and intensive therapy (IT). This level is necessary for those patients who cannot respond to the standard new sex therapy approach described, and require a clinician who is appropriately trained in his discipline for intensive psychotherapy. Some therapists employ these levels sequentially, starting from the simplest and moving to the more complex only as necessary, which is the approach suggested by Annon. Others screen patients in this framework to determine the level likely to be most effective in treating the individual patient. In both instances the objective is to relieve the problem effectively in the simplest and most economical manner. These therapists maintain that to do more is unjustified.

The individual physician, as indicated at the outset of this chapter, has the freedom and right to choose the extent to which he or she wishes to incorporate sex therapy into his or her own medical practice. *The physician does not have the right to ignore the problem presented,* directly or indirectly, by the patient. Whether comfortable with it or not, the physician is viewed as an appropriate and knowledgeable authority in this area. At the very least he or she must be sufficiently comfortable with his or her own sexuality, as well as with that of the patient, and sufficiently knowledgeable in sexual behavior and dysfunction to recognize the problem and make an appropriate referral. Many problems are resolved by the physician by simply removing the physical source, and the sexual function aspects may or may not ever be recognized. But in cases in which these persist despite successful medical treatment, either further treatment of the sex problem or referral is indicated. The physician may very well choose to treat some or even most of the patients with sexual function disorders seen in his or her practice.

Giving permission basically requires only the physician's satisfaction and comfort with his or her own sexuality and tolerance for the sexuality of others. Lack of breadth of knowledge in the sexual area is the only limitation to *adding limited information.* These two functions can be done in rather short time spans in the physician's office. To employ *specific suggestion,* the physician must add breadth of knowledge in the treatment approaches developed by Masters and Johnson and others, as well as the therapeutic skills and experience necessary to apply them. Unless he is a psychiatrist, the physician will always refer patients who require *intensive therapy.*

SEXUAL OBJECT CHOICE DISORDERS

Sexual Orientation Disturbance

HOMOSEXUALITY. Homosexuality consists of sexual orientation toward other persons of the same sex, and is not considered a psychiatric disorder in itself. *Sexual orientation disturbance* is a diagnostic term applied to those homosexual persons who are disturbed by, in conflict with, or wish to change their sexual orientation. Homosexual contacts have been observed in both males and females of many species of mammals, and in the case of males the mounting animal not infrequently reaches orgasm. Homosexual relationships between human males have at times been widely accepted and practiced both in civilized cultures and primitive tribes. Homosexual behavior involving human females, also known as lesbianism or sapphism, has also been widely practiced at times, although it has generally been considered both less frequent than male homosexuality and less likely to arouse social censure. In recent years there has been considerable discrepancy between attitudes toward male homosexuality in different localities, and Bernard Glueck (1956) noted that New York State reduced a homosexual offense between two adult males from a felony to a misdemeanor at the same time that California was increasing the maximum penalty for the same offense from 10 to 20 years. Nevertheless, the occurrence of mutual masturbation with others of the same sex is a widespread phenomenon during adolescence.

Alfred Kinsey and associates (1953) reported that by the age of 45 years, approximately 37 percent of males and 13 percent of females have had some homosexual experience to the point of orgasm. Among single persons in the age group 36 to 40 years, 40 percent of males and 10 percent of females reported current involvement in active homosexual relationships. It is among members of the latter group that there is likely to be a high proportion of exclusively homosexual individuals with true *psychosexual inversion.* The majority of such persons have neither been convicted of homosexuality in court nor consulted a psychiatrist voluntarily. Those who do seek psychological or psychiatric assistance are more apt to do so on account of neurotic anxiety or depression than any great desire or expectation of changing their basic homosexual orientation.

Heterosexual Pedophilia

Heterosexual pedophilia includes any sexual activity by a mature male with a female partner who has not started to show pubertal changes. In their study of male sex offenders in Sing Sing prison, Glueck and his associates found that men in this group tended to be middle-aged or older, to have poor marital adjustment, and to have considerable disturbance in reality perception, particularly when under the influence of alcohol. Mohr and his associates (1964) found a distinct trimodal age distribution among heterosexual pedophiles referred to an outpatient clinic, with peaks occurring in adolescence, and in the fourth and sixth decades. Their adolescent group was characterized by retardation in psychosexual and social development. The middle-aged group was characterized by regression, with severe marital and social maladjustment, often compounded by alcoholism. The older group was characterized by loneliness and actual impotence or concern about impotence.

Homosexual Pedophilia

Homosexual pedophilia involves any sexual activity by a mature male with a prepubertal boy. Glueck reported that these men showed the greatest amount of psychiatric disturbance among all the groups of offenders in the Sing Sing study, and a high proportion of them were diagnosed as frankly psychotic. They showed marked impairment of reasoning and judgment, and the only individuals with whom they could successfully relate were boys. In their study of offenders referred to an outpatient clinic, Mohr and co-workers found that the homosexual pedophiles showed the same trimodal age distribution as the heterosexual pedophiles, but that they showed a much greater tendency to seek orgasm during their sexual activities with the child. Orgasm was sought by over 50 percent of the homosexual pedophiles as compared with only 6 percent of the heterosexual pedophiles. Furthermore, over half the offenses of heterosexual pedophiles occurred in the home of either patient or victim, whereas the homosexual pedophiles had a greater tendency to seek out the victim and set up the situation for the offense.

Zoophilia

Zoophilia, or bestiality, involves any form of sexual gratification obtained through contact with an animal. In the case of males, Kinsey and associates reported a cumulative frequency of 8 percent, occurring mainly during adolescence and generally consisting of coitus with a female animal. In the case of females, they reported a cumulative frequency of 3.6 percent, occurring during both adolescence and adult life, and consisting mainly of general body contact.

Fetishism

Fetishism is a form of erotic symbolism in which sexual stimulation and gratification are obtained only through some special part of the body or some inanimate object that has acquired special sexual significance. Such fetishes or sexual symbols are frequently exciting to the normal male, and may be objects of special significance in heterosexual foreplay. The parts of the body most frequently sexualized include the buttocks, thighs, legs, feet, breasts, and hair, while inanimate objects most apt to become fetishes include female underwear, stockings, shoes, silk garments, furs, and gloves. College administrators may encounter simple forms of mass fetishism in the form of panty raids on girls' dormitories, and military censors have sometimes intercepted large quantities of women's underwear and other fetish objects sent from home at the request of enlisted men serving overseas. In severe forms of fetishism, however, inanimate objects with no power to arouse most persons sexually become the only means through which the individual can obtain sufficient excitement to achieve orgasm. Such fetishists may be arrested by the police because of snipping hair or compulsively stealing fetish objects. The latter constitutes one form of *kleptomania;* in other forms there is compulsive stealing without any conscious sexual gratification being achieved. Similarly, *pyromania* consists of compulsive fire-setting, which constitutes a form of fetishism when it is done to obtain sexual gratification, although here again some forms of pyromania do not involve conscious sexual motivation.

Transvestitism

Transvestitism, or transvestism, consists of dressing in clothing appropriate to the opposite sex, and has been practiced by both men and women since antiquity. As in other forms of sexual deviation, however, males have attracted most of the attention, and it is apparently to his data on males that Hirschfeld was referring when he stated that about 35 percent of transvestites are heterosexual, an equal percentage homosexual, about 15 percent bisexual, and the remaining 15 percent either restricted to autoerotic activities or completely asexual. This variety of sexual orientations in transvestites, however, is probably equally true of women who dress as men. Among both sexes there would appear to be three major categories of transvestitism: (1) a form of fetishism, in which the individual is predominantly heterosexual or autoerotic; (2) a predominant homosexual orientation, in which transvestitism represents mainly a means to an end, namely, attracting homosexual partners; (3) a form associated with *transsexualism,* involving a conscious desire to change into a member of the opposite sex.

Transsexualism

Transsexualism is a form of *gender role disorder,* evident since early childhood, in which there is both *psychosexual inversion* (i.e., a reversal of gender identity) and a desire for *surgical transformation* of bodily sex organs to conform with the psychological sexual orientation. Usually the transsexual person has also been a transvestite, and has lived and passed as a member of the opposite sex. Often he or she has engaged in overt homosexual behavior, consistent with the inverted psychosexual identification. Many surgical procedures have been undertaken to change external anatomy from male to female. The contrary procedure, from anatomical female to male, has been attempted far less frequently. Such procedures do not always have a happy outcome, and there should always be intensive psychiatric and psychological evaluations before any surgical transformation is attempted.

SEXUAL SITUATION DISORDERS

Exhibitionism (Male Genital Exhibitionism)

Exhibitionism may be defined as the exposure of the male genital in public and in sight of a female person as a final sexual aim. This final sexual aim distinguishes the act from exposure of the male genital for other motives which have been recorded since antiquity. Thus, Theophrastus (about 300 B.C.) wrote that "the buffoon is one that will lift his shirt in the presence of a free-born woman," and Christoffel (1956) drew attention to genital exposure in primitive cultures as a form of aggression or defense (i.e., counterattack) against women. In our society, male genital exhibitionism constitutes one of the most frequent sexual deviations to be recognized, amounting to as high a proportion as one-third of all sexual offenses coming to court in some jurisdictions. Since the offender is likely to be placed on probation, exhibitionists constitute a small fraction of imprisoned sexual offenders but a relatively high proportion of those receiving psychiatric treatment as outpatients.

In an excellent study of exhibitionists attending an outpatient clinic, Mohr and his associates (1962) stressed the need to distinguish between exhibitionists exposing themselves to girls as a final sexual aim, and pedophiles doing the same thing preparatory to further sexual activities with the child. They found that the girls and women to whom the exhibitionists exposed themselves were almost always strangers, and that the act itself might range from showing the penis without an erection or conscious sexual feelings, to masturbation with the use of obscene language in an intense sexual experience. Exhibitionism has frequently been regarded as closely related to voyeurism, and this group found that voyeurism was in fact the only other form of deviation that was at all common among exhibitionists. The age distribution of their sample of exhibitionists showed an interesting bimodal distribution, with the first peak culminating in adolescence and the other culminating in the twenties. Those in the adolescent group were unmarried, but nearly all those in the young adult group had married before the onset of exhibitionism. However, one-third of the latter group had been married less than a year, and the two outstanding factors related to exposing themselves seemed to have been impending or recent marriage and impending or recent birth of a child. Such data suggest that the urge to expose himself occurs at a time when the patient is caught in a conflict with a female: the mother in adolescence and the wife or future spouse in early adulthood. It has also been remarked that the wife of the exhibitionist frequently appears to be a mother substitute, and that the patient himself is usually self-effacing and not at all exhibitionistic or aggressive in most other respects.

Voyeurism, or Scopophilia

Voyeurism consists of obtaining sexual gratification through looking at the genitalia or sexual behavior of others. The use of visual stimuli to increase sexual excitement is, of course, a normal partial aim, and the Kinsey surveys indicated that on the whole such visual stimulation was very much more important to males than to females. Society has long catered to the male desire for visual and other sensual stimulation through a variety of art forms, including painting, sculpture, photographs, magazines, books, plays, movies, and impromptu or special performances in brothels. It has sometimes been considered acceptable (or sophisticated) for a man to take his wife or mistress to a brothel to watch the show, and even to have her engage in sexual activity with another partner so that he may be further stimulated to normal heterosexual gratification. In contrast with such practices, the true voyeur obtains a maximum of sexual excitement from watching others, and orgasm occurs under these circumstances either spontaneously or through masturbation. The typical Peeping Tom is a socially isolated schizoid individual who prowls respectable neighborhoods after dark, looking through lighted windows for women who are in various stages of undress but who rarely are engaged in sexual activities. A minority of voyeurs are primarily interested in watching deviant behavior, such as sadistic acts carried out on others.

Sexual Masochism

Sexual masochism consists of sexual gratification obtained through suffering bodily or mental pain, and is derived from the name of Leopold von Sacher-Masoch (1836-1895) who subjugated himself as a "slave" to women. His first great sexual experience was with Anna von Kottwitz, who was a dominating woman several years older than he and the model on whom he based two books, *Venus in Furs* and *The Divorced Woman or the Erotic Story of an Idealist*. A much more frequent and less deviant form of masochism involves the woman in a primitive society or subculture of our own society who provokes her mate into abusing her so that he may then or later show her how much he loves her.

In the seventeenth and eighteenth centuries a number of English women became addicted to flagellation, or whipping, which may well have been related to the treatment they had previously received at the hands of their parents and teachers. Magnus Hirschfeld quoted a contemporary description of a feminine flagellation club whose members were mostly married women who met once a week to whip each other. Similar homosexually oriented masochistic practices were widespread in monasteries, convents, and boarding schools. However, the origin of heterosexual masochism in males has frequently been attributed to a combination of punishment and sexual stimulation by sadistic females during their childhood. In their adult years, male masochists have been able to indulge their perversion in brothels equipped with a variety of ingenious machines on which they could be flagellated or tortured. Attempts to inflict pain on themselves have not infrequently led to genital mutilation, castration, or even death. Other forms of extreme masochism include the ingestion of excreta, and certain aspects of necrophilia. The more extreme the deviant behavior, the greater is the probability that the person will show evidence of psychosis.

Sexual Sadism

Sexual sadism involves the attainment of sexual gratification through inflicting bodily or mental pain on others. This disorder is named after the

Marquis de Sade (1740-1814) who practiced or fantasied a wide variety of perversions that he recorded, among other places, in his novel *Justine and Juliette, or the Curse of Virtue and the Blessing of Vice.* He was repeatedly arrested but released because of his social position. Following one of his orgies, at which two prostitutes died from an overdose of cantharides (an irritant, formerly used as an aphrodisiac to increase sexual stimulation), he was sentenced to death but soon afterwards was reprieved and set free.

It was not long before another woman was found unconscious after he had cut open her veins at several points and lacerated the skin all over her body. He was then taken to the Bastille, and later to a lunatic asylum where he eventually died. It is of some interest to note that extreme sadism was recognized as evidence of insanity as long ago as the beginning of the eighteenth century, although some societies have continued to tolerate or even institutionalize the sadistic treatment of minority groups up to the present time. Such sadism, of course, had its origin in antiquity, and has tended to be preserved most strongly in totalitarian, militaristic, and patriarchal cultures. Flogging or torture was frequently the lot of animals, captives, slaves, servants, children, and wives or concubines. Such treatment tended to become a male prerogative, and it is not surprising that in his sexual relationships the male should sometimes obtain additional pleasure from inflicting suffering on his partner. In civilized societies the infliction of pain before or during intercourse is generally minimal, and confined to such acts as will also intensify the pleasure of the partner, such as biting, scratching, and squeezing. However, there are some deviant individuals for whom the infliction of severe pain, the sight of blood, or even death may constitute the only means by which they may attain the maximum of sexual pleasure. The greater the degree of sadism necessary to obtain sexual gratification, the greater the probability that the individual is psychotic.

Sexual Assault Disorder

In his study of male sexual offenders in Sing Sing prison, Glueck found this group to have a more aggressive, outgoing, impulsive type of personality than any other group of sexual offenders. They were the youngest of the groups and contained a higher proportion of blacks than other groups. The assault itself frequently occurred when control was diminished by alcohol or by a combination of sexual frustration and temptation. It is relevant in this connection that the antisocial personality, even when sober, has a low tolerance of frustration, and can resist anything but temptation. When the victim is known to the assailant, interpersonal factors may be highly significant. For example, a woman may knowingly arouse a man sexually with the conscious intention of frustrating him, only to find that he will not be denied what she had in effect promised him. Alternatively, through unconscious denial of sexuality, a woman with a hysterical or other neurotic disorder may unwittingly provide the temptation and provoke the sexual response that she consciously rejects.

BIOLOGICAL AND PSYCHOSOCIAL DETERMINANTS OF SEXUAL BEHAVIOR

It has often been assumed that normal and deviant sexual behavior must bear a close relationship to *endocrine function.* In lower animals, sexual activity may be consistently decreased by castration, or increased and generalized to include homosexual as well as heterosexual activity by administration of male hormones to male animals. In humans, however, there is a poor correlation between blood hormone levels and overt sexual behavior. In females the marked changes in endocrine activity during puberty and menopause may be unaccompanied by any change in current sexual behavior. In males the sharp increase in hormone levels accompanying normal or precocious puberty are not necessarily accompanied by overt behavioral changes, and castration during adult life may have relatively slight effects on established patterns of sexual behavior. Following castration there is a tendency for sexual behavior to decrease in quantity, but for no change to occur in the direction of the sexual aim. Similarly, no consistent abnormalities of endocrine function have been found in any group of persons with sexual deviation.

In their extensive comparison of sexual behavior in many species of animals and in 190 human societies, Ford and Beach noted that humans are less dependent on sex hormones than are subhuman primates, and that the latter in turn are freer of hormonal control than lower mammals. They concluded that in the course of evolution the extent to which gonadal hormones control sexual behavior has been progressively relaxed, with the result that human behavior is relatively independent of this source of control.

Hampson, Money, and their associates provided extensive evidence on the relative significance of biological and psychosocial determinants in the development of adult psychosexual orientation and behavior. Their findings were based on an intensive study of persons with a variety of endocrine or hermaphroditic disorders. *True hermaphroditism* involves the presence of both ovarian and testicular tissue in the same person, and is extremely rare. *Pseudohermaphroditism* involves various types of genital malformation and is much more frequent, as is *masculinization in females,* resulting from excessive production of male hormones by an overactive adrenal cortex. In such persons it is possible to distinguish among seven variables relating to their sex, any one of which might be incongruent with some or all of the other variables. These are as follows: (1) chromosomal sex; (2) gonadal sex; (3) hormonal sex; (4) internal accessory organs; (5) external genital appearance; (6) assigned sex and rearing; and (7) adult gender role, or psychological sex.

These workers found that the last variable of *adult gender role, or psychological sex, invariably corresponded with assigned sex and rearing,* regardless of existing contradictions with respect to any of the five preceding variables. Hampson concluded that gender role, or psychological sex, is learned, and stated: "In place of a theory of innate constitutional psychologic bisexuality such as that proposed by Freud, we would substitute a concept of psychosexual neutrality in humans at birth. Such neutrality permits the development and perpetuation of diverse patterns of psycho-

sexual orientation and functioning in accordance with the life experiences each individual may encounter and transact."

In the normal child there is a strong positive *identification* with the parent of the *same* sex, which leads to early and permanent adoption of the attributes and behavior that are culturally sanctioned in members of that sex. In persons with *psychosexual inversion,* by contrast, there is a decisive childhood identification with a parent or parent surrogate (for example, an older brother or sister) of the *opposite* sex. The intensity of the latter identification, and the age of the child when it first develops, are significant determinants of the degree of sexual inversion shown in adult life. Among those persons with extreme psychosexual inversion, and an exclusive preference for homosexual relationships throughout adult life, identification with the parent or surrogate of the *opposite* sex has been evident since early childhood. The reasons for this identification, however, have not been easy to establish retrospectively.

In an extensive comparison of 106 homosexual males and 100 heterosexual males undergoing psychoanalysis, Bieber and his associates reported that the majority of homosexuals had overly close relationships with their mothers, and mutually hostile relationships with their fathers. Almost half of the mothers of the homosexuals were dominant wives who debased their husbands. Most of these mothers were explicitly seductive, and about two-thirds of them openly preferred their homosexual sons to their husbands, and allied with the sons against the husbands. In about half of these cases the patient was the mother's confidant. However, it should be recognized that these homosexual males were in psychoanalytic therapy, and therefore not typical of all males with homosexual preferences.

Well-adjusted parents tend to reinforce normal psychosexual attitudes and behavior, and to extinguish (i.e., not reinforce) deviant behavior in their children. Maladapted parents, on the other hand, may reinforce inappropriate identifications and deviant sexual behavior while extinguishing normal sexual curiosity and exploration. Various forms of sexual deviation may arise as substitute phenomena when normal development toward heterosexuality meets with extreme frustration or actual punishment.

The diversity of deviant sexual behavior suggests that many different experiences are likely to contribute to its development. Following his study of the Sing Sing male sexual offenders, Glueck remarked: "We could not demonstrate one specific traumatic episode in the sexual development of most of the men. There appeared to be a continuously traumatic, prohibiting and inhibiting attitude towards sexual behavior throughout the developmental years that was reflected in the serious distortions of the adult sexual patterns." Most of these sexual offenders showed a marked lack of knowledge about sexual activity and normal patterns of sexual behavior. Those with the greatest deviation in sexual aim correspondingly gave a history of the greatest modesty during childhood, and similarly showed the greatest difficulty in approaching the adult female. The typical sexual offender is *not* aggressive but, rather, overly inhibited in his other sexual activities. Admittedly he fails to show consideration for the person against whom he commits the offense, but often he himself doesn't even obtain satisfaction from the deviant sexual activity.

Forty-four percent of Glueck's sample of sexual offenders remained unmarried at the time of the study (at a median age of 33.5 years), and gave such reasons as economic insecurity, sexual difficulties, and personality difficulties. Nearly half of those who were married stated that they were not usually satisfied by their marital sexual relationships. The disturbance in their ability to relate to other adults, illustrated in their relationships with their wives and other sexual partners, was further emphasized by their isolation in general areas of adult socialization. Those involved in the most deviant behavior tended to be the most shy and timid, and were also the most likely to show overt symptoms of schizophrenia or other psychosis. A considerable proportion used alcohol to excess, and this behavior tended to intensify the pathological patterns of adaptation.

Characteristic of most persons with sexual deviation is a profound lack of information concerning normal sexual activities, a diminished ability to achieve gratification from any form of sexual activity, and unsatisfactory interpersonal relationships with other adults. These characteristics are related to excessive prohibition and inhibition of sexual behavior during the developmental years. Traditionally, members of upper and middle socioeconomic classes have been taught a greater degree of control over sexual and aggressive impulses than members of lower classes. Among the latter, the prevailing pattern has tended to consist of stereotyped sex with a variety of heterosexual partners. Among the former, the prevailing pattern has more often included a variety of sexual behaviors with the same partner. Differences in social learning have therefore been held responsible for the relatively higher frequency of deviant sexual behavior at upper and middle socioeconomic levels, in contrast with the relatively higher frequency of sexual assault at lower socioeconomic levels.

REVIEW QUESTIONS

226. The most effective technique for treating premature ejaculation is:
    (A) attention diversion
    (B) changing the frequency of intercourse
    (C) application of a local anesthetic to the penis
    (D) use of a condom
    (E) the squeeze technique

227. Transsexualism is:
    (A) the desire to be transformed into the opposite sex
    (B) wearing the clothes of the opposite sex
    (C) attraction to and sexual contact with members of both sexes
    (D) latent homosexuality
    (E) hermaphroditism

228. In the treatment of homosexuality, the most important of the following factors in determining prognosis is:
    (A) motivation
    (B) history of parental relationships
    (C) treatment method

    (D) environment

    (E) ability to relate to the opposite sex

229. The typical exhibitionist is:

    (A) impotent

    (B) defending against latent homosexual impulses

    (C) schizophrenic

    (D) past age 50

    (E) lonely, shy, and insecure

230. Which of the following has been found to be the most important determinant of gender role (psychological sex) in adult life?

    (A) chromosomal sex

    (B) external genital appearance

    (C) assigned sex and rearing

    (D) hormones

    (E) internal reproductive organs

SELECTED REFERENCES

1. Annon, J.S. (1974). *The Behavioral Treatment of Sexual Problems. Vol. I: Brief Therapy.* Honolulu: Enabling Systems, Inc.

2. Bieber, I., et al (1962). *Homosexuality.* New York: Basic Books.

3. Cole, T.N. (1975). Sexuality and the spinal cord injured. In R. Green (Ed.), *Human Sexuality.* Baltimore: Williams & Wilkins Co.

4. Cormier, B.M., Kennedy, M., and Sangowicz, J. (1962). Psychodynamics of father-daughter incest. *Canadian Psychiatric Association Journal,* vol. 7, pages 203–217.

5. Ellis, A., and Abarbanel, A. [Eds.] (1961). *The Encyclopedia of Human Sexual Behavior.* New York: Hawthorne Books.

6. Ford, C.S., and Beach, S.A. (1951). *Patterns of Sexual Behavior.* New York: Harper & Row.

7. Glueck, B.C., Jr. (1956). *Final Report, Research Project for the Study and Treatment of Persons Convicted of Crime Involving Sexual Aberrations.* Albany: New York State Department of Mental Hygiene.

8. Hampson, J.L. (1963). Determinants of psychosexual orientation (gender role) in humans *Canadian Psychiatric Association Journal,* vol. 8, pages 24–34.

9. Hirschfeld, M. (1944). *Sexual Anomalies and Perversions.* New York: Emerson Books.

10. Kaplan, H.S. (1974). *The New Sex Therapy.* New York: Brunner/Mazel.

11. Kaplan, H.S. (1975). *The Illustrated Manual of Sex Therapy.* New York: Quadrangle/The New York Times Book Co.

12. Karpman, B. (1954). *The Sexual Offender and His Offenses.* New York: Julian Press.

13. Kinsey, A.C., Pomeroy, W.B., and Martin, C.E. (1948). *Sexual Behavior in the Human Male.* Philadelphia: W.B. Saunders Co.

14. Kinsey, A.C., Pomeroy, W.B., Martin, C.E., and Gebhart, P.H. (1953). *Sexual Behavior in the Human Female.* Philadelphia: W. B. Saunders Co.

15. Lorand, S., and Balint, M., [Eds.] (1956). *Perversions: Psychodynamics and Therapy.* New York: Random House.

16. Masters, W.H., and Johnson, V.E. (1966). *Human Sexual Response.* Boston: Little, Brown and Co.

17. Masters, W.H., and Johnson, V.E. (1970). *Human Sexual Inadequacy.* Boston: Little, Brown and Co.

18. Mohr, J.W., Turner, R.E., and Jerry, M.B. (1964). *Pedophilia and Exhibitionism.* Toronto: University of Toronto Press.

19. Pauly, I.B. (1965). Male psychosexual inversion: Trans-sexualism. *Archives of General Psychiatry,* vol. 13, pages 172–181.

20. Pion, R.J., and Annon, J.S. (1975). The office management of sexual problems: Brief therapy approaches. *The Journal of Reproductive Medicine,* vol. 15, pages 127–144.

19. Disorders of Childhood and Adolescence

L. EUGENE ARNOLD, M.Ed., M.D.

The childhood shows the man,
as morning shows the day.
John Milton, Paradise Regained

Whether the logical place to discuss psychiatric disorders of adolescence is in a chapter on childhood disorders, in a completely separate chapter, or in parts of the chapters about adult disorders, is a dilemma that typifies many of the frustrations that seem to plague adults who don't know what to do with adolescents. Many disorders in adolescents, particularly older adolescents, can be appropriately diagnosed and treated within the conceptual framework of adult psychopathology (e.g., the schizophrenias, depression, and many anxiety and hysterical disorders). However, the inclusion of adolescent disorders within a chapter on childhood disorders seems justified on the following grounds: (1) Some disorders of adolescents, particularly early and middle adolescents, more closely resemble disorders of younger children than those of adults. (2) Adolescents by and large still share with younger children economic and to some extent psychological dependence on their parents. (3) Adolescence is still legally classified as part of childhood in most localities, and even in nonlegal contexts adolescents are still sometimes referred to as children. (4) The end of adolescence represents an important landmark in a developmental continuum beginning with conception and ending at death.

DEVELOPMENTAL PERSPECTIVE

The developmental perspective is one of the chief concepts distinguishing child psychiatry. Without it no reasonable diagnosis or treatment plan could be formulated. Many behaviors or feelings that are normal at certain stages of childhood would be viewed as regressive and perhaps as prima facie evidence of psychopathology in an adult. For example, it should not be considered unusual for a 4-year-old boy to show his penis or a 5-year-old girl to climb on her father's lap and say, "Daddy, put your hand on my hiney," but the same behavior in an older person would likely lead to a diagnosis. The same speech dysfluencies that suggest severe anxiety in a stuttering adult represent a normal stage of speech development in most 3-year-olds. Similarly, toddlers go through a normal obsessive-compulsive stage that need not be diagnosed as a neurosis; preschoolers often suffer unrealistic fears (e.g., darkness or dogs) that are usually transient and need not always warrant a diagnosis of phobia; and children under the age of 3 or 4 years can wet the bed without incurring a diagnosis of enuresis.

Even when a symptom is not age-appropriate, its seriousness may be mitigated by chronological proximity to the appropriate age. A "2-year-old tantrum" is not normal in an 8-year-old, but it is certainly less ominous than in a 14-year-old. Symptoms such as enuresis, smearing, and mutism, which would constitute severe regression in an adult, perhaps symptomatic of psychosis, may represent only a very short step backward for a youngster. The well-trained 4-year-old who begins soiling or wetting at the birth of a sibling is usually manifesting only a transient situational disturbance that will respond well to brief supportive intervention. Naturally, assessment of such situations should take into account age, the time elapsed since passing through the appropriate developmental stage, and the intensity and duration of the symptoms.

Even when there is obviously serious disturbance, the prognostic implications may not be equally serious, because of the child's psychobiological flexibility, plasticity, and adaptability, as well as constitutionally variable rates of development. Children, as immature developing organisms, can compensate amazingly for physical, psychological, and social trauma when appropriate intervention gives them a second chance. Even in the absence of outside intervention, the child is sometimes given a "second chance" by his constitutionally variable rate of development.

Developmental patterns may vary in three ways: among individuals, over time for a given individual, and among various parameters within the individual. Most children do not develop in a smooth progression, at least not in all aspects (physical, cognitive, and emotional). There tends to be a steplike series of plateaus, sometimes with physical development surging ahead of mental development or vice versa. In terms of age-specific averages, a given child may be chronologically 10 years old, mentally 12, emotionally 8, and physically 14, while another 10-year-old might be mentally 10, emotionally 12, and physically 9. Some of these differences may persist as adult individual differences, aptitudes, or weaknesses. On the other hand, a child lagging behind his age mates in some respect may catch up and even surpass them eventually. An obvious example is the "runt" whose growth spurts in the late teens. The same phenomenon can occur in cognitive and affective development. Furthermore, a child may vary even within a given developmental parameter, such as cognitive development. Thus he may be far advanced or retarded in social intelligence or spatial intelligence compared to his other intellectual abilities. Again, such variations may persist into adult life as aptitudes or disabilities, or they may "even out" over time.

The ultimate outcome is influenced by both constitutional and environmental factors, including what other assets or liabilities the child has. Strengths in other areas can "prop up" and assist development in the deficit areas, or problems in several areas can synergistically compound each other. It also sometimes happens that very gratifying assets in one area may reduce motivation for the child to compensate, adapt, and develop in a less gratifying deficient area. For example, if a child has a musical or artistic talent, he and his parents may use the stereotype of a temperamental artist as an excuse for his not learning to control his temper or relate to peers adequately. This is also an example of *self-fulfilling prophecy,* an extremely important dynamic element in child development which will be discussed more fully below.

In order to assess psychopathology in children and distinguish it from age-appropriate immaturity, the diagnostician should be familiar with the highlights of the normal developmental continuum as presented in Table 19-1.

COMPREHENSIVE APPROACH TO CHILDREN'S PROBLEMS

Comprehensiveness might also be called a systems approach because it considers the child to be a thinking, feeling, metabolizing organism in dynamic equilibrium internally and externally, interacting through various feedback loops as both agent and recipient with his own internal biological and psychological systems as well as with external people, things, and events. Although the factors thus influencing and comprising a child's emotional development and adjustment are myriad, most of them can be organized under five major categories: neurological factors, constitutional factors, parental expectations and family dynamics, life events, and school and community.

Neurological Factors

Neurological and other "organic" factors are relatively more frequent in psychiatric disturbances of children than in those of adults. This is especially true for the more serious disturbances. Hertzig and Birch, in their studies of 200 adolescents in psychiatric hospitals, found over half showing two or more neurological indicators, such as audiovisual integration deficits or motor overflow. With younger children, even outpatient problems may involve substantial neurological components. One-half of elementary school—aged children referred to child psychiatry clinics manifest some degree of minimal brain dysfunction (MBD), at least as a complicating factor. A high proportion of epileptic children manifest emotional and behavioral symptoms, which may be doubly caused, both psychologically through body-image impairment and neurologically from the same cause as the epilepsy. Other chronic illness and physical handicaps, such as diabetes, asthma, rheumatic fever, deformity, and disfigurement, can also affect a growing child's emotional adjustment. Fortunately, the presence of an organic factor in a child's psychiatric disturbance does not

Table 19-1. Developmental Highlights

Age	Developmental landmarks	Freud's psychosexual stage	Erikson's developmental task stage*	Piaget's cognitive stage	Salient dynamics, defenses, and reactions	Critical concerns
0 Early Infancy	Smile by 2 mo., vocalizes, attends visually by 3 mo.	Oral	Basic trust vs. mistrust	Sensori-motor (manipulation of objects, beginning use of symbols, development of object permanence & imagery).	Introjection, projection, incorporation, symbiosis.	Stimulus & affect deprivation.
½ year Later Infancy	Sits, shy with strangers. Transfers by 8 mo. "Mama, dada" by 10 mo. Walks by 14 mo.				Attachment, dependency, individuation.	Separation from caretaker.
1½ year	3 words besides mama, dada.	Anal	Autonomy vs. shame & doubt		Power of words, negativism to assert autonomy, denial.	Overcoercion or oversubmission.
Toddlerhood	Runs, climbs steps, kicks ball, scribbles by 2 yr. Follows directions, toilet trained.			Pre-operational (animism, magic, egocentricity).		
3 years	Pedals trike, copies circle, separates from mother.	Phallic-oedipal	Initiative vs. guilt		Displacement, curiosity, assertiveness, repression, identification	Loss of same-sex parent, seduction, fear of mutilation.
Pre-school	Full name and copies cross by age 4. Buttons up, square, 3 colors age 5.					
6 years	Draws 6-part man.	Latent	Industry vs. inferiority	Concrete operations (conservation, seriation).	Sublimation, obsessive-compulsiveness, regression, rules, skill mastery.	Incompetence (e.g., learning disability), low self-esteem.
Elementary School	Interest in peer group, games with rules, speech of adult clarity, (although simpler).					
Puberty	Secondary sex characteristics.	Genital	Identity vs. role diffusion	Formal operations (abstraction, science).	Body image, autonomy, ambivalence, altruism, identification, sublimation, intellectualization.	Acting out of previously repressed conflict; mastery of increasing drives; identity, career choice.
Adolescence	Peer loyalties over family. Interest in politics, philosophy, and social issues as well as celebrities and heroes.					

carry as grave a prognosis as it would for an adult, because the child's plasticity, adaptability, and incomplete development may allow him to compensate for many organic impairments.

Constitutional Factors

Constitutional factors present at birth are closely related to the preceding set of biological considerations. These are mostly considered hereditary, and include potential maximum intelligence, temperamental traits, and appearance, including hair, skin, and eye color, regularity of features, potential height, and relative size of nose, feet, or other body parts. All of these affect the child's acceptance in various cultures and influence his self-image and self-esteem through verbal and nonverbal feedback from other people.

Constitutional *temperamental traits* are a particularly important consideration, especially with infants and very young children. Thomas, Chess, and Birch described nine temperamental traits that they were able to identify from the first few weeks of life, in many cases in the newborn nursery, before the parents had had a chance to influence the child interpersonally. They described these traits as: activity level, rhythmicity or regularity, quality of mood, adaptability, persistence, distractibility, approach-withdrawal spectrum, intensity, and threshold of stimulation. Individual children manifest various combinations and degrees of these traits, providing an almost infinite variety of infantile temperaments. However, about two-thirds of children can be roughly classified into three categories: "easy child" (the largest group), "difficult child," and "slow-to-warm-up child." No particular constellation of temperamental traits is good or bad in itself. The important consideration is the congruence or dissonance between the child's temperament and the parents' temperaments, expectations, and comfort in dealing with various temperamental manifestations of the child. For example, one parent may find his child's persistence a nuisance because of difficulty in getting him to cease unwanted behavior, while another parent may admire and take pride in the same trait in his child.

Parental Expectations and Family Dynamics

From infancy the child's temperamental traits and other constitutional factors are being modified by interaction with parents, sibs, culture, and physical environment. Parents who value a particular trait, such as activity level or persistence, will tend to reinforce its manifestations, thereby increasing its degree and frequency (see Chap. 5). Converse considerations apply to unacceptable traits. Parental values and expectations tend to shape the child's behavior in the expected direction. Cultural and familial patterns of personality are thus superimposed over the child's basic constitution, often by means of deviation-amplifying feedback loops (vicious and virtuous cycles) functioning as *self-fulfilling prophecies*. A good example is gender identity. Boys may be expected to be tough, active, and aggressive, and are reinforced for such behavior (see Chap. 5), thereby increasing its frequency, confirming the parental expectation that it is appropriate, and leading to still more reinforcement. In addition to such operant influences there appears to be an inherent tendency for young children to try to meet parental expectations perceived consciously or unconsciously, even if they are not objectively desirable or what the parents overtly claim they want.

Fortunately, most parental expectations are *constructive*. However, they can be just as effective and just as self-fulfilling when they are *destructive*. A good example of this would be a boy who is expected to be a liar and thief because he looks like one of his uncles who happened to be a liar and a thief. The parents may treat such a child with anxious distrust, communicating to him that he is untrustworthy, and subtly undercutting the self-esteem required for honesty and openness. They may also implicitly give permission to lie and steal because being "destined for it" makes it not really his fault. If neurotically invested in their prediction, they may even unconsciously encourage the boy's lying and stealing by making excuses for him, rationalizing, and protecting him from the consequences. Sometimes destructive expectations are inadvertently set up by physicians or other professionals. A common cause of immature, anxious dependence in an overprotected child is the parents' projected fear and expectation of the child's vulnerability dating from a childhood illness when a physician mentioned the possibility that the child could die. Perhaps the physician neglected later to reassure the parents that the danger was over, or perhaps the reassurance was given but not "heard." In child psychiatry clinics, a common explanation by new patients and their parents for impulsiveness or other behavior problems is, "I can't help it because I'm hyperkinetic" (or "brain damaged," or "epileptic," etc.). A diagnosis made years before becomes an excuse for the child to quit trying to control himself and for the parents to stop setting limits. Thus the expectation of uncontrollability can become a self-fulfilling prophecy.

Sometimes such *problem-labeling* fills a family need to escape responsibility for behavior, to act out against authorities through the child, or to project unacceptable impulses into the child identified as having the problem. In the latter case a true *scapegoating* process may evolve, with all the "good" siblings having an investment in the problem child's remaining "bad." As one 14-year-old said in family therapy, "You have to have some bad guys in the family. If you didn't have bad guys to compare to, you wouldn't know that you're a good guy." More about early learning experiences in the family can be found in Chapter 5.

Family expectations are often shaped by culture or subculture, such as those regarding sex-specific personality characteristics or whether children should be seen and not heard. Problems may arise for the child when his family's or subculture's expectations conflict with those of the larger society or culture. The youngster who manifests genteel manners to please his parents may be teased or rebuffed by classmates who consider him snobbish or standoffish for those same manners. Sometimes the problem can be resolved by developing different standards for home and the rest of the world, but such duplicity does not always come naturally to children.

Life Events
Life events such as birth, death, illness, separation,

and relocation tend to affect children even more than adults. Even such a benign occurrence as trading the family car for a new one can be traumatic for a toddler, who may grieve for a couple of days because he wants "*my* car, not that one!"

Birth of younger siblings, regarded by most adults and even by many older siblings as a happy event, may require some difficult adjustments for the preschooler, even when his parents handle it well. In addition to facing the problems of being displaced as the favored baby, the youngster must adjust his orientation to the "world" that is his family. Counting heads may become a temporary preoccupation, with much discussion of how many people are now in the family. A reevaluation of self-image is in order because his relative size, strength, intelligence, and other assets no longer rank him at the bottom of the totem pole. He may also have some cognitive difficulty integrating the idea that the barely animate lump of protoplasm in the crib is really a person like himself and that he himself was that small at one time. Unfortunately, the birth of a sibling is usually associated with a temporary absence of mother from the home, which in itself may be rather traumatic. In fact, the presence of the new arrival may be less significant than the more serious trauma of mother's absence. It is not unusual for preschoolers to show some temporary regression at such times. In many cases, of course, especially with parental support, preparation, and understanding, the challenge of the adjustment promotes psychological growth.

Absence of a parent through divorce, separation, death, or illness can also be quite traumatic, and the youngster will often blame himself for the unfortunate occurrence, compounding his anxiety and grief with guilt. He may behave in such a way as to bring punishment on himself as expiation. Serious illness in the child himself can also precipitate maladaptive behavioral or emotional reactions, which can be aggravated by parental response to the same threat. The emotional sequellae of illness or surgery tend to be worse when they necessitate hospitalization or other separation from home and parents. Changes of residence or school, especially frequent ones, may disrupt the child's sense of security and stability and abort his attempts to form peer relations.

School and Community

School functioning for the child is analogous to job functioning for the adult. Failure to achieve and behave at school should be considered as ominous a sign for a child as a similar occupational failure is for an adult. Additionally, school provides one of the more objective assessments of peer relations and group behavior. *Neglecting to obtain information from the school is probably one of the most common pitfalls for the inexperienced diagnostician.* In almost all cases school information can clarify, confirm, and provide a check on emotionally colored parent-supplied information. For a few common diagnoses, it is absolutely essential. For example, hyperkinetic reaction or attention-deficit syndrome should not be diagnosed without information on the child's school functioning (assuming that he is of school age). With the parents' consent, it is best to obtain such information directly from the school by letter, phone call, or personal visit, rather than accepting secondhand information from the parent about what has happened in school.

Important issues about which teachers and other school personnel can provide information are peer relations, number and intensity of friendships, temperamental traits, abilities, handicaps, differences in relating to male and female authorities, reaction to success and frustration, characteristic behavior, consistency of behavior, and circumstances affecting behavior and achievement. Examples of the latter are time of day or week, weather, social setting (group vs. individual, peers vs. authorities, task orientation vs. social orientation), and physical setting (classroom, corridor, cafeteria, playground). Observations by school personnel tend to be valid and reliable because they have had experience in dealing with children; they have many normal "controls" with whom to compare the child in question; they see the child over a much longer period of time than does the diagnostician; and they are usually able to take a more objective emotional stance toward their observations of the child than are the parents.

PREVENTION — GENERAL CONSIDERATIONS

Children present unique opportunities for prevention. As developing organisms they are vulnerable on the one hand but plastic and adaptable on the other. The foundations of adult mental health are laid in childhood, even as far back as in utero.

Prenatal and *perinatal* factors have been demonstrated to exert a marked influence on the child's later performance and behavior, which have been shown to correlate with quality of adult adjustment. These factors include such obstetrical considerations as health of the mother, gestational nutrition, in utero exposure to infections or toxins, complications of labor and delivery, etc. Some obstetrical practices, such as induction of labor for convenience, and some pediatric practices, such as isolation of premature infants in incubators, may need to be reexamined with more rigorous follow-up. A few studies suggest that provision to "premies" and other newborns of such "natural" stimuli as the sound of a heartbeat, random movement (vestibular stimulation), and skin contact has a soothing effect, promoting weight gain and normal development. In fact, there is some evidence that the well-documented initial weight loss of normal newborns, for which ad hoc physiological explanations have been advanced, may actually be an artifact of the separation of infants in newborn nurseries from the maternal heartbeat.

Every child has a right to be born wanted. Adequate *family planning* resources may be one of the most efficient means of promoting mental health in both children and parents. This should include adequate education, both biological and ethical, for teenagers, who contribute a disproportionate share of unwanted pregnancies, unwanted children, and unhappy parents.

Once the child has arrived, whether wanted or not, *his parents need help and support* with his rearing. Methods need to be worked out to provide in our mobile society of nuclear families the social support formerly provided by the extended family and small, stable communities. One of the easier and more acceptable areas in which to do this is health education, *including mental health education.* This should be on a face-to-face (preferably group) basis, not relying merely on books or television. In fact, books on child rearing can sometimes interfere with parents' natural good judgment by confusing them or making them hesitate when firm decisiveness is needed.

Because practically all children after the age of five spend a significant proportion of their time in school, *school consultation* provides a prime avenue of prevention. With appropriate consultative help, teachers and other school personnel can learn to provide parents some of the needed support discussed above, and form a cooperative working alliance which can bring more stability and order to the child's environment. Most schools have already made commitments to health education, including the areas of sex, mental health, and drugs. Many educators are as aware of the need for mental health consciousness in the schools as are psychiatrists, and welcome consultation to that end. Of course, there is some danger of promoting the trend for schools to take over more and more of the responsibilities of the family. However, there are many areas of school where mental health can be promoted without usurping the responsibilities of families. For example, it falls well within the purview of schools to individualize programs in such a way that each child experiences success at some level. Another example would be promotion of peer cooperation. Much can be accomplished by modification of the present system rather than by addition of new things.

Legal Aspects

Whatever is done to promote child mental health will, of necessity, have to operate within the constraints of the law. Three areas of law concern children at the most elementary level of basic mental health — their security and sense of belonging. These areas are: (1) *divorce law,* particularly the questions of custody and visitation rights; (2) *adoption and foster care;* and (3) *child abuse* (including

neglect and exploitation). Unfortunately, in the past the law has tended to see children as the property of the parents. It has paid more attention to the property rights of the parents than to the rights of children to live with someone who loves them, whom they love, and who can provide the optimum psychosocial environment. One welcome legal advance has been the almost universal enactment of *child abuse legislation,* which requires reporting of suspected child abuse by anyone who has occasion to suspect it and provides legal immunity from suit for such bona fide reporting. Interestingly, some abusing parents welcome the surveillance of the court or social agency and are able to refrain from abuse under such a structure. More such emphasis by the law and the courts on the best interest of the child could do much toward alleviating distress of children.

However, efforts to revise laws that affect children need to be thought out seriously. Past attempts to improve the lot of children through legislation have sometimes backfired. For example, establishment of separate juvenile courts, originally intended to protect children from harsh adult-type justice, has actually resulted at times in more severe treatment without the protection of due process. Such abuses have led to a current tendency to apply adult constitutional rights to children. The danger is that if carried far enough this may result in children being protected from their parents' active love and concern by a strict application of adult constitutional rights to their situation. The concept of "developmental rights" needs to be considered. For example, a child's right to have someone love him enough to help him curb his impulses may be more important to him at a particular stage of development than the right to freedom of movement. The whole issue requires further study.

In addition to these general considerations, specific opportunities for prevention will be discussed under specific disorders in the following pages.

INTERVIEW AND TESTING

Depending on the age of the child and on the personnel available, various interview options may be adopted. One of the traditional approaches has been for a therapist to interview the child while a social worker interviews the parents. If the same person will be interviewing both, some experts prefer to have the parents of *young children* come alone for an initial interview. They can then help the parents formulate a plan for preparing the child for his first visit. In the case of *adolescents,* many experts turn this around and interview the adolescent alone first. They then ask his permission to see his parents, explaining that what he told the interviewer will be kept confidential unless it concerns some kind of danger, such as suicide plans, about which the parents need to know to take effective steps for safety and welfare. If the adolescent seems hesitant, he can be offered the option of attending the interview with the parents. It is rare for an adolescent to refuse permission for an interview with parents, and most choose not to sit in when given the option. In rare cases, the adolescent may be so untrusting, even after adequate discussion and explanation of the necessity for seeing the parent, that it may be necessary to have a third party interview the parents.

The method favored at the Ohio State University Child Psychiatry Clinic for nearly all children and adolescents, whether one or several professionals are available for the interview, is the following:

If either the youngster or the parents show up alone for the first appointment, he, she, or they are interviewed and helped to formulate plans for involvement of the missing party. If it is the parents who have come alone, they are warned not to use any deceit in bringing the youngster to the next appointment and are helped to plan what to tell him. If it is the youngster who has come alone, it is explained that his parents' consent must be obtained before any treatment can be given. If the parents refuse to come in, they can mail their written consent. However, all applicants are encouraged to have all three, the child and both parents, present at the first session.

Ordinarily all family members are first seen together for a brief period, the exact length depending on how productive this joint interview seems.

This provides an opportunity to observe parent-child interaction and how the presence of the other members of the family alters each individual's mental status as compared with that noted in later, private interviews. It also provides an opportunity to assess the feasibility of family therapy as a treatment modality. Further, it gets the problem out into the open so that later the child will know that the interviewer knows that the child knows that the interviewer knows what the problem is, thereby aborting denial. In this sense the ice is broken.

For this procedure to be most effective, *the initial questions should be directed to the child,* who is always treated with respect. Many times the child will frankly state the problem, possibly because he knows that if he doesn't, his parents will, and he wants to say it his way first. After he has finished, the parents can then be asked if they have anything to add or if they have any other concerns besides what he brought out. If the child indicates reluctance to talk, or says that he doesn't know the reason for coming, the interviewer can express puzzlement that he would not inquire about it, and can offer to help him with this inquiry. At this point the interviewer, as the child's ally (but not hostile to the parents), can inquire what light the parents can shed on the situation. At various times during the parents' story the interviewer can turn to the child to check details in a respectful, trusting manner. If the parents start maligning or accusing the child destructively, the interviewer can modulate, limit, or split them immediately for separate interviews. At the end of the parents' story, the child is asked if anything has been left out or if he wishes to add anything. Efforts should be made throughout the joint interview to build a common basis of agreement about what the problem is.

If two or more interviewers are present, the group can then split up in the interest of more efficient information gathering and to allow all parties a chance to speak more frankly in private. If there is only one interviewer, the child and parents can be sequentially interviewed alone. In the latter case, the most common practice is to interview the child alone and then the parents, but this order may be reversed if the child seems to have difficulty trusting, so that he will know that the interviewer is not "reporting" to the parents after his interview. In this case, the final summary and recommendations to the parents need to be made in the presence of the child (which is usually desirable anyway).

Information to be elicited from parents includes whatever they had been reluctant to say in front of the child, problems in the marriage or family, parents' personal psychiatric problems, and the child's family and developmental histories as outlined in Chapter 3. The latter includes review of developmental milestones and their psychological significance to parents and child. Naturally, the parents also need to be given an opportunity to verbalize any spontaneous concerns.

PRIVATE INTERVIEW WITH CHILD. When the child is seen alone, establishment of rapport should be the first order of business. This may involve engaging the child in some discussion about sports, clothes, pets, or some other interest. In the case of very young children, especially preschoolers, some comic or other unorthodox approach may be in order. Sometimes informal psychological tests, discussed below, can help in building rapport, particularly if they involve tasks in which the child can feel he has succeeded or can get positive reinforcement for his performance. Such play materials as dolls and puppets may help the very young child to express himself. For older children and adolescents, of course, adult-type verbal interviews may be very appropriate, including an adult mental status examination. With prepubescent children, their natural cognitive immaturity needs to be distinguished from thought disorder or impairment of intellectual function. In addition to the usual interview techniques, including inquiries about dreams, there are some special techniques helpful with children:

One useful modality is *projective questioning,* such as the "three wishes" question mentioned in Chapter 3. It is important to state this in such a way that the child is not led into the restricted tendency to ask only for material objects. Some-

times it is necessary to clarify that he can wish *to be something,* or *to do something,* or *that something be changed;* however it is often sufficient merely to use the open-ended terminology, "What would you wish?"

Another projective technique is *asking the child to complete a story* about three birds: A mother bird, a father bird, and a baby bird were living in a nest at the top of a tall tree until a strong wind came along and blew them all out of the nest, and blew the nest out of the tree, and blew the mother bird that way (pointing), and the father bird that way (pointing another direction), and the baby bird that way (pointing a third direction). Healthy endings to this include: The father bird finds the mother bird and baby bird and they all go back together to rebuild the nest; or the mother bird finds the baby bird while the father bird rebuilds the nest. Such deviant responses as that a cat ate the birds, that the baby bird found the mother and father bird, or that the baby bird went back and rebuilt the nest himself, are revealing of the way the child sees the world, his parents, and his relationship to them.

In *the mutual storytelling technique,* the child is invited to a make-believe television panel show in which there is a contest to make up the most original and interesting story. With appropriate television-announcing jargon, the child is introduced as a guest star who will be allowed to have the first try at making up an original story. The story must have a moral, which is often as revealing of the child's affective functioning as the story itself. (The interviewer can make up a story with a therapeutic purpose in return.)

Psychological Tests for Children

For preschoolers, the *Denver Developmental Screening Test* or some other developmental test can help assess the child's functioning, or at least his need for more sophisticated psychological testing.

One psychological test that can be easily administered during the interview to children aged 5 years and over is the *Bender Visual-Motor Gestalt Test.* This test can provide information about the degree of neurological involvement in the child's problem as well as clues to perfectionism, motivation, impulsiveness, anxiety in task situations, and other "emotional" aspects of the child's functioning. Koppitz's *The Bender Gestalt Test for Young Children* provides a scoring system, but Bender herself advocates a more qualitative assessment. Familiarity with children's typical performance at various ages can sharpen the diagnostic usefulness of this test.

An alternative to the Bender test, especially for younger children, is to request *drawings of common geometric figures.* If the child cannot draw these on command, he should be shown the figures and allowed to copy. At 3 years of age he should be able to draw a circle, at age 4 a cross, at age 4½ a square, at age 5 a triangle, and at 7 a diamond.

The *Peabody Picture Vocabulary Test* (PPVT) and *Quick Test* (QT) are fairly quick and easy intelligence tests that can be administered and scored for immediate information during an interview. They involve having the child identify pictures.

The *Draw-a-Person Test* (DAP) can yield a mental age estimate without the child's knowing he is being tested. Three years' mental age credit is given for at least a scribble on the paper. An additional 3 months is awarded for each part or feature, such as head, neck, trunk, arms, legs, shoulders, eyes, pupils, brows, nose, nostrils, hair, clothing, chin and forehead, joints, fingers, symmetry, etc. Correctly proportioned and two-dimensional parts are scored double. For children 3 to 10 years old, this test can yield a mental age usually within 10 percent of standardized, more sophisticated intelligence tests. In addition, it can yield projective information about body image and other concerns. It is ordinarily assumed that the first person drawn by the child is a projection of his own self-image, even though he is merely asked to draw "a person." After the first drawing, he can be asked to draw a person of the opposite sex, which can yield further information about his sexual identity and view of his two parents.

Probably a better technique for the latter objective is the *Kinetic Family Drawing.* A child is given the instruction, "Draw a picture of your whole family, including yourself, doing something. Try to make them look as much like real people as possible, not cartoon characters or stick figures. And remember, have everybody doing something." With a little experience and familiarity with the principles in Burns and Kaufman's *Kinetic Family Drawings: Action, Styles and Symbols,* such drawings will virtually speak to the interviewer, revealing family pathology in a surprisingly explicit manner.

To check academic achievement when immediate feedback is needed without waiting for school information, such tests as the *Durrell Reading Test,* the *Gray Oral Reading Test,* the *Wide Range Achievement Test,* or the *Peabody Individual Achievement Test* can be used.

From the interview techniques and simple tests mentioned above, along with information from parents and teachers, adequate data can be obtained about most children for formulation of a rational treatment plan. However, in some cases more sophisticated psychological testing, such as that described below, is indicated. (Many of these tests are described in more detail in Chapter 4.)

Projective tests include the *Children's Apperception Test* (CAT), the *Blacky Test* (a similar test using pictures of dogs in various situations), and the *Rorschach.*

Adolescent norms for the *Minnesota Multiphasic Personality Inventory* (MMPI) have recently been developed, and this test will probably be more widely used for adolescents, although not for preadolescents.

One of the more popular intelligence tests is the *Wechsler Intelligence Scale for Children* (WISC). To get the maximum information from this, it is important to evaluate the subtest scores as well as the full scale, verbal, and performance IQs. The *Stanford-Binet* is still used, especially for children below age 6, but there is also a *Wechsler Preschool and Primary Scale of Intelligence* (WPPSI).

For more sophisticated evaluation of learning-disabled children, the *Illinois Test of Psycholinguistic Ability* (ITPA) is sometimes used. This test yields specific information valuable to educators in planning a child's remedial program. Other tests useful in evaluating children's perceptual deficits and other educational handicaps include the *Wepman Test of Auditory Discrimination, Slingerland Test of Language Disabilities, Rutgers Test,* and the *Silver-Hagin SEARCH battery.*

SPECIFIC DISORDERS

Many disorders of childhood and adolescence can and should be appropriately diagnosed in the same categories as for adults even though there may be age-specific frequency differences (see Chap. 9). Such disorders as conversion hysteria, anxiety, and phobia are as common among children and adolescents as among adults. Other disorders, such as manic-depressive illness, paranoia, schizophrenias, and alcohol dependence, occur less commonly in children. Personality disorders should be diagnosed conservatively in adolescents and hardly ever in younger children because of the instability of the developing personality. On the other hand, some diagnoses such as somnambolism may be made more frequently in children than in adults. Finally, there are some diagnoses that are ordinarily made *only* in children and adolescents, such as behavior and conduct disorders. Most of the diagnoses that are more common in children and adolescents than in adults concern disorders of development (failure to attain age-appropriate functioning in one or more areas of ability or behavior). Examples would be specific reading disorders, articulation or language disorders, enuresis, and attention deficit syndrome (hyperkinesis).

Disorders of Attachment and Separation

In the normal course of human development, the infant makes an affective attachment to the mother (or mother surrogate) as a primary love object from whom he derives basic feelings of security, stability, and worth, which enable him gradually to separate from her in increasingly riskier, lengthier, and more distant excursions, eventually involving attachments to other people. Several things can go wrong during this process.

MATERNAL PRIVATION. Maternal privation is the absence of adequate opportunity for enjoying attachment to a mother figure. It is often called *maternal deprivation,* although the latter term technically is the premature withdrawal of the mother figure. The results of either situation may be very similar. In its extreme forms it can result in physical disease and death, but more often it produces stunting of cognitive and emotional development (as described in Rene Spitz's famous report). The infants he studied apparently suffered some stimulus privation as well as privation of maternal affection, but there seems no doubt that human infants need something besides adequate nutrition, warmth, sanitation, and physical comfort for normal development. The implications for prevention are obvious.

SEPARATION ANXIETY. Separation anxiety arises when the contact with mother is abruptly or prematurely disrupted after the infant has formed an attachment — *maternal deprivation* proper. John Bowlby described three stages of a child's reaction to loss of mother: (1) *active protest* (motivated by separation anxiety), with crying, calling for mother, rejection of other caretakers, tantrums, etc.; (2) *despair* ("anaclitic depression"), with mournful passivity; and (3) *detachment,* with denial of desire for mother. Prolonged absence of the mother figure, especially without other psychological supports, can cause severe psychopathology. The most vulnerable age range appears to be 6 months to 2 years (the lower age being the time at which an infant learns to distinguish his mother from other people). Normal amounts of separation anxiety are ordinarily resolved by youngsters returning to "check" on mother periodically during their fledgling excursions. Unexpected absence of mother or long separations can leave a residual of separation anxiety, which can cause problems from time to time in later life.

ATTACHMENT FAILURE. Attachment failure refers to the inability of an individual to form deep or lasting relationships. Possible etiologies include constitutional inability, lack of opportunity to form attachments during critical stages of infancy, and abrupt or premature disruption of attachments, leading to a learned association of separation anxiety with attachment situations.

TREATMENT. Treatment of attachment and separation disorders requires first of all environmental structuring to provide the needed care and affection from a consistent, stable caretaker. For some patients, this in itself is sufficient to reverse the disorder. In others, especially older children and adolescents, psychotherapy may be indicated. Recent primate research indicates that antianxiety agents may be useful adjuncts to therapy of the maternal (de)privation syndrome. Unfortunately, some patients that have progressed to the "affectionless" stage may be intractable to any treatment.

PREVENTION. Prevention is based on an understanding of these disorders. The following should be kept in mind: (1) Each child needs a consistent, stable, loving, affectionate caretaker. (2) That caretaker should not abruptly be absent for long periods, especially when the child is between 6 months and 2 years old. (3) If a long absence is anticipated, the child should be prepared by short absences to allow him to develop secure dependence on a secondary caretaker. (4) When the primary caretaker is away, the child should be cared for in familiar surroundings by someone he already knows. Sibs should be kept together, especially for the sake of the younger ones.

Pervasive Developmental Disorders and Child Psychoses

Such syndromes as early infantile autism, childhood schizophrenia, symbiotic psychosis, atypical child, and childhood psychotic brain syndrome are far less common than adult psychoses. Such diagnoses should be made only when buttressed by thorough evaluation. They carry such serious prognostic import that a "false positive" can be extremely destructive to the mental health of the whole family.

The names, syndromes, and categories of childhood psychoses remain an area of controversy. Some experts still believe that autism and symbiotic psychosis are subtypes of childhood schizophrenia. However, most at present appear to accept a distinction between schizophrenia and *early infantile autism,* or *Kanner's syndrome.*

AUTISM. This disorder is ordinarily diagnosed during the preschool years, with the signs first noted by parents during the first year or two of life. The characteristics include: (1) extreme autistic aloneness (difficulty mixing with other children); (2) failure to use language for meaningful communication (echolalia, preference for gestures); (3) failure to distinguish between people and inanimate objects, or treating people as if they were inanimate objects; (4) need for preservation of sameness (routine or surroundings); (5) resistance to learning new things; (6) fascination with objects; (7) preoccupation with twirling or spinning; (8) a feylike quality, as if from another world; (9) odd or bizarre play; (10) failure as an infant to cuddle or mold to the adult caretaker when being held; (11) standoffish manner; (12) overactivity; (13) acting as if deaf (with normal audiometry); (14) heedlessness of real danger; (15) inappropriate laughing or giggling; (16) lack of eye contact. A child does not need to show every one of these characteristics to be diagnosed autistic, but does need to show several (half of them, according to one author). Many of the characteristics are found in other disorders, such as deafness or minimal brain dysfunction, and occasionally (in milder degree) in normal children. Autistic children in general do not show hallucinations or delusions.

CHILDHOOD SCHIZOPHRENIA. By contrast, schizophrenic children, usually first diagnosed above kindergarten age, may show hallucinations, delusions, affect intensely inappropriate to their verbal communication, and intense ambivalence, in addition to bizarre speech, thought, or behavior. They attempt to use speech for meaningful communication, although they may show echolalia or neologisms. They are thought to be suffering an early expression of the same disorder as affects adolescents and adults and should be diagnosed by the same criteria.

SYMBIOTIC PSYCHOSIS. This failure to differentiate from the mother may be a variant of autism. Such a child shows an inability to function autonomously, perhaps reacts with panic when separated from the mother.

ETIOLOGY. The etiologies of child psychoses and pervasive developmental disorders remain unclear. There may well be multiple causations, undoubtedly including a strong constitutional or other organic predisposition. Two recent diagnostic advances have been the finding of biochemical, particularly serotonin, abnormalities in children who clearly meet stringent diagnostic criteria for autism, and the development of a diagnostic behavioral questionnaire by the Institute for Child Behavior Research.

PROGNOSIS. Although the prognosis is generally guarded for childhood psychoses and pervasive developmental disorders, it tends to be improved by: (1) IQ above 70; (2) development of meaningful speech by the age of 5; (3) symbiotic features in early childhood; (4) a good home that can meet the excessive needs; (5) absence of frank organic disorder such as epilepsy; and (6) intensity, duration, and variety of therapeutic intervention, and responsiveness to these.

TREATMENT. Treatment for child psychoses and pervasive developmental disorders tends to be long and arduous. Adolescent psychoses have a favorable drug response rate comparable to that of adults, but neuroleptic drugs are not as successful in treating childhood psychoses, especially in autistic children. Nevertheless, there are enough patients who do respond to warrant a trial of the medication when other approaches fail. The most successful chemotherapy for autistic children is that directed at target symptoms shared by non-autistic children, such as hyperactivity or aggression. Since childhood psychoses often involve a failure to progress rather than regression, educational or habilitative approaches are often helpful. Special remedial help for such accompanying problems as learning disabilities, speech disorders, per-ceptual deficits, and incoordination can help the child's overall adjustment. Sign language has been reported helpful for some patients. Systematized, well-planned programs of behavior modification can sometimes shape the child's behavior in a more normal direction even when intense, less systematic efforts of the parents have been unsuccessful. Some encouraging results from psychotherapy have been reported by a few brilliant psychotherapists, but those results have not been generally replicable in any consistent fashion, a problem common to most treatments suggested for childhood psychoses. The treatment program generally needs to be individualized for each child; finding the right treatment and techniques can often be accomplished only on a trial-and-error basis.

Parents need to be enlisted in the design and execution of a treatment program, especially for autistic children. At the same time, parents need counseling and help in preserving some time, energy, and resources for their other children and for themselves, as well as help in accepting the child's handicap and resolving their feelings about it.

Attention Deficit Disorders (MBD, Hyperkinesis, Learning Disability)

This very common syndrome (or group of syndromes), afflicting 5 percent of elementary school children by conservative estimate, has a variety of names. Some of the more common are: *minimal brain dysfunction (MBD), hyperkinetic syndrome, hyperkinesis, hyperactivity, hyperkinetic impulse disorder, developmental delay, maturational lag, psychoneurological integration deficit,* and *learning disability.* These terms and concepts are overlapping rather than congruent, as the Venn diagram in Figure 19-1 shows for the three most common ones. While most hyperkinetic children are also learning disabled, learning disability is more prevalent, affecting perhaps 10 to 20 percent of elementary school children.

Although overactivity, restlessness, and other motor disturbances are among the most salient characteristics of many of the affected children, overactivity is not a requirement for the diagnosis. Many experts believe that the attention impair-

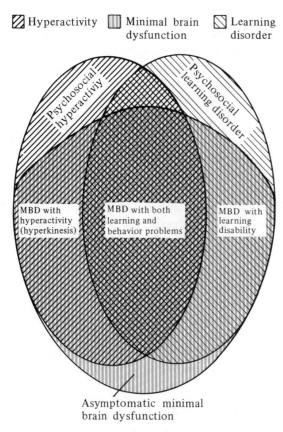

Hyperactivity   Minimal brain dysfunction   Learning disorder

Psychosocial hyperactivity

Psychosocial learning disorder

MBD with hyperactivity (hyperkinesis)

MBD with both learning and behavior problems

MBD with learning disability

Asymptomatic minimal brain dysfunction

Figure 19-1. Relationship among the concepts of hyperactivity, minimal brain dysfunction, and learning disorder. (Adapted from Arnold, L. E. [1976]. Minimal brain dysfunction: A hydraulic parfait model. Diseases of the Nervous System, vol. 37, pages 171-173. Reproduced by permission.)

ment (e.g., short attention span or distractibility) is the more basic problem, but it is not even clear that this needs to be present for the diagnosis to be made. No one symptom is either necessary or sufficient. For the diagnosis to be justified, the child should manifest several of the following: restlessness or overactivity, unpredictable variability, impulsiveness, irritability or low frustration tolerance, lability or explosiveness, short attention span, distractibility, inability to work in a group while performing well on a one-to-one basis, underachievement despite acceptable motivation and normal intelligence, and "soft" neurological signs

such as poor coordination and perceptual deficits (e.g., visual-motor deficit). The latter can be recognized either by psychological testing or by careful neurological examination. Such psychological test findings as visual-motor impairment on the Bender Gestalt or a scatter on subtests of the WISC, especially with poor performance on the subtests associated with attention or "organic" impairment, help support the diagnosis.

The most important source of diagnostic information, however, is the report of adult caretakers who have long experience with the child, such as teachers and parents. The most valuable reports are of concrete, specific observations and comparisons to other children, rather than global statements that the child is hyperactive. Rating scales can help the adult caretakers attempt more objective assessment. A history of gestational or early developmental abnormality is supportive of the diagnosis but neither necessary nor conclusive.

ETIOLOGY. Etiology is controversial and may involve several factors. Besides true brain damage, the following have been advanced by various authors as contributing etiological factors in at least some children: deprivation or privation of various sorts (maternal, cultural, stimulus); genetic predisposition; hypersensitivity (allergy and food or food-additive intolerance); disorders of nutrition and metabolism (vitamins, iron, carbohydrates); environmental poisoning (lead, insecticides); radiation (fluorescent lighting, television); emotional stress; and training. Such a diversity of proposed etiologies may reflect a diversity of nosological entities subsumed under this category. This disorder may actually be a collection of syndromes that have not yet been adequately delineated and distinguished from each other. Support for this idea comes from physiological studies such as galvanic skin response, electroencephalogram, and electropupillogram, all of which seem to distinguish a subgroup of such children who are *underaroused* physiologically even though their overt behavior appears overactive. There also appear to be children who are *overaroused* physiologically as well as behaviorally.

PROGNOSIS. No good longitudinal controlled studies have been done, but the few follow-up studies available indicate that many such children continue to have problems through adolescence and into adulthood. The learning and perceptual problems in particular seem to persist, although the restlessness and overactivity in most cases abate with maturation. Some familial studies suggest a correlation between childhood hyperkinesis and adult sociopathy or hysterical personality, but it has not been proved through longitudinal studies that the former develops into the latter. Nevertheless, many clinicians feel that hyperkinetic children are at high risk for developing delinquency and adult personality disorder. There may also be a higher risk for development of adult schizophrenia. Certainly adolescent psychiatric populations include a disproportionate percentage of adolescents who have a history of hyperkinesis in earlier childhood. In any event, the large number of children suffering from some manifestation of this syndrome represents a large pool of vulnerable personalities.

TREATMENT. Treatments proposed are as varied as proposed etiologies. Some of the treatments bear a logical relation to a hypothetical etiology, such as an elimination diet based on food or additive hypersensitivity. However, some of the more effective treatments, such as behavior modification and drug therapy, are empirical attacks on target symptoms. A good treatment plan should be comprehensive, flexible, optimistic, and oriented to gradual improvement over a period of time. It usually includes parent guidance, teacher consultation, structuring activities, reorientation of the child's expectations and explanation of his handicap, appropriate educational remediation such as a learning disability tutor or a learning and behavior disorder class, and perhaps some supportive psychotherapy. The latter may need to be expanded to more intensive psychotherapy if secondary emotional problems have developed, such as despair, depression, low self-esteem, resentment, or reactive hostility. Behavioral management paradigms can enlist the child's cooperation in planning, selection of reward, and charting. Contracting and reality therapy are often helpful, especially with older children and adolescents.

If there is an allergic history or if there are such signs of allergic diathesis as nose or eye rubbing, rings around the eyes, or a history of food intolerance as an infant, a trial of an elimination diet may be helpful. In the case of preschoolers and any child with a history of tactile or vestibular stimulus deprivation, it may help to encourage the parents to hold, cuddle, and rock the child, even if he resists. In the latter instance, he should be held until he gives in and accepts cuddling and stroking for a few minutes. Identification of specific perceptual deficiencies, followed by structured tutoring designed to strengthen the deficient channels, has been found to reduce significantly the later manifestation of academic and behavioral problems.

Chemotherapy can be a useful adjunct to (not substitute for) the other interventions described above. Almost every psychotropic drug has been reported to be efficacious for children with these problems. Most experts favor the *stimulant-antidepressant group,* including amphetamine, methylphenidate, pemoline, amitriptyline, and imipramine. These drugs appear to improve concentration and performance, calm restlessness, allow the child better impulse control, and make him more responsive to reward and punishment. They have two main disadvantages: They do not work for all such children (although another drug in the same general group may help if the first one tried does not) and their use has become so politicized as to lead to consternation among many parents. The inclusion of the stimulants on schedule II as "dangerous" drugs by the Federal Drug Enforcement Administration because of their addicting properties in adults has added to the confusion and consternation. A nondefensive consultative disclosure of all pertinent facts will help the parents to make a rational, informed decision. When a stimulant or tricyclic antidepressant has been found ineffective, a major tranquilizer may be useful. Occasionally anticonvulsants help, especially if there is an episodic, intense quality to the behavior problem. In refractory cases, drugs of two types may be combined, but it is usually better to try to find one effective drug for the child, titrate to the minimum effective dosage, and try "weaning" him during school vacations.

PREVENTION. Prevention possibilities are as varied as etiological theories and treatment methods. Although few of the following preventive possibilities are supported by well-controlled research, most of them are compatible with common-sense clinical impression: (1) adequate prenatal and perinatal care, including maternal nutrition; (2) encouragement of breast feeding to delay exposure of the immature organism to potential allergens and food additives and to promote mother-child interaction, with accompanying vestibular, tactile, and auditory stimulation; (3) bringing the child into interaction with the mother at the earliest possible opportunity, including skin-to-skin contact in the delivery room, rooming-in procedures, and avoidance of incubator any longer than absolutely necessary; (4) provision of appropriate tactile, vestibular, and auditory stimulation within the incubator when use of the incubator is necessary (e.g., random rocking, audio tape of heartbeat); (5) encouragement of parents to hold, cuddle, and talk to even those infants who seem to dislike it, since they may need it even though they cannot at first respond positively to it; (6) all the measures described previously under Disorders of Attachment and Separation for prevention of maternal deprivation syndrome; (7) insistence on speech in addition to nonverbal communication when the child becomes capable of talking; (8) ridding the environment of toxins (such as heavy metals) and other dangers to physical health; (9) kindergarten and first grade remediation of specific deficient perceptual skills; and (10) gearing task demands to a child's individual developmental ability level.

Other Behavior Disorders (Unsocialized Aggressive, Delinquent, and Runaway)

The appropriate classification and grouping of behavior disorders constitutes a challenge. There is a good deal of overlapping, and many behavior-disordered children manifest signs and symptoms of more than one category. Even the distinction between the attention deficit disorders and these other behavior disorders is not clearcut. Some unsocialized aggressive children, for instance, seem more like hyperkinetic children than like runaways or even delinquents. They may even respond well to stimulant medication. Both unsocialized aggressive and delinquent youngsters can have underlying minimal brain dysfunction. Often the choice of specific diagnosis depends on the most salient symptoms noted at the time. The same child can be diagnosed hyperkinetic in kindergarten, unsocialized aggressive in third grade, delinquent in high school, and antisocial personality in the Army. (This example is not meant to imply that such progression is usual.) Some experts have questioned whether it is reasonable even to attempt classifications, arguing that actually the behavior disorders constitute a spectrum. Others feel that attention deficit disorders with or without hyperactivity should be distinguished from the other behavior disorders. There is some justification from factor analysis of behavior checklists for distinguishing the behavior problems of inattention, hyperactivity, unsocialized aggression, and antisocial behavior (delinquency and running away).

UNSOCIALIZED AGGRESSION. Unsocialized aggressive children may be described as "out of control." perhaps due to inherently poor impulse controls (MBD?), or inadequate limit-setting by parents, or both. Some might be described as "spoiled brats" while others appear to be reacting to parental rejection or modeling of violence. There are tendencies to disregard rights of other people, to resort to physical violence when frustrated, to deny personal responsibility, and to project blame onto other people. Except for inappropriate aggression and quick temper, behavior may be rather well patterned and organized. This diagnosis may be made at any age from toddler to teen but is more frequent in younger children.

DELINQUENCY AND RUNNING AWAY. These are generally considered teenage problems, but they have in recent years been filtering down into lower age groups. Running away has often been considered a special form of delinquency that girls favored in lieu of the more aggressive forms practiced by boys. This sex distinction has eroded in recent years, but another distinction has been made in the law. Acts that would not be a crime if committed by an adult, such as running away, truancy, curfew violations, and refusal to obey parents ("status violations") are being classified as "unruly" rather than "delinquent." While this distinction seems worthwhile legally, ethically, and perhaps prognostically, it is not clear that the teenagers themselves make this distinction. To a troubled adolescent, any rule that at the moment happens to be interfering with his wishes may appear as arbitrary as status laws. Whether he is considered unruly or delinquent may depend on the most salient offenses at the time.

Runaways and delinquents have in common an orientation toward action rather than verbalization and a tendency to avoid or escape unpleasant situations or feelings through action. A runaway tends to do this through open flight, whereas delinquents may resort to counterphobic attack or attempts to master feelings by demonstrating mastery of the situation in destructive ways.

The delinquent youth may range from an ineffectual, learning-disabled, poorly socialized dropout who gravitates to delinquent behavior because of inability to do anything more constructive, to a well-socialized, well-organized, intelligent gang leader who develops ulcers because of the heavy responsibility he feels toward his gang and who engages in delinquent behavior only because of peer or subculture sanction. The latter could be characterized as a socialized delinquent or group delinquent and has a better prognosis, since the problem is mainly one of values. The former is more likely to engage in solitary delinquency. He is also more likely to slip into a lifelong pattern of maladjustment, especially if he does not receive intensive help, including basic competency-oriented skill development. Between these two extremes are numerous variants, including neurotics with superego lacunae resulting from parental sanction of specific types of antisocial behavior.

PROGNOSIS. Although antisocial behavior in childhood and adolescence increases the risk of serious adult psychiatric disturbance (schizophrenia, depression, sociopathy), this is not an inevitable outcome. Even without help, some behavior-disordered youngsters learn from experience and eventually "straighten up." More importantly, clinical experience suggests that many such youngsters can be helped.

TREATMENT. Treatment requires structure and firm limits, often in a residential or inpatient treatment setting. Underlying psychotic, neurotic, or neurological problems need to be evaluated and treated appropriately. Constructive peer relations need to be encouraged. Much of therapy will take place through identification with appropriate adult models who can frankly and nondefensively share their own values and feelings about issues important to the youngsters without pressuring them to accept those values. The therapeutic approach should be compatible with such values of the youngster as "looking out for number one," peer loyalty, getting other people to do what you want, staying out of trouble or out of jail, and so on. Unless the main problem is thought to be neurotic, psychotherapy should in most instances be concrete and directed to solution of problems whose definition the therapist and patient mutually agree on. Reality therapy is particularly good for delinquents. Most behavior-disordered youngsters suffer low self-esteem and need to be convinced of their own worth by any means available, including positive reinforcement for saying realistically good things about themselves.

PREVENTION. Prevention includes: (1) all of the things suggested for prevention of maternal (de)privation and attention deficit syndromes; (2) early treatment as symptoms first appear; (3) elimination of social and economic stresses statistically associated with high delinquency rates; and (4) debunking the myths extant among some parents and even some professionals that firm limits may thwart a child's initiative or warp his personality.

Stress Disorders (Adjustment Reactions)

The diagnoses of adjustment reaction of childhood or adolescence have been abused (overused) in the past. The age of the patient is not sufficient grounds to make this diagnosis. There must be an acute or transient disturbance obviously in reaction to some stressful circumstance, usually some life event such as illness, moving, separation, or death in the family. Also, the disturbance should not take the form of a well-delineated disorder diagnosable under some other category, such as conversion hysteria, depression, or schizophrenia.

Often an adjustment reaction implies basic good health. It may be a natural response of an otherwise healthy personality to some pathogenic stimulus, and represents attempts at coping with the circumstance. Therefore, it generally carries a good prognosis, at least with appropriate crisis intervention. The diagnostician-therapist, however, needs to keep in mind that an adjustment reaction may accompany a more serious problem. In fact, children with other, more serious disturbances are more vulnerable to adjustment reactions than are normal children.

TREATMENT. Treatment of choice is crisis intervention with brief supportive psychotherapy, parent guidance, and promotion of communication between parent and child so that the parent can assume a more supportive role.

PREVENTION. Prevention of adjustment reactions is very similar to their treatment except for the timing. For anticipated stressful life events, such as moves, beginning school, birth of siblings, or elective surgery (of child or family member), the child can be prepared psychologically by supportive explanation and an opportunity to talk out or play out his feelings. Books about other children of similar age undergoing the same life event and managing it successfully are usually helpful. Questions from the child should be answered truthfully, and he should not be assured that it will not hurt. Unsolicited assurance about absence of pain will merely raise the child's suspicions. If the child asks about pain, the question should be answered in a straightforward, matter-of-fact way. If pain is anticipated, the adult may often add a truthful qualification like "a little bit" or "for a little while." Often the anticipated sensation can be honestly reinterpreted as tightness, coldness, numbness, stinging, etc., which may be less anxiety-provoking. For unfortunate life events that cannot be anticipated, such as unanticipated death or illness, or hospitalization of a family member or of the child himself, the child's successful adjustment can be facilitated by an immediate explanation at his level of understanding and by the attention of a supportive, understanding adult.

Presence or acquisition of a *handicap* can cause secondary adjustment problems that may result in neuroses affecting body image, self-esteem, and sense of security or vulnerability. For the parents of handicapped children to be supportive and helpful in preventing these secondary emotional problems, they may need the help of a professional in resolving their own emotional reaction to having a handicapped child.

Regression, Passive Aggression, and Oppositional Behavior

Closely related to adjustment reactions are three ways of reacting to stress or pressure so common among children as to be considered normal under many circumstances: regression, passive aggression, and oppositional behavior. The child's unconscious choice of these ways of reacting appears related to his status as an unstable, developing individual with very little power vis-à-vis the adults with whom he must deal.

REGRESSION. This results from the fact that newly learned social skills are not yet second nature and are easily lost under stress. This can be dealt with by supportive understanding and positive expectation, as well as by paying some attention to the source of stress, relieving it where appropriate.

PASSIVE AGGRESSION. This remains one of the few ways in which a weak, powerless child can express hostility safely or exert some control over the situation. The appropriate treatment for this is difficult for many adults, involving patience, understanding, refraining from coercion or struggle, reinforcing more active behavior (especially cooperation), and providing other avenues for expressing hostility or exerting some control.

OPPOSITIONAL BEHAVIOR. This resembles passive-aggressive behavior, but seems less an expression of hostility or an attempt to control the environment, and more of a struggle for psychological autonomy. It can be dealt with by demonstrating a respect for the child's autonomy and reinforcing his sense of self-direction, thereby decreasing his psychological need for the behavior.

Anxiety and Hysterical Disorders (Neuroses)

Anxiety seems to be a universal equalizer, for neuroses (anxiety and hysterical disorders) constitute the group of diagnoses in which the least distinction needs to be made between children and adults. Most adult neuroses are also found frequently in children, in recognizable form meeting the usual diagnostic criteria. Conversion disorders, especially those involving headache or bellyache, often go undiagnosed.

SCHOOL PHOBIA. School phobia (or school refusal) is actually a form of *separation anxiety*. The child becomes extremely anxious at school and insists on staying at home with the mother because he is afraid something will happen to mother while he is away. This is usually related to maternal anxiety about the child's welfare and about being a good mother, with a need for the child's approval. Depression can also be found in the clinical picture. The anxiety and depression are often converted to gastrointestinal or other somatic symptoms that bring the child to the pediatrician and have the secondary gain of keeping the child home or getting him sent home. The prognosis is generally thought to be good for younger school phobics, but for the small percent who have a recurrence in adolescence, the prognosis is much graver. Approximately half of the latter group have an underlying psychosis and often need hospitalization.

Treatment of school phobia involves a combination of crisis intervention and follow-up, with a family and community orientation. The following steps should be taken: (1) Evaluate the problem adequately both psychiatrically and medically (assuming that there are physical complaints); (2) in children with an underlying psychosis, prescribe appropriate medication as indicated; (3) involve both parents (if available) in the intervention; (4) explain the problem to the child, both parents, and some responsible person at the school; (5) return the child immediately to school ("We can't teach you to swim unless you're in the water"); (6) make sure that all parties understand that there is no psychiatric or medical reason for the child not to attend school, setting up the expectation that the child will attend *(home tutoring is contraindicated)*; (7) see that a responsible person is designated to guarantee that the child gets to school and stays in the building (not necessarily in the classroom); (8) offer family therapy and flexible individual psychotherapy for parents and child, on a frequent basis at first (for most younger children it is more important for the mother, or occasionally the father, to have psychotherapy than for the child, and most mothers are accepting of this). In refractory cases addition of imipramine has sometimes been helpful.

Treatment for most other children's neuroses closely parallels that for adult treatment. Psychotherapy may need to be through the medium of play. Parents' support, and possibly participation in therapy, needs to be enlisted. If parental psychopathology is causing or perpetuating the child's neurosis (as in the case of school phobia), the parent may also need to have psychotherapy. Occasionally minor tranquilizers are helpful for short periods, but the indications are more stringent than for adults.

Mood Disorders (Depression)

In the past, depression was thought not to occur in young children and rarely in adolescents. Besides the possibility that it was less frequent in the past, there are two possible explanations for its being unrecognized: Adults tend to deny such problems in children, having a need to remember childhood as a happy time; and children and adolescents have a tendency to mask their depression with either behavioral acting-out or conversion symptoms.

Treatment is similar to that for neuroses or adjustment reaction, depending on severity and duration of the depression. Occasionally antidepressant drugs are indicated.

Suicide Threats

Suicide, although less frequent in younger children, is one of the five leading causes of death in teenagers. In addition, far more suicide threats, gestures, and attempts are made than actual suicides committed. One problem with assessing suicide risk in youngsters in the large amount of manipulativeness and acting out of anger involved. In fact, it is very common for a teenager to state frankly that the reason he attempted suicide was because he was angry with someone. The proportion of anger involved in a suicide threat or attempt seems inversely proportional to age. However, there can also be a large element of desperation. In many instances, the youngster is acting out the family's implicit message that he is expendable.

All suicide threats should be taken seriously, and if the youngster persists in the threat after appropriate attempts to negotiate a "no suicide" contract, he should be hospitalized. If the threat is manipulative or an expression of anger, the idea of hospitalization is usually aversive enough to prevent this from becoming a habitual method of acting out, whereas failure to take the threat seriously may challenge the youngster to prove that he is not bluffing. Opportunities for expressing anger in other ways and offers of help in working out stressful life situations usually result in defusing of the suicide potential. Although the incidence of endogenous depression is low in those under the age of 18, reactive depression (problems with family, loss of girlfriend or boyfriend, school failure, etc.) is common and does carry suicide potential. Psychosocial treatment, as opposed to antidepressant medication or electroconvulsive therapy, is of more relative importance with suicidal children and adolescents than with adults.

Specific Symptom Disturbances (Specific Developmental Disorders)

ENURESIS. Enuresis is one of the most common problems of childhood; the incidence of wetting in children over the age of four exceeds 10 percent Only a small percentage of cases are due to infection or anatomical defect. A larger percentage are psychogenic, but the most common cause, accounting for over half the cases of primary enuresis, is maturational lag or neurophysiological dysfunction. Secondary (acquired) enuresis, occurring after a period of being dry, is more likely to be psychogenic, although such problems as infection or onset of diabetes need to be ruled out.

Sometimes enuresis is a presenting symptom of a neurosis or adjustment reaction and should be treated accordingly. Enuresis as a target symptom can be successfully treated by a variety of procedures, none of which is effective in all cases. For younger children, bladder stretching by daytime fluid forcing and holding as long as possible, perhaps combined with evening fluid restriction, is often helpful. Some boys of latency age respond well to an explanation of bladder sphincter function and attempts to strengthen the sphincter by retaining as long as possible during the daytime or stopping repeatedly in midstream while voiding. Behavior modification paradigms appear to work well, even such a simple thing as a star chart, keeping track of wet and dry nights. Often it is not even necessary to offer any kind of tangible reward, just the good marks on the chart. More intelligent youngsters can sometimes carry this whole procedure out themselves without involving their parents. In many cases, though, it is helpful to have the support and supervision of a parent. Often it is useful to have the child change or help change the wet bedding.

Various gimmicks are also useful. One such is to have the child set an alarm clock for himself for two hours after going to sleep so that he can awaken and go to the bathroom. By setting the clock a half hour later each night he can eventually be dry the whole night. Another is a mechanical device that rings a buzzer or bell or administers a mild shock when the sheets are wet. *Imipramine,* which has strong anticholinergic effect on the detrusor and which reduces the amount of stage 4 sleep, has also been found helpful; if used, it can usually be discontinued after 6 weeks. Whatever approach is used, the assumption needs to be made by therapist and parents that the child wants to gain control over his own sphincters. Parents may need help in taking a supportive rather than punitive attitude.

ENCOPRESIS. This is another symptom for which parents may need help in taking a supportive rather than punitive attitude. Soiling after the age of 3 years usually has a strong psychogenic component. It may be that the child is caught in a vicious cycle of large, hard, painful stools which he then postpones, making the next one equally large and painful. This results in a "leakage around an impaction" phenomenon. The retention may also be part of a passive-aggressive, hostile, withholding relationship with the parents. Repeated passing of well-formed stools into the pants with no leakage in between suggests either neurological loss of control, severe lack of training, or deliberate voluntary acting out of hostility indicative of a severe parent-child disturbance.

Treatment of encopresis depends on a careful determination of the kind of encopresis and the child's and parents' attitudes toward it, as well as an assessment of the total parent-child relationship. When retention is part of the picture, medical intervention with stool softeners or suppositories to give the rectum a chance to resume its normal size will unfortunately be necessary. When the parent-child relationship is basically sound and a vicious cycle of retention alone seems to be the main problem, directing the parents in a supportive attitude and setting up a specific plan of management with the child's cooperation may be sufficient. When passive aggressiveness, hostile interaction, punitiveness, and coerciveness are present in the family, the parents will need to be helped to respect the child's autonomy and allow him other avenues for expressing anger and resentment. Some parents may require psychotherapy to facili-

tate this flexibility. In many cases the child will also need psychotherapy. One axiom sometimes advanced for therapy is: "If he's dirty, clean him; if he's clean, dirty him." This means that an obsessive, neat, withholding encopretic can usually benefit from encouragement for such "dirty" activities as fingerpainting or making mudpies, whereas a sloppy encopretic with poor personal hygiene needs training in basic cleanliness.

SPEECH DISORDERS. Speech disorders that are not anatomical are of two main types: articulation deficits and fluency problems (stuttering). An unusual variant is a congenital delay in which the child's normal speech development is delayed until the age of 3 or 4 years, but then proceeds normally. *Articulation problems* often reflect a neurophysiological immaturity and usually respond well to group instruction, practice, and drill, especially if buttressed by contingent rewards. Many schools offer speech therapy that is adequate for correction of articulatory defects. Even without help, many articulation problems tend to improve with maturation.

Stuttering, or pathological dysfluency, is a more serious problem, usually requiring individual attention and some sort of psychotherapy. It needs to be distinguished from the normal maturational dysfluency of a toddler who, in his development of verbal skills, may sound much like an adult stutterer but does not have the associated anxiety. Frequent dysfluencies persisting to school age, especially if associated with obvious anxiety, require intervention to prevent a lifelong disability. Parents' support needs to be enlisted. For young children, the most effective intervention may be to demonstrate to the parents how to read to the child with concomitant tactile contact to desensitize him to words. The older child needs both specific techniques to deal with the stuttering habit and psychotherapy for the underlying anxiety.

DEVELOPMENTAL LANGUAGE DISORDER. This may accompany learning disorders (see next page). Some authors even conceive of this as the primary problem, with the specific learning disorders being a secondary manifestation. Such children show problems with concept formation, abstraction, logical reasoning, associations, or syntax. Patient, supportive encouragement for practice is helpful. There is a suggestion that stimulant medication may be helpful, but this is not as well documented as for the accompanying behavior disorders.

LEARNING DISORDERS. Learning disorders (reading disorders, learning disabilities, LD) are common school-age problems, with a prevalence of about 10 to 20 percent. Some learning disorders are psychogenic, but the majority are basically neurophysiological ("perceptual deficits," maturational lag), with secondary emotional problems because of frustration, failure, and disappointment. Many learning-disordered children also have behavior problems and could be classified as having attention deficit syndrome (minimal brain dysfunction, hyperkinesis).

The prognosis for improvement with maturation is good if the child can be kept motivated in the meantime. He needs support from parents and teachers with an optimistic expectation of gradual improvement through small steps. His circumstances need to be arranged so he can experience some success at his level of capability. This can be done through either special classes or special tutoring adjunctive to a regular class taught by a flexible, understanding teacher who can help structure the child's activities in the direction of success experiences. Medication with the stimulant-antidepressant group of drugs is not as clearly helpful for learning disorders as it is for the accompanying behavior problems (hyperkinesis), but some authors recommend it even for hypoactive learning-disabled children.

COORDINATION DISORDER. This may accompany learning disorder as part of the neurophysiological deficit or maturational lag, or may occur as the primary problem. It can be thought of in some ways as a learning disorder in the motor sphere. As with a reading disorder or an arithmetic disorder, one of the dangers is that the child will quit trying, thereby losing the opportunity to learn. Extra physical education and even some physical medicine rehabilitation can help such children develop an acceptable level of coordination. Here again, small successes at the child's level of ability are necessary to maintain motivation and interest.

SLEEP DISORDERS. These are not unusual among children. *Insomnia* is not the most common of these, but can occur, especially in hyperkinetic children. More common complaints are *colic* in the infant and *night terrors* or *somnambulism* in the preschooler or young school-age child.

Colic is characterized by nocturnal screaming, as if the child is in pain, and is usually aggravated when the child is held by an anxious parent and usually abates when he is held by a more objective adult. It may be a symptom of autonomic instability, but also appears to be influenced by the security and stability the infant senses from the environment. One pediatrician reported reducing the incidence of colic in his practice from 10 percent to 2 percent by having the obstetrician lay the newborn on the mother skin-to-skin for a few minutes in the delivery room.

Night terrors and *somnambulism* occur during stage 4 sleep and need to be distinguished from *nightmares,* or bad dreams, which are thought to occur during REM sleep. A youngster can be easily awakened or may waken spontaneously from a nightmare, which he can remember afterwards and which will usually bear some content relation to a waking concern. Youngsters experiencing night terrors or sleepwalking are very difficult to waken, usually cannot remember what they said, did, or experienced, and are confused about where they are. Persistent nightmares may be an indication for psychotherapy, but occasional nightmares in an otherwise healthy-appearing child may warrant merely reassurance and watchful waiting. For night terrors and sleepwalking, education of parents is important. This education should include securing the house for a sleepwalker. In extreme cases night terrors and possibly somnambulism may be helped by medication that lightens stage 4 sleep, such as tricyclic antidepressants or benzodiazepines.

Tic Disorders

Tics are involuntary intermittent contractions of a muscle or group of muscles. They may result from neurological disorders, emotional disorders, or a combination of these. They are distinguished from chorea by the similarity of each contraction to the previous one and from tremors by their irregularity. Many tics of childhood disappear spontaneously or with treatment of an underlying emotional disorder, while some persist into adult life.

Tic de Gilles de la Tourettes, or *maladie des tics,* is a syndrome of more ominous prognosis than other tics. Its onset is progressive, usually during latency or early adolescence. It presents at first as involuntary spasmodic grunts, which gradually become articulated into obscenities (coprolalia) as the disease progresses. Other parts of the body are eventually involved; some patients show whole-body tics. Various etiologies have been proposed, but currently the best evidence favors a neuro-chemical disorder: brain dopamine overactivity. Therefore, the treatment of choice is haloperidol or other potent dopamine-blocking medication. Behavior modification has also been found helpful in suppressing the more disabling manifestations, and supportive psychotherapy can help the patient learn to live with the problem.

Eating Disorders

Pica, the eating of nonfood materials such as dirt, paint, plaster, etc., can be a manifestation of an adjustment reaction that carries a severe risk in environments polluted with heavy metals or other toxins. Supervision of the child's ingestion should be part of the treatment plan. *Food fads,* whether part of a peer culture phenomenon in adolescence or a manifestation of finickiness at a younger age, are usually transient, but if persistent and severe they should be evaluated. A more severe problem is the generally poor dietary pattern followed by many youngsters with the availability of junk foods. The latter may be related to the increasing problem of *obesity* among teenagers, which deserves further study.

The opposite problem, *anorexia nervosa,* actually appears to be related to obesity. Typi-cally, a pubertal youngster (usually female) goes on a weight-losing diet because of some plumpness and cannot stop losing once she reaches the ideal weight. Weight loss continues, and a frequent result without intervention (sometimes even despite intervention) is death. In the hospital the weight loss can usually be reversed by behavior modification and milieu treatment. Family therapy and psychotherapy are needed for the underlying family and psychodynamic problems. Low-potency major tranquilizers have been used, especially in the acute stage.

Psychogenic dwarfism may be related to pica or poor food intake. The psychogenically "turned off" pituitary resumes secretion again when the child is removed from the family.

Gender Disorders in Childhood

Gender disorders, treated more fully in Chapter 18, usually trace their roots to early childhood. The exact origin is unclear, possibly being partly biological, but more likely involving either separation anxiety (or other emotional conflict) or reinforcement patterns and other nonverbal messages from parents. Gender disorder should be distinguished from a "liberated" attitude. The latter may involve pursuing activities, occupations, and pastimes of both sexes while retaining a firm identification with and satisfaction with one's own biological sex. The child who not only pursues activities of the opposite sex but actively avoids activities of his or her own sex or otherwise expresses dissatisfaction with his or her biological assignment may be manifesting a problem that requires intervention to prevent more serious problems in later life. In contrast to the situation with adults, there is a good chance in young children of reversing a transsexual identity or resolving the child's dissatisfaction with his biological sex, especially when the parents are cooperative. Both behavior modification and group therapy with age mates of the same sex have been found helpful.

SPECIAL THERAPEUTIC CONSIDERATIONS FOR CHILDREN

Among several ways in which therapy of children differs from therapy of adults, the importance of

involving the parents is preeminent. With children, transference issues are not merely residues of the past; they are vital current reality, with the child returning home to his parents after each therapy session. The child spends far more time with his parents than with the therapist and the parents are far more important to the child, thereby exerting far more psychological influence. Therefore no therapeutic program can hope to succeed without at least the passive cooperation of the parents. The chances of success are enhanced by more active cooperation and even participation of the parents. The relative importance of *family therapy* and *parent guidance* is inversely proportional to the child's age. For preschoolers, parent guidance will usually be the main therapeutic vehicle, sometimes without even any further contact with the child after the initial evaluation. For older children and adolescents family therapy is more commonly used. With older adolescents who live away from home or who are otherwise psychologically divorced from their families, family therapy may be contraindicated.

Another important part of the environment of children and adolescents is the peer group. Their natural propensity for groups makes **group therapy** an important modality. In fact, for many adolescents group therapy is the treatment of choice, not just a cheaper substitute for individual psychotherapy. Often a combination of group therapy with either family therapy or individual psychotherapy is helpful. One of the advantages of group therapy is that some children can use it as a substitute for family therapy, re-creating within the group the family issues that they need to work through, while other children can use it for working through intrapsychic problems they wish to handle separately from concomitant family therapy. Thus it can complement either individual or family therapy as well as being the main therapeutic modality. Groups should be led by male-female cotherapist couples, especially in the case of adolescents, for whom identification with appropriate adult models is a prime therapeutic mechanism.

Chemotherapy is not as important for children, relative to psychosocial therapy, as it is for adults.

However, judicious temporary use of drugs in selected cases can expedite therapy if used as *part of a comprehensive approach.*

There are two **developmental considerations** affecting therapy of children: (1) Therapeutic communication needs to be at the developmental level of understanding of the child. Nonverbal communication, concrete communications, and such mediums as play and activity therapies assume relatively more importance with children than with adults. (2) Therapy needs to be geared to complement and aid the healing power of the child's appropriate developmental level. For example, a 6-year-old girl manifesting regression at the birth of a new sibling could be encouraged through play therapy or counseling of the parents to assume the role of assistant mother, congruent with the identification with mother which she should be experiencing at this age as part of the resolution of her oedipal situation. While misapplied psychotherapy can further interfere with natural psychological development, appropriate psychotherapy can "unhook," or release, the child to resume normal development.

REVIEW QUESTIONS

231. The concept of superego lacunae is associated with:
    (A) infantile autism
    (B) anaclitic depression
    (C) juvenile delinquency
    (D) anxiety neurosis
    (E) childhood schizophrenia

232. A major difference between the functional psychoses of early childhood and those of adulthood is:
    (A) the former are regressive while the latter are not
    (B) the former are improved and the latter exacerbated by stimulant medication
    (C) the former are much more often reactive to situational stress
    (D) the former are almost never followed by residual psychiatric impairment
    (E) none of the above is true

233. In obtaining a psychiatric history of a child,

both parents should be interviewed if possible. The most important reason for this is:

(A) it increases the reliability of the information obtained

(B) to avoid future legal problems involving treatment of the child

(C) to be sure that the parents' complaints are not a purely imaginary product of their own psychopathology

(D) because children with psychiatric problems nearly always have parents with psychiatric problems

(E) to obtain an impression of the nature of the relationship between the parents and the manner in which they individually respond to the child

234. The usual emotion behind a runaway reaction is:

(A) depression

(B) mania

(C) fear

(D) arrogance

(E) revenge

235. Which of the following conditions is more common in females than males?

(A) dyslexia

(B) hyperkinetic reaction

(C) schizophrenia, childhood type

(D) mental retardation

(E) none of the above

236. A 15-year-old boy has become increasingly critical of his parents, especially their political and religious views. At times he manifests dependency on them but at other times he proclaims his independence and expounds certain altruistic views. He spends considerable time in front of a mirror applying acne cream to his face but resists bathing or changing clothes. His school work is good despite his insistence on rock music while studying. The physician should:

(A) request psychological testing to rule out serious psychopathology

(B) suspect drug abuse

(C) institute a series of family therapy sessions

(D) reassure the parents that such behavior is common during adolescence

(E) encourage the parents to spend more time with the boy

237. Parents of autistic children are typically:

(A) schizophrenic

(B) mentally retarded

(C) ghetto residents

(D) Jewish of Eastern European origin

(E) upper- or middle-class college graduates

238. The adverse consequences of maternal deprivation are clearly demonstrated by:

(A) Kanner's study of autistic children

(B) Harlow's monkey studies

(C) Piaget's study of cognitive development

(D) Freud's study of "Little Hans"

(E) Erikson's study of identity crisis

239. An 8-year-old child attending an inner city school is reported to have an IQ of 80. In interpreting this score, it would be correct to state that:

(A) the child has mild mental retardation

(B) the child has a mental age of 10 years

(C) this child requires remedial tutoring

(D) all intelligence testing at this age has poor predictive value

(E) none of the above is justified

240. A symptom which would *not* be associated with a childhood or adolescent adjustment reaction is:

(A) pica

(B) paranoid delusions

(C) delayed language

(D) nightmares

(E) enuresis

241. School phobia is usually due to:

(A) separation anxiety

(B) mental retardation

(C) hyperkinetic behavior disorder

(D) stranger anxiety

(E) fear of failure

242. In a psychiatric examination of a 6-year-old child, a good principle to follow is:

(A) to have one or both parents present at all times

(B) to avoid asking the child about anything which he does not bring up himself

(C) to have toys present in the interview room

(D) to offer the child a reward for answering all your questions

(E) to assure the child that whatever he tells you will be kept secret from his parents

243. Which of the following is *least* characteristic of anorexia nervosa?
   (A) lowered vital signs when the weight is low
   (B) denial of illness
   (C) history of obesity
   (D) decreased physical activity
   (E) episodes of bulimia, followed by vomiting

244. A 13-year-old suddenly develops marked weakness in one arm, about which he seems unconcerned. Physical and neurological examinations reveal no associated abnormalities. Among the following, the most likely diagnosis is:
   (A) psychophysiological disorder
   (B) drug experimentation
   (C) adjustment reaction
   (D) conversion hysteria
   (E) intracranial neoplasm

245. The Swiss psychologist Jean Piaget:
   (A) wrote the first formal description of the syndrome of infantile autism
   (B) studied the effects of maternal deprivation by rearing monkeys in isolation or with "surrogate mothers" made of wire or cloth
   (C) wrote *Childhood and Society*
   (D) proposed a four-stage model of cognitive development
   (E) invented play therapy as a psychotherapeutic modality suitable for very young children

---

Summary of Directions

A	B	C	D	E
1, 2, 3 only	1, 3 only	2, 4 only	4 only	All are correct

---

246. A 2-year-old is likely to manifest regressive behavior when:

(1) left with a sitter
(2) fatigued
(3) a new sibling is born
(4) not feeling well

247. Drugs likely to be helpful in treating a child with minimal brain dysfunction and attention-deficit syndrome (hyperkinetic reaction) include:
   (1) chlorpromazine (Thorazine)
   (2) methylphenidate (Ritalin)
   (3) detroamphetamine
   (4) phenobarbital

248. Suicide during adolescence:
   (1) is attempted three times as frequently by girls as by boys
   (2) is the most common cause of death
   (3) is successfully completed three times as frequently by boys as by girls
   (4) is more frequent in those of lower than higher intelligence

249. A 4-year-old girl is hospitalized for surgery to correct a congenital heart defect. To minimize lasting emotional trauma, it would be advisable to:
   (1) explain to the child before the operation what will happen and what it will be like postoperatively
   (2) insist that no one discuss the impending operation with the child lest she become frightened
   (3) encourage the mother to remain with the child during the day and, if possible, overnight
   (4) sedate the child heavily immediately when admitted so that she will not know what is happening

250. Symptoms which might be indicative of a depressive neurosis in an 11-year-old include:
   (1) delinquent behavior
   (2) running away from home
   (3) sexual acting out
   (4) suicide attempt

251. Early infantile autism (Kanner's syndrome) almost always involves:
   (1) extreme aloneness starting at birth
   (2) failure to use language for communication

(3) an anxiously obsessive desire for sameness

(4) a fascination for objects accompanied by poor or absent relationships with persons

252. Treatment of school phobia usually involves:
   (1) psychotherapy for child and parents
   (2) antidepressant medication
   (3) investigation of the child's school environment
   (4) temporary removal from school and tutoring at home

253. A diagnosis of adjustment reaction should *not* be made:
   (1) when the patient is less than 2 years old
   (2) when organic factors cannot be definitely ruled out
   (3) when developmental disturbances are the only symptoms
   (4) when a precipitating stress cannot be found

254. The temperament of a child:
   (1) is defined as his inborn predisposition to react to stimuli in a certain way
   (2) has a strong effect on his environment
   (3) may predispose him to adjustment reactions and certain other illnesses
   (4) is relatively easy for parents to modify

255. In the case of a 3½-year-old child who is not yet speaking intelligible words, the physician should seriously consider the possibility of:
   (1) mental retardation
   (2) deafness
   (3) autism
   (4) parental overindulgence and overprotection

SELECTED REFERENCES

1. Adams, P.L. (1974). *A Primer of Child Psychotherapy.* Boston: Little, Brown and Co.

2. Arieti, S. [Ed.] (1974). In G. Caplan (Ed.), *American Handbook of Psychiatry* (2nd ed.). Vol. 2. New York: Basic Books. Chapters 1 to 26.

3. Arnold, L.E. (1976). *Mental Health Consultation to Schools.* Teaneck, N.J.: Behavioral Science Tape Library, Sigma Information.

4. Arnold, L.E. [Ed.] (1977). *Helping Parents Help Their Children.* New York: Brunner/Mazel.

5. Berlin, I.N., and Szurek, S.A. [Eds.] (1969). *Learning and Its Disorders.* Palo Alto: Science and Behavior Books.

6. Berlin, I.N. (1975). *Advocacy for Child Mental Health.* New York: Brunner/Mazel.

7. Burns, K.C., and Kaufman, S.H. (1972). *Actions, Styles, and Symbols in Kinetic Family Drawings.* New York: Brunner/Mazel.

8. Chess, S., and Thomas, A. (annual). *Annual Progress in Child Psychiatry and Child Development.* New York: Brunner/Mazel.

9. Coddington, R.D., Arnold, L.E., Leaverton, D.R., and Rowe, M. (1973). *Child Psychiatry Case Studies.* Flushing, New York: Medical Examination Publishing Co.

10. Di Leo, J.H. (1970). *Young Children and Their Drawings.* New York: Brunner/Mazel.

11. Erikson, E.H. (1964). *Childhood and Society.* New York: Norton.

12. Fraibourg, S. (1975). Ghosts in the nursery. *Journal of the American Academy of Child Psychiatry,* vol. 14, pages 387–421.

13. Freud, A. (1965). *Normality and Pathology in Childhood Assessments of Development.* New York: International Universities Press.

14. Gardner, R.A. (1971). *The Boys' and Girls' Handbook About Divorce.* New York: Bantam Books.

15. Gardner, R. (1971). *Therapeutic Communication with Children: The Mutual Storytelling Technique.* New York: Science House.

16. Goldstein, J., Freud, A., and Solnit, A.J. (1973). *Beyond the Best Interests of the Child.* New York: Free Press.

17. Harrison, S.I., and McDermott, J.F. [Eds.] (1973). *Childhood Psychopathology.* New York: International Universities Press.

18. Johnson, A., and Szurek, S.A. (1952). Genesis of antisocial acting out in children and adults. *Psychoanalytic Quarterly,* vol. 21, pages 323–343.

19. Joint Commission on Mental Health of Children (1973). *Mental Health: From Infancy*

Through Adolescence. New York: Harper & Row.

20. Kessler, J.W. (1966). *Psychopathology of Childhood.* Englewood Cliffs, N. J.: Prentice-Hall.

21. Kohlberg, L. (1968). The child as a moral philosopher. *Psychology Today,* September, pages 25–30.

22. Koppitz, E.M. (1963). *The Bender Gestalt Test in Young Children.* New York: Grune & Stratton.

23. Lewis, M. (1973). *Clinical Aspects of Child Development.* Philadelphia: Lea & Febiger.

24. Miller, D. (1974). *Adolescence: Psychology, Psychopathology, and Psychotherapy.* New York: Aronson.

25. Patterson, G., and Gullion, M.E. (1976). *Living With Children.* Champaign, Illinois: Research Press.

26. Piaget, J. (1967). In D. Elkind (Ed.), *Six Psychological Studies.* New York: Vintage.

27. Rimland, B. (1968). *Diagnostic Checklist for Behavior-Disturbed Children.* San Diego: Institute for Child Behavior Research.

28. Safer, D.J., and Allen, R.P. (1976). *Hyperactive Children: Diagnosis and Management.* Baltimore: University Park Press.

29. Salk, L. (1973). The role of the heartbeat in the relations between mother and infant. *Scientific American,* vol. 228, no. 5, pages 24–29.

30. Shaw, C.R., and Lucas, A.R. (1970). *Psychiatric Disorders of Childhood.* New York: Appleton-Century-Crofts.

31. Stone, L.J., and Church, J. (1973). *Childhood and Adolescence: A Psychology of the Growing Person.* New York: Random House.

32. Thomas, A., Chess, S., and Birch, H. (1968). *Temperament and Behavior Disorders in Children.* New York: Brunner/Mazel.

33. Toman, W. (1969). *Family Constellations.* New York: Springer.

34. Wender, P. (1968). Vicious and virtuous cycles: The role of deviation-amplifying feedback in the origin and perpetuation of behavior. *Psychiatry,* vol. 31, pages 309–323.

35. Yale University Press (annual). *The Psychoanalytic Study of the Child.* New Haven: Yale University Press.

20. Mental Retardation

There are three kinds of brains; one understands itself, another can be taught to understand, and the third can neither understand itself nor be taught to understand.
Niccolo Machiavelli

DEGREES OF MENTAL RETARDATION

Mental retardation consists of significantly below-average intellectual functioning, which may be present at birth or become evident later in the developmental period, and which is associated with impaired adaptive behavior that is reflected in maturation, learning, or social adjustment. Emotional disturbance is often present, and may involve other major psychiatric disorders such as anxiety, depression, or schizophrenia. However, mental retardation becomes evident during childhood (relative to the development of peers) and persists throughout the remainder of the person's lifetime.

The degree of retardation is expressed in terms of the intelligence quotient (IQ), which originated as a ratio of mental age (established for a normative peer group) divided by chronological age. The IQ range of each diagnostic category of retardation corresponds with the standard deviation of IQ in the general population; i.e., 16 IQ points. Since intellectual development is completed by a chronological age of about 16 years, levels of mental retardation also imply a maximum mental age that will be attained during the adult's lifetime. (These concepts were discussed more fully in Chapter 4.)

The degrees of mental retardation are defined as follows:

Borderline: IQ 68 through 83 (i.e., between 1 and 2 standard deviations below the mean), corresponding with a maximum adult mental age of about 11 to 13 years. This category numbers roughly 15 percent (almost one in every six persons) of the general population, and is excluded from further consideration in the remainder of this chapter. All other degrees of mental retardation, with IQ less than 68, number less than 3 percent of the total population.

Mild: IQ 52 through 67 (between 2 and 3 standard deviations below the mean), corresponding with a maximum adult mental age of about 8 to 11 years.

Moderate: IQ 36 through 51 (between 3 and 4 standard deviations below the mean), corresponding with a maximum adult mental age of about 5½ to 8 years.

Severe: IQ 20 through 35 (between 4 and 5 standard deviations below the mean), corresponding with a maximum adult mental age of about 3 to 5½ years.

Profound: IQ under 20 (more than 5 standard deviations below the mean), corresponding with an adult mental age no greater than that of the average 3-year-old child.

The educational potential of mentally retarded children corresponds roughly with these levels or ranges of retardation. The profoundly retarded (IQ less than 20) are *totally dependent.* They number only one in a thousand of the general population, and represent only 3 percent of all mentally retarded persons, but roughly 30 percent of the institutionalized retarded.

The severely retarded (IQ 20 to 35) are *trainable* but cannot learn academic skills. However, the moderately retarded (IQ 36 to 51) are *educable* to about the fourth grade level by their late teens. These two groups (severely and moderately retarded) constitute about three per thousand of the general population, and only 11 percent of all retarded persons, but roughly 50 percent of the institutionalized retarded population.

Mildly retarded children with IQs of 52 through 67 are also educable to about the sixth grade level by their late teens. They number roughly 3 percent of the general population, and represent 85 percent of all mentally retarded persons, but only 20 percent of the institutionalized retarded population.

The implications of various degrees of retardation for adaptive behavior during three age periods (preschool, school age, and adult) are summarized in Table 20-1.

Table 20-1. Adaptive Behavior Classification for Various Degrees of Mental Retardation According to Chronological Age

Degree of Retardation	Preschool Age 0 to 5 Years Maturation and Development	School Age 6 to 18 Years Training and Education	Adult 18 Years and Over Social and Vocational Adequacy
Profound IQ below 20	Gross retardation; minimal capacity for functioning in sensorimotor areas; need nursing care	Some motor development present; cannot profit from training in self-help; *totally dependent*	Some motor and speech development; totally incapable of self-maintenance; need complete care and supervision
Severe IQ 20 to 35	Poor motor development; speech is minimal; generally unable to profit from training in self-help; little or no communication skills	Can talk or learn to communicate; can be trained in elemental health habits; cannot learn functional academic skills; profit from systematic habit training (*trainable*)	Can contribute partially to self-support under complete supervision; can develop self-protection skills to a minimal useful level in controlled environment
Moderate IQ 36 to 51	Can talk or learn to communicate; poor social awareness; fair motor development; may profit from self-help; can be managed with moderate supervision	Can learn functional academic skills to approximately 4th grade level by late teens if given special education (*educable*)	Capable of self-maintenance in unskilled or semi-skilled occupations; need supervision and guidance when under mild social or economic stress
Mild IQ 52 to 67	Can develop social and communication skills; minimal retardation in sensorimotor areas; rarely distinguished from normal until later age	Can learn academic skills to approximately 6th grade level by late teens; cannot learn general high school subjects; need special education, particularly at secondary school age levels (*educable*)	Capable of social and vocational adequacy with proper education and training; frequently need supervision and guidance under serious social or economic stress

Adapted from Sloan, W., and Birch, J. W. (1955). A rationale for degrees of retardation. *American Journal of Mental Deficiency, 60*:258–264.

MILD (PHYSIOLOGICAL OR PRIMARY) VS. SEVERE (PATHOLOGICAL OR SECONDARY) RETARDATION

Mental retardation has become a matter of concern to many professional disciplines. Two major categories of mental retardation are distinguishable according to the professionals traditionally first involved: school teachers or physicians. Whether the child has an IQ above or below 50 correlates highly with a number of other significant factors including: (1) the age at which retardation becomes evident, (2) the presence or absence of gross brain pathology, (3) the probability of retardation in other close relatives, and (4) the probable need for institutional care (as well as the age and reasons for admission to institutions).

Mild Retardation

Mild retardation is about eight times as frequent as all three more severe degrees of retardation combined. These children usually look normal, and show no signs of congenital malformations or physical handicaps. They often live in underprivileged neighborhoods, and have siblings who are also mildly retarded. Such factors combine to make it unlikely that mild retardation will be recognized until after the child starts school and is identified as a slow learner. The absence of brain pathology has led to mild retardation being described in such terms as *physiological, aclinical, residual, primary, endogenous,* and *cultural-familial.*

At first it may seem paradoxical that the frequency of mental retardation among the close relatives (parents and siblings) of the *mildly* retarded is *higher* than among relatives of those with more severe degrees of retardation. It is true that some forms of the latter are known to result from conditions transmitted by simple mendelian inheritance. However, *mild retardation should be regarded as the lower end of the normal Gaussian distribution curve of intelligence in the general population.* Hence heredity and environmental factors are just as important in determining mild mental retardation as in contributing to the overall determination of intelligence (see Chap. 7). Such hereditary factors are probably *polygenic* (the cumulative effects of multiple minor genes), and have often been underestimated. In any event, they are often associated with, and compounded by, concurrent malnutrition (prenatal or postnatal) and psychosocial deprivation, both familial and cultural.

Moderate, Severe, and Profound Retardation

Moderate, severe, and profound retardation are associated with brain disease, and often with congenital malformation and physical handicaps. The more severe the retardation, the more obvious it will be to nonprofessional observers, and the greater the probability of associated physical disabilities. Hence medical advice is likely to be sought earlier than in the case of mild retardation. Such disorders as Down's syndrome, microcephaly, and hydrocephaly may be easy to identify early, but it is extremely important to recognize disorders that may not be so grossly obvious but are *treatable,* such as cretinism, phenylketonuria (PKU), galactosemia, and hypoglycemosis, in order to obtain the best possible results. *The lifelong level of adaptation may be dependent on prompt recognition and appropriate intervention.*

Most forms of severe mental retardation are environmental (including the intrauterine environment), and have also been referred to as *secondary* or *exogenous.* However, there are a large number of forms attributable to simple monogenic autosomal inheritance (each form being rare in itself). Severe retardation also results from autosomal anomalies (e.g., Down's syndrome), in contrast with mild degrees of retardation that may be associated with anomalies of the sex chromosomes. The next sections contain a summary of the *major clinical categories of mental retardation,* as published in the manual sponsored by the American Association on Mental Deficiency (1973 revision)

CLINICAL CATEGORIE

1. Infections and Intoxications

PRENATAL INFECTIONS. The four most frequent prenatal infections resulting in mental retardation are rubella, syphilis, cytomegalic inclusion disease, and toxoplasmosis.

Rubella has replaced syphilis in recent years as the most frequent cause of congenital anomalies and mental retardation associated with maternal infection. The incidence and severity of damage are directly related to the stage of pregnancy during which the infection occurs: If it occurs during the first trimester about 10 to 20 percent of infants will be affected, with the figure rising to as high as 50 percent if it occurs during the first month. The abnormalities typically involve the eyes, ears, and heart, but may also result in brain damage, sometimes with microcephaly.

Syphilis was formerly the most frequent form of maternal infection resulting in fetal abnormalities, but has declined in recent years as a result of routine serological testing of pregnant women and prompt treatment with penicillin. The onset of symptoms in the child may occur at any time from birth to adolescence, and prompt treatment may arrest the infection, with resulting near-normal intelligence or only mild retardation, rather than severe retardation and death.

Cytomegalic inclusion body disease is a viral infection that is usually mild in the mother but may produce severe brain damage in the fetus. Diagnosis is based on the finding of inclusion bodies in various tissues, or in the cellular components of urine, cerebrospinal fluid, or blood.

Toxoplasmosis results from infection by a protozoan which has a worldwide distribution among various species of animals; it is usually acquired by drinking contaminated water. Infection acquired prenatally from the mother may result in a variety of brain lesions, including hydrocephaly or microcephaly and leading to epilepsy or mental retardation.

POSTNATAL CEREBRAL INFECTION. This may result from any form of encephalitis or meningitis occurring during infancy or childhood.

INTOXICATION. It is believed that retardation may rarely be attributable to severe and prolonged *toxemia of pregnancy*. It may certainly result from other maternal intoxications such as carbon monoxide, lead, arsenic, quinine, and ergot.

Hyperbilirubinemia is often caused by Rh incompatibility between fetus and mother, but may also be caused by ABO or other incompatibilities, or any other condition producing a sufficiently high level of serum bilirubin (e.g., prematurity or severe neonatal sepsis). There may be yellow staining of basal ganglia and other brain areas *(kernicterus),* with demyelination, gliosis, and other changes, usually resulting in cerebral palsy, deafness, and mental retardation, often with choreoathetosis.

Postimmunization encephalopathy results when antitetanus serum, or vaccines such as smallpox, rabies, and typhoid, affect the peripheral nerves, or more rarely the central nervous system. There may be convulsions, stupor, coma, and motor dysfunction, followed by permanent damage resulting in behavior disorders, dyskinesias, seizure disorders, and mental retardation.

Other encephalopathies due to intoxication include permanent brain damage resulting from many toxic agents as already summarized in Chapter 11. *Lead* has been the most significant of these in causing mental retardation in young children. Sources of lead include paint, toys, lead acetate ointment, and cosmetics. Blue lines on the gums, punctate basophilic staining of red blood cells, and a lead line on bone x-rays confirm the diagnosis.

2. Trauma, Physical Agent, and Hypoxia

PRENATAL INJURY. This is probably rare, but includes prenatal irradiation, and asphyxia due to maternal hypoxia, anemia, or hypotension.

MECHANICAL INJURY AT BIRTH. Intracranial hemorhage and brain damage may result from various obstetrical complications, such as disproportion, postmaturity, malpresentation, and precipitate delivery. Brain damage may result in gross neurological disability and mental defect, or more subtle disorganizations of motor, sensory, perceptual, emotional, and integrative behavior.

PERINATAL HYPOXIA. This may be difficult to identify in humans, and impossible after the passage of time. However, guinea pigs and monkeys have been subjected to varying degrees of asphyxia at birth, which were followed by changes in neurological structure and function, including the development of epileptic seizures, and impairment of memory and learning.

POSTNATAL HYPOXIA AND INJURY. As in adults, a chronic brain syndrome may result from severe hypoxia or trauma in infancy or childhood, with prolonged unconsciousness and subsequent regression or arrest in development.

3. Metabolism or Nutrition

NEURONAL LIPID STORAGE DISEASES. *Infantile cerebral lipidosis (Tay-Sachs disease)* was formerly known as *infantile amaurotic family idiocy.* The disorder, a *ganglioside storage disease,* is inherited by a single pair of recessive genes (both parents are heterozygous carriers), and most cases are from Jewish families. It becomes evident during the first year of life, with motor weakness, blindness, and developmental regression. Retinal examination shows degeneration of the macular area, with a "cherry-red spot." Death usually occurs within 1 to 3 years. There is a specific deficiency of the enzyme hexosaminidase A.

Late infantile cerebral lipidosis (Bielschowsky-Jansky disease) is a lipofuscin storage disease, and is transmitted by a single pair of recessive genes. The onset is a little later than with Tay-Sachs disease (after the second or third year of life), and there is optic atrophy rather than the cherry-red spot in the macula. Otherwise, the course is similar, with paralysis, mental deterioration, and blindness, progressing to death in a few years.

Jansky disease) is a lipofuscin storage disease, *Vogt disease)* is also a lipofuscin storage disease, transmitted as an autosomal-recessive characteristic. The disease becomes evident between the ages of 5 and 10 years, with incoordination, paralysis, seizures, and pigmentary degeneration of the retina, leading to blindness and death within 5 to 10 years.

Late juvenile cerebral lipidosis (Kuf's disease) is another lipofuscin storage disease, inherited as an autosomal-recessive trait. It usually becomes evident between the ages of 15 and 25 years as a chronic organic brain syndrome, with progressive dementia, motor disability, and seizures. It is associated with mental retardation only when the onset occurs in childhood (earlier than usual for this disorder).

Glycolipidosis of kerasin type (Gaucher's disease) is more common in Jewish children, and is characterized by deposition of kerasin in the reticuloendothelial cells of the spleen, liver, and other organs. Diagnosis is by splenic puncture, aspiration of bone marrow, or biopsy of a lymph node which shows Gaucher cells. The nervous system is not usually involved, except in infants, in which case there is developmental regression and progression of the disease, and a fatal outcome within a few years of onset. The metabolic abnormality is due to diminished activity of glucocerebrosidase.

Glycolipidosis of phosphatide type (Niemann-Pick disease) is inherited as a simple mendelian recessive characteristic, and has its onset during infancy. There is often deafness and cerebromacular degeneration, sometimes with a cherry-red spot similar to Tay-Sachs disease. It is distinguished from the latter by deposition of lipophosphatides in the reticuloendothelial system, particularly the liver and spleen. Biopsy of spleen, bone marrow, or lymph nodes shows characteristic foam cells. It occurs predominantly in Jewish infants.

Hurler's disease (gargoylism, or lipochondrodystrophy) is another glycolipidosis with neuronal involvement. Two forms have been recognized, both of which involve recessive inheritance, one form being autosomal and the other sex-linked. (The latter is sometimes called *Hunter's syndrome.*) Both result in widespread connective tissue involvement and typical skeletal deformities. There is a large head with protruding forehead (far out of proportion to the stunted body), and mental retardation is usually severe, leading to death before adolescence.

CARBOHYDRATE DISORDERS. *Galactosemia* is a congenital error of carbohydrate metabolism, transmitted by a single pair of autosomal-recessive genes, and resulting in accumulation of galactose in the bloodstream. The infant is unable to metabolize milk, and there is usually vomiting and jaundice. There is malnutrition in spite of an insatiable appetite. Urinalysis with Benedict's reagent shows the presence of reducing substances, that may be identified as galactose by chromatography or fermentation tests. Generalized metabolic failure *will lead to death if milk is not removed from the diet.* Delay in recognition and treatment may also result in irreversible mental retardation, associated with cataracts and cirrhosis of the liver. Either of two different enzyme deficiencies may produce this disorder.

Glycogenosis (von Gierke's disease) is another inborn error of carbohydrate metabolism transmitted by autosomal-recessive inheritance. There is a deficiency in any one of several glycogen-metabolizing enzymes, and deposition of glycogen in various organs including the brain.

Hypoglycemia may result from a variety of conditions and lead to mental retardation associated with epileptic seizures. There is a familial variety transmitted by autosomal-recessive inheritance, characterized by a deficiency of alpha cells in the pancreas. Diagnosis may be confirmed by glucose tolerance tests, and *early recognition and treatment are essential if permanent mental retardation is to be prevented.*

AMINO ACID DISORDERS. *Phenylketonuria (PKU)* is a metabolic disorder, inherited by a single pair of autosomal recessive genes, preventing the normal conversion of dietary phenylalanine into tyrosine by absence of the enzyme phenylalanine hydroxylase. Phenylalanine accumulates and is metabolized into phenylpyruvic acid, which gives a musty odor to the urine, and results in a vivid green color on adding ferric chloride solution. Affected children are often blond and blue-eyed, with a history of eczema and dermatitis. Parents are heterozygous carriers, having moderate elevation of phenylalanine in the blood, but no adverse effects. *The mental retardation associated with PKU may be greatly reduced in severity or prevented altogether through early diagnosis and intervention* with a diet low in phenylalanine.

There are many rare disorders involving other amino acids, including tyrosine, methionine, cystine, tryptophan, valine, leucine, and isoleucine.

MINERAL DISORDERS. *Wilson's disease (hepatolenticular degeneration)* is inherited as a simple recessive trait. There is an inability of ceruloplasmin to bind copper, which shows a decreased level in the bloodstream, and an increased concentration in liver, brain, and other organs. The basal ganglia are particularly affected, and there is a nodular cirrhosis of the liver. Most patients eventually develop a Kayser-Fleischer ring of greenish-brown pigment, deposited in the cornea adjoining the sclera (seen on slit lamp examination). There are two forms of this disorder (inherited separately), one with onset in childhood (between the ages of 7 and 15 years and resulting in mental retardation) and the other in adulthood (producing a chronic brain syndrome).

ENDOCRINE DISORDERS. *Hypothyroidism (cretinism)* causes generalized reduction in growth and metabolism. The body length is reduced, and the appearance is puffy and dull, with cold, dry skin. Lips are thick, and the tongue protrudes. Apathy is frequent, and there is often constipation, slow pulse, and generalized neurological deficits (ataxia, hyporeflexia, rigidity, and tremors). There is usually hypochromic anemia, with elevation of blood cholesterol, accompanied by reduced protein-bound iodine, and reduced radioactive iodine uptake. *Early diagnosis and treatment are essential to reduce permanent retardation and attain maximum intellectual function.*

NUTRITIONAL DISORDERS. Mental retardation may result from dietary deficiencies of various essential nutrients, particularly protein and members of the vitamin B complex. Nutritional disorders also result from idiosyncratic diets, metabolic disorders, parasitism, debilitating disease, excessive intake of vitamins, and various feeding problems. This form of mental retardation is relatively frequent at the lowest socioeconomic levels and in underdeveloped countries.

4. Gross Brain Disease (Postnatal)

NEUROCUTANEOUS DYSPLASIA. *Neurofibromatosis (von Recklinghausen's disease)* is inherited by an autosomal-dominant gene, with reduced penetrance and variable expressivity. The usual manifestations include pigmentation of the skin (café au lait patches), with fibromatous tumors of the skin, peripheral nerves, and central nervous system. There are often epileptic seizures, and variable intelligence, from normal to severely retarded.

Trigeminal cerebral angiomatosis (Sturge-Weber-Dimitri's disease) involves a port wine stain, or angioma, on the skin of the face, usually in the area supplied by the trigeminal nerve. There is a corresponding vascular malformation over the meninges of the parietal and occipital lobes. There is variable neurological involvement, which may include epilepsy or mental retardation.

Tuberous sclerosis (epiloia or *Bourneville's disease)* is transmitted by a dominant autosomal gene with reduced penetrance. There are multiple gliotic nodules in the central nervous system, and adenoma sebaceum of the face, with tumors of other organs. There are variable neurological signs, epileptic seizures, and mental retardation.

CEREBRAL WHITE MATTER, DEGENERATIVE. There are a group of similar conditions, characterized by diffuse demyelination of the white matter of the brain, and associated sclerosis of the glia. They are often familial, and mental deterioration is associated with a variety of neurological deficits, with frequent convulsive seizures. The most common forms are as follows:

1. *Sudanophilic leukodystrophy.*
2. *Sudanophilic leukodystrophy of Pelizaeus-Merzbacher type* (aplasia axialis extracorticalis congenita).
3. *Progressive subcortical encephalopathy* (encephalitis periaxialis diffusa, Schilder's disease).
4. *Spinocerebellar ataxia* (Friedreich's ataxia)

involves cerebellar degeneration, with onset between the ages of 2 and 15 years, accompanied by variable dementia (or mental retardation when the onset is early).

5. Unknown Prenatal Influence

CEREBRAL MALFORMATIONS. *Anencephaly* and *hemianencephaly* are among the most common congenital brain malformations, invariably resulting in death at birth or shortly thereafter due to absence of one or both cerebral hemispheres or even greater portions of the central nervous system.

Malformations of gyri include agyria, macrogyria, and microgyria. The latter is a relatively common pathological finding in the severely mentally retarded.

Congenital *porencephaly* is characterized by large funnel-shaped cavities occurring anywhere in the cerebral hemispheres.

CRANIOFACIAL ANOMALIES. *Primary microcephaly* is transmitted by a single pair of autosomal-recessive genes, and invariably associated with moderate to severe retardation. Microcephaly may also be *secondary* to exogenous lesions, resulting from infections, trauma, or asphyxia. The term is reserved for adults with a head circumference of 17 inches or less; or children with a head circumference of less than 13 inches at 6 months, 14 inches at 1 year, or 15 inches at 2 years.

Macrocephaly (megalencephaly) is a rare condition involving increased size and weight of the brain, due partly to a proliferative type of gliosis.

Craniostenosis involves an unusually shaped skull, which is sometimes genetically transmitted and sometimes, but not invariably, associated with mental retardation. The two most common forms consist of *acrocephaly* (oxycephaly) or steeple-shaped skull; and *scaphocephaly* or boat-shaped skull.

Laurence-Moon-Biedl syndrome is transmitted as a simple mendelian recessive characteristic that is usually autosomal but may sometimes be sex-linked. The four cardinal features of the syndrome are retinitis pigmentosa, adiposogenital dystrophy, polydactyly, and mental retardation.

Congenital hydrocephalus consists of an increased volume of cerebrospinal fluid within the skull. When there is increased volume *without increased pressure,* it is merely compensatory to atrophy or hypoplasia. When there is an *increase in pressure,* it is due to disturbance in absorption, formation, or circulation of the cerebrospinal fluid. Obstruction is much more frequent than failure of the absorption mechanism. There is great variation in accompanying neurological impairment and mental retardation.

6. Chromosomal Abnormality

SHORT ARM DELETION OF CHROMOSOME 5 *(Cri du chat).* This is a rare disorder, resulting from absence of part of the fifth chromosome. Affected children are severely retarded, show multiple congenital abnormalities, and utter a characteristic catlike cry during infancy. The latter is due to laryngeal abnormalities that diminish with increasing age so that the cry disappears.

DOWN'S SYNDROME (MONGOLISM). This is the most frequent of all the clinical or pathological types of moderate and severe mental retardation. By far the majority of patients with mongolism have trisomy of chromosome 21 in group G, which results in a total of 47 chromosomes. A small proportion of cases have been attributed to mosaicism or to translocation. Down's syndrome is the only common form of mental retardation due to autosomal abnormality (since other forms are relatively rare or lethal). Mongoloids are often the lastborn offspring of older mothers, and the risk of having such an offspring is roughly 100 times as great for mothers past the age of 45 years as for mothers under the age of 20. Mongoloids have characteristic facial features, palms, and fingerprints. The two main creases running transversely across the palm may be replaced in mongoloids by a single crease (simian line). Fingerprints are characterized by L-shaped loops instead of the usual whorls. As in other forms of severe mental retardation, there is a tendency for the patient to be sterile. However, the few mongoloid mothers that reproduce

give birth to about 50 percent normal and 50 percent mongoloid children (due to transmission of the entire extra chromosome).

X AND Y CHROMOSOME ABNORMALITIES. These disorders tend to be associated with *mild* mental retardation, or sometimes with normal intelligence. The only disorder in this category that occurs with any significant frequency is Klinefelter's syndrome. The usual karyotype is XXY, and the condition appears about once in 800 male births. There are small, atrophic testes, usually accompanied by sterility and by gynecomastia after puberty. Such patients constitute roughly 1 percent of all mentally retarded males in institutions.

7. Gestational Disorders

PREMATURITY. This is a residual category for retarded patients who had a birth weight of less than 2,500 gm (5.5 lbs) or a gestational age of less than 38 weeks at birth, and who do not fall into any of the preceding categories. However, premature birth exposes the infant to an increased risk of brain damage from mechanical trauma and asphyxia, with vulnerability to neuropsychiatric abnormality increasing progressively as the birth weight of the infant decreases. Among infants with a birth weight of less than 1,500 gm, roughly 50 percent have a neurological or intellectual defect, and some of these also have a major visual handicap.

8. Retardation Following Psychiatric Disorder

Childhood schizophrenia leads to cognitive impairment and may result in failure of language development and other signs of mental retardation. However, childhood schizophrenia has been divided into two groups, according to the presence or absence of recognizable organic brain disease. This diagnostic category does *not* include psychoses associated with known brain disease, but only those cases of mental retardation secondary to major psychiatric disorder in early childhood.

9. Environmental Influences

This is a large category encompassing the many

cases of mental retardation that have no clinical or historical evidence of organic pathology. Logically, it should include most persons with mild retardation (IQ 52 through 67), which has also been known as primary, physiological, aclinical, or residual mental retardation. However, the category was narrowed by including only those persons in whom there is a positive family history of mental retardation, or reduction in environmental stimulation due to sensory impairment. The group was therefore subdivided, according to the presence of one of these two sets of factors:

PSYCHOSOCIAL DISADVANTAGE (CULTURAL-FAMILIAL MENTAL RETARDATION). This category should logically include a very large number of the mildly retarded, who constitute the lower end of the normal curve for distribution of intelligence in the general population. However, the definition specifies that evidence of retardation must be found in at least one of the parents and in one or more siblings, "presumably because some degree of cultural deprivation results from familial retardation." In fact, mental retardation among other family members is an empirical finding for which there may be various explanations, including similar heredity, inadequate nutrition during prenatal or early postnatal development, other similar biological stress or deprivation, adverse learning, or similar socioeconomic and cultural deprivation.

SENSORY DEPRIVATION. Mental retardation may also result from deprivation of normal environmental stimulation in infancy and early childhood. This may result from severe sensory impairment such as blindness and deafness, and may be more severe than cultural-familial retardation.

EDUCATION, TRAINING, AND TREATMENT
Early recognition and diagnosis of various forms of potentially severe mental retardation will permit specific and effective intervention that may need to be continued throughout the person's lifetime. Such treatment may: (1) be life-saving; (2) prevent much more severe retardation than would otherwise result; and (3) sometimes enable the person

to attain a normal level of intellectual and social functioning.

Appropriate antibiotic therapy may prevent many of the unpleasant effects of congenital syphilis, or of postnatal meningitis. Several inborn errors of metabolism may be minimized by changing the diet. Thus phenylketonuria (PKU) requires a diet free of phenylalanine, whereas galactosemia requires a diet free from milk. Other metabolic disorders requiring prompt intervention include both hypoglycemia and hypothyroidism (cretinism).

The administration of anticonvulsant medication is an important factor in minimizing mental retardation associated with epileptic seizures. Similarly, the potentialities of partially paralyzed, mentally retarded persons can often be increased by active physiotherapy. Numerous nonspecific forms of medical treatment have been applied in unsuccessful attempts to increase intellectual function. These include the administration of vitamins, hormones, and brain stimulants.

Other psychiatric disorders of all types may occur in conjunction with mental retardation. Unfortunately, recognition of functional symptoms in the severely retarded may be hampered by a tendency to attribute all behavioral deviations to the known organic pathology. Such errors may deprive a patient of effective treatment for the only aspect of his condition that will improve significantly. Although a brain-damaged patient may have increased vulnerability to drug side effects, judicious use of psychotropic medications may provide considerable benefit.

Mental retardation due to deafness or blindness may be overcome by appropriate training. Retardation due to emotional deprivation is at least partly reversible when prompt action is taken to provide adequate parental care and educational opportunities.

Socialization programs differ according to the degree of retardation and age of the person. In the mildly retarded, socialization involves two distinct problems, namely scholastic inefficiency and social ineptitude. The scholastic problem is a matter of teaching basic and relevant content in an interesting manner that maintains motivation, together with training in speech, manual and occupational skills, and the development of vocational interests. The problem of attempting to overcome the patient's social ineptitude requires guidance and reeducation, with application of group techniques of psychotherapy as indicated. Techniques of behavior therapy have found wide application in all aspects of training of the mentally retarded.

REVIEW QUESTIONS

256. Severely retarded persons (IQ less than 52) are *more likely* than mildly retarded persons (IQ 52 to 67) to have:
    (A) a mentally retarded parent
    (B) mentally retarded siblings
    (C) retardation attributable to transmission by a simple mendelian mechanism
    (D) all of the above
    (E) none of the above

257. Phenylketonuria:
    (A) is due to a single pair of autosomal-recessive genes
    (B) occurs only in the offspring of two parents who metabolize phenylalanine abnormally
    (C) is amenable to treatment
    (D) all of the above
    (E) none of the above

258. The major cause of mental retardation and congenital malformation resulting from maternal infection is:
    (A) syphilis
    (B) toxoplasmosis
    (C) rubella
    (D) hepatitis
    (E) influenza

259. Jewish infants of Eastern European extraction have greater than average predisposition for:
    (A) Tay-Sachs disease
    (B) cri-du-chat syndrome
    (C) Turner's syndrome
    (D) phenylketonuria (PKU)
    (E) tuberous sclerosis

260. Patients exhibiting "sociocultural" retardation:
    (A) come from well-to-do families about as often as they come from impoverished families
    (B) typically have IQ scores below 50
    (C) adapt reasonably well to situations other than school
    (D) usually have average vocabulary
    (E) are usually retarded as a result of genetic transmission

Summary of Directions

A	B	C	D	E
1, 2, 3 only	1, 3 only	2, 4 only	4 only	All are correct

261. Conditions more likely to be associated with severe mental retardation than with mild retardation include:
    (1) chromosomal anomaly
    (2) gross brain pathology
    (3) physical deformities
    (4) mental retardation in siblings

262. Clinical findings in patients with Down's syndrome usually include:
    (1) dry, pale, coarse skin
    (2) IQ less than 50
    (3) delay in ossification
    (4) single palmar (simian) crease

263. Inherited disorders of fat metabolism which produce mental retardation include:
    (1) Tay-Sachs disease
    (2) Gaucher's disease
    (3) Niemann-Pick disease
    (4) Wilson's disease

264. Physical findings often associated with a diagnosis of phenylketonuria include:
    (1) musty odor to urine
    (2) dermatitis
    (3) blond hair
    (4) hydrocephalus

265. Which of the following are associated with tuberous sclerosis (Bourneville's disease)?
    (1) brain glioma
    (2) adenoma sebaceum of the face
    (3) pulmonary and renal cysts
    (4) short stature, webbed neck

266. Which of the following are true of neuro-

fibromatosis (von Recklinghausen's disease)?
(1) café au lait spots and skin polyps frequently found
(2) may have normal intelligence
(3) may have optic and acoustic gliomata
(4) inherited as a recessive autosomal trait

267. Incidence of mental retardation would be reduced by:
(1) rubella immunization
(2) genetic counseling
(3) prenatal care programs
(4) postnatal pediatric care

268. Most cases of mental retardation:
(1) can be ascribed to monogenic inheritance
(2) result from birth trauma, infection, or inborn errors of metabolism
(3) require institutional care
(4) are either idiopathic or associated with psychosocial deprivation

269. The frequency with which mental retardation is diagnosed:
(1) is higher in males than in females
(2) is highest during school age
(3) depends on social class
(4) does not vary between urban, suburban, and rural areas

270. Both genetic and environmental factors lead to the development of mental deficiency in:
(1) Down's syndrome
(2) galactosemia
(3) Klinefelter's syndrome
(4) phenylketonuria

SELECTED REFERENCES

1. Adams, M. (1971). *Mental Retardation and Its Social Dimensions.* New York: Columbia University Press.

2. American Medical Association (1974). *Mental Retardation: A Handbook for the Primary Physician* (2nd ed.). Chicago: American Medical Association. No. OP-314.

3. American Association on Mental Deficiency (1973). *Manual on Terminology and Classification in Mental Retardation* (1973 revision). New York: American Association on Mental Deficiency. Special Publication No. 2.

4. Birch, H.G., Richardson, S.A., Baird, D., et al. (1970). *Mental Subnormality in the Community: A Clinical and Epidemiologic Study.* Baltimore: Williams & Wilkins Co.

5. Carter, C.H. (1971). *Handbook of Mental Retardation Syndromes* (2nd ed.). Springfield, Illinois: Charles C Thomas.

6. Heber, R.F. (1970). *Epidemiology of Mental Retardation.* Springfield, Illinois: Charles C Thomas.

7. Holmes, L.B., et al (1972). *Mental Retardation: An Atlas of Diseases with Associated Physical Abnormalities.* New York: Macmillan Co.

8. Kindred, M., et al [Eds.] (1976). *The Mentally Retarded Citizen and the Law.* New York: The Free Press, Division of Macmillan Co.

9. Knobloch, H., Rider, R., Harper, P., and Pasamanick, B. (1956). Neuropsychiatric sequelae of prematurity. *Journal of the American Medical Association,* vol. 161, pages 581–585.

10. Kolb, L.C., Masland, R.L., and Cooke, R.E. [Eds.] (1962). *Mental Retardation.* Baltimore: Williams & Wilkins Co. (Research Publications for the Association for Research in Nervous and Mental Disease, vol. 39.)

11. Masland, R.L., Sarason, S.B., and Gladwin, T. (1958). *Mental Subnormality: Biological, Psychological, and Cultural Factors.* New York: Basic Books.

12. Penrose, L.S. (1973). *The Biology of Mental Defect* (3rd ed.). New York: Grune & Stratton.

13. Sloan, W., and Birch, J.W. (1955). A rationale for degrees of retardation. *American Journal of Mental Deficiency,* vol. 60, pages 258–264.

14. Stevens, H.A., and Heber, R. [Eds.] (1964). *Mental Retardation: Review of Research.* Chicago: University of Chicago Press.

15. Tredgold, A.S., and Soddy, K. (1963). *A Textbook of Mental Deficiency* (10th ed.). Baltimore: Williams & Wilkins Co.

16. Woollam, B.H., and Millen, J.W. (1956). Role of vitamins in embryonic development. *British Medical Journal,* vol. 1, pages 1262–65.

Answers and Comments to Review Questions

CHAPTER 1 (pp. 12–14)

1. **D** The correct answer is *sublimation*, which is the unconscious diversion of unacceptable instinctual drives (sexual or aggressive) into personally and socially acceptable channels (p. 10).

2. **A** *Repression* is usually regarded as a common denominator or prerequisite for all unconscious defense mechanisms, which may lead to the formation of neurotic symptoms (p. 8).

3. **C** The correct answer is *identification*, the unconscious patterning of oneself after another person (p. 9). It should be contrasted with *imitation*, which is a conscious process.

4. **B** *Object relations* are defined as "emotional attachments between one person and others, as opposed to the feelings that one has for oneself." They are not present at birth, but first appear during the oral phase as the infant becomes aware of his dependency on another person (the mother figure).

5. **A** The answer is *aggression* (p. 5). Freud's final formulation contrasted sexual instincts (corresponding with libido or *Eros* and serving the pleasure-pain principle) with aggressive drives (corresponding with *Thanatos* and serving the repetition-compulsion principle).

6. **E** Freud's model of paranoia was derived from his study of an autobiography by a famous jurist named Schreber, who described the development of an elaborate system of paranoid delusions. The interpretation may be summarized as follows: The psychosexual development of the paranoid patient is fixated at the oedipal (phallic) phase, resulting in *unconscious homosexual feelings.* Because it is con-sciously unacceptable, the patient's feeling "I love him" is strongly *repressed;* by the mechanism of *denial* it is transformed into "I do not love him; I hate him." The latter is equally unacceptable, and is therefore *projected* as "He hates me," and eventually reemerges into consciousness in the elaborated form of "I am persecuted by him." Freud had few clinical experiences with paranoid patients and in fact never met Schreber. Subsequent analytic interpretations have deemphasized latent homosexuality, but have continued to view projection as the defense mechanism most directly involved in paranoid delusions.

7. **E** The unrelated process is *isolation*, which is the separation of an idea from its related affect (p. 11). The superego results from *internalization* of the ethical standards of society, and develops by *identification* with parents and significant others. The latter includes the more primitive processes of *introjection* and *incorporation* (p. 9). In certain circumstances (e.g., deviant subcultures) this process may produce an adequate and functional superego which nevertheless is in conflict with the standards of the larger society.

8. **D** The most likely answer is *rationalization* (p. 9).

9. **E** The best answer is *nocturnal dreaming* (p. 7).

10. **E** This concept is defined on p. 4. The other alternatives refer to: (A) *transference;* (B) *countertransference;* (C) *resistance;* and (D) *regression.* See pp. 10–11.

11. **B** The *ego* is the executive part of the personality. The first four alternatives refer to structural theory (p. 7), whereas the preconscious is a concept from Freud's earlier topographic theory (p. 7).

12. **D** *Transference* is one of the basic concepts of psychotherapy (pp. 5 and 10).

13. **E** Sudden and unexpected bereavement may

result in intense feelings of frustration and anger. It is difficult to be angry at the deceased and unacceptable to be angry at God. The man described has *displaced* his emotions onto a more acceptable substitute, the intern (p. 10).

14. A The answer is *suppression,* which is a *conscious* decision to control and postpone dealing with feelings (p. 8). This man is not described as redirecting an instinctual drive (*sublimation,* p. 10), as disavowing his grief (*denial,* p. 8), as replacing grief with euphoria (*reaction formation,* p. 8), nor as seeking out feared situations (*counterphobic behavior,* p. 9). The latter processes involve unconscious efforts and are therefore full-fledged defense mechanisms.

15. A Secondary process thinking is a function of the *ego,* whereas primary process thinking and all other items listed are associated with the id (p. 7).

16. A Nonverbal communication is universal throughout life and in all cultures. Exchange of nonverbal messages does not usually involve conscious awareness on the part of either sender or receiver (p. 12).

17. B Defense mechanisms of the ego against anxiety are automatic, unconscious (by definition), and universal (pp. 7–8).

18. A Anal characteristics dating from the first to third years of life include the triad of stubborness, excessive neatness, and parsimony, or stinginess (p. 6). These are generally considered a subset of obsessive-compulsive personality traits, which also include rigidity, perfectionism, indecisiveness, overconscientiousness, and over-inhibition. Low tolerance for frustration is a nonspecific finding in many forms of psychiatric disorder and is not associated with any specific phase of psychosexual development.

19. B Choices (1) and (3) are correct (p. 10). Paranoid ideation is based on *projection*

(p. 9); compulsive rituals involve the mechanism of *undoing* (p. 11).

20. E All choices are correct. Psychoses are viewed as narcissistic regression and disruption of relationships with other persons (object relations). Psychotic conflicts are external (environmental) whereas neurotic conflicts are internal (intrapsychic).

CHAPTER 2 (pp. 25–27)

21. D The answer is *perseveration* (p. 17). *Echolalia* involves parrotlike repetition of another's utterances (p. 21); *coprolalia* is the persistent use of vulgar, obscene, or "dirty" words, and is often seen in Gilles de la Tourette's syndrome; *coprophilia* is a morbid, excessive preoccupation with filth or feces. The term *fixation* is a psychoanalytic concept referring to arrest in psychosexual development (p. 6).

22. A This is most likely to be an *illusion,* which is a distorted perception of a real external sensory stimulus; a *hallucination* is a perception without external basis (p. 16). *Delusions* are disorders of thought rather than perception (p. 18). *Fausse reconnaissance* is a form of paramnesia in which the patient subjectively feels certain that he is correctly recalling something that is patently inaccurate. *Agnosia* is a loss of ability to correctly interpret certain sensory stimuli and the significance of related memory impressions; it is associated with organic brain syndromes, and sometimes with chronic schizophrenia or hysterical disorders.

23. B The most specific answer is *delusion of reference,* since this is a fixed false *belief* involving misinterpretation of others' motives (resulting from the mechanism of projection); see p. 18. Distortion of perception (hallucination or illusion) does not appear likely. *Xenophobia* is a seldom used term meaning morbid, illogical fear of strangers.

24. C A *delusion of influence* is a fixed irra-

tional belief that one is being controlled by an external agent (p. 18).

25. E The best answer is *formication,* a form of haptic hallucination in which the patient feels insects crawling on or under the skin (p. 16). Somatic delusions may or may not be present but the situation described clearly involves sensory perception of non-existent external stimuli. *Micropsia* involves seeing real external visual stimuli reduced in size (p. 16). *Akathisia* is a form of involuntary motor restlessness which occurs as an extrapyramidal side effect of neuroleptic drugs (pp. 107–108).

26. B The phenomenon described is *depersonalization* and is seen in a variety of syndromes, including hysteria, schizophrenia, and epileptic auras. A similar symptom is *derealization* (loss of the sense of reality concerning one's situation or surroundings).

27. B The literal meaning of the term is "beautiful indifference." This is seen in patients with conversion hysteria, who often show an inappropriate lack of concern about their disabilities. It is not synonymous with *shallowness* or *flatness* of affect, which refers to diminution or absence of reactivity in all external feeling tone; the latter is characteristic of chronic schizophrenia and some organic brain syndromes (p. 20).

28. A *Anaclitic depression* is an acute, severe impairment of an infant's physical, social, and intellectual development that sometimes occurs following sudden deprivation of the mother figure. It may lead to a state called *marasmus,* in which the infant stops eating, wastes away, and dies.

29. B The symptom described is *flight of ideas;* by contrast, pressure of speech is continuous, compulsive speech that is difficult to interrupt (p. 17). The two symptoms often occur together in manic or hypomanic states. *Bulimia* refers to compulsive gorging with food.

30. A The key word is *functional,* which means "abnormal function that is not attributable to changes in metabolism or structure." This rules out choices B, C, and D. Functional amnesia is a major form of *dissociative* reaction (p. 11).

31. E The major classification is based on severity of impairment (i.e., estimated IQ). Subclassification is based on a combination of etiology and pathology (p. 21).

32. D Delusions are pathognomonic of psychosis, and therefore rule out a primary diagnosis of personality disorder (deeply ingrained maladaptive pattern of behavior which impairs adjustment to the vicissitudes of life, but does *not* involve neurotic symptoms caused by anxiety nor psychotic distortions of reality). Organic brain syndromes may or may not involve delusions or other evidence of psychosis.

33. C The correct answer is C. Blocking (also called *thought deprivation*) occurs occasionally in normal experience, but is also seen in a variety of mental disorders, and most often in schizophrenia (p. 17).

34. E The patient is not coining new words (neologisms) but rather changing his sequence of thought on the basis of the sounds of words as he speaks them (p. 17).

35. E Delusions of reference are paranoid rather than depressive delusions (p. 18). However, depression may have associated paranoid ideation in some psychoses, (e.g., schizoaffective, involutional, or organic).

36. A Disturbances of affect may involve: (a) tone or prevailing mood (euphoria, depression, fear, rage, etc.), or (b) reactivity or responsivity (apathy or lability).

37. B Mental retardation implies arrest in intellectual development. *Dementia* consists of irreversible deterioration in previously developed intellectual function, resulting from permanently altered brain structure or metabolism. *Dementia praecox* is an obsolete term referring to schizophrenia.

38. C   *Magical thinking* is the belief that thinking something is the same as doing it, and ignores logical relationships between cause and effect. It is frequent in childhood, in dreams, in primitive cultures, and in certain mental disorders — particularly psychoses and obsessive-compulsive neurosis (p. 17).

CHAPTER 3 (pp. 40–41)

39. E   Loss of health due to parkinsonism or other progressive disease usually leads to various combinations of denial, depression, and anger. A physician is negligent if he fails to evaluate the potential for suicide in any depressed patient. Following direct discussion there will be a basis for deciding about referral to a psychiatrist and/or admission to hospital.

40. C   The best response is C, which encourages the patient to elaborate and clarify the basis for her hostility. A represents premature interpretation; B involves inappropriate and gratuitous reassurance; D may be perceived by the patient as hostile and judgmental; E represents rejection.

41. E   The best answer is E. A is premature and probably inappropriate reassurance, B is an unwarranted attack that invites defensiveness, and C is a weak, premature, and impractical attempt to solve the problem. Answer D is nonempathetic, judgmental, and destructive of rapport.

42. E   The major advantages of hospitalization for this patient, who is currently psychotic (regressed and autistic), include: (1) constant observation and protection from physical harm; (2) attention to food and fluid intake; (3) withholding of any drug he may have been abusing; (4) ensured regular dosage with antipsychotic medication and observation for side effects; and (5) potential reduction of alienation from friends, which may result from excessive demands on their time, energy, and good will.

43. D   The physical safety of patients (including this patient) and staff overrides all other considerations, and the physician must not endanger others in order to avoid being viewed as a "bad guy." Every effort should be made to get the patient's cooperation in surrendering the knife, but all alternatives except D involve unacceptable risks. In addition, E involves deceit, which would probably be discovered and damage the physician-patient relationship more than honest confrontation.

CHAPTER 4 (pp. 49–50)

44. B   The WAIS includes several verbal and several performance subtests which measure *current* intellectual function and which may be impaired to different degrees (i.e., selectively) by organic brain syndromes or other severe psychopathology (pp. 44–45).

45. E   The term *reliability* refers to consistency of results, while *validity* is concerned with whether the test really measures what it is intended or claimed to measure (p. 43).

46. A   Administration and scoring of the MMPI require less training than does interpretation. The validity of the test may be reduced by various factors, including poor motivation (e.g., minimizing or exaggerating symptoms). It provides most relevant data on current mental status rather than unconscious dynamics, and is better able to discriminate among various functional syndromes than to differentiate functional from organic (pp. 47–49).

47. A   The MMPI is not useful for young children, since reading and general language ability of at least sixth grade level are necessary. The DAP and CAT are frequently used in formal psychological evaluations of preadolescents; the DAP, modelling clay, and finger painting can be used in clinical situations where less formal evaluation will suffice. Each of these latter four tests can be considered a projective technique (pp. 45–47).

48. B The formula relating IQ with mental age (MA) and chronological age (CA) is given on p. 44. However, a value of 16 should be used for CA whenever the person in question is age 16 or older. Thus, an MA of about 4 years corresponds to an IQ of 25 for all persons past age 16.

49. C The concept of mental age is not applied when chronological age exceeds 16 and IQ exceeds 100. Instead the *percentile rank* may be used to interpret IQ scores, as described on p. 44. Whether this woman's intellectual functioning was impaired at the time this IQ score was obtained cannot be determined without additional data.

50. C The distribution of IQ scores approximates the normal curve, with mean = 100 and standard deviation = 16. Thus 50% of the population will be within about 2/3 of one standard deviation unit of the mean (i.e., between 90 and 110).

51. E Denial of psychopathology may produce elevations on the L and K scales, but the F scale is likely to be low. Each of the other conditions listed might produce a higher than average tendency to endorse items such as "Evil spirits possess me at times," which are scored on the F scale. See p. 47.

52. A The Shipley-Hartford Test compares vocabulary (verbal) with abstract thinking, and permits a numerical estimate of IQ (useful range, 75 to 125). There is selective impairment of abstract thinking in many patients with organic brain syndromes, but this is also associated with severe functional disorders (pp. 44–45).

53. C The Bender-Gestalt Test does not measure verbal or abstract thinking, but rather perceptuomotor performance. Certain characteristic patterns of defects in the latter are more likely to be associated with organic brain syndromes than with functional disorders. A numerical estimate of IQ is not provided. A secondary use of the test is as a projective technique, particularly in children (p. 45).

54. E Each of the factors is important. Excessive anxiety may impair performance, but moderate anxiety may enhance motivation and result in better performance than if anxiety were completely absent.

55. C Projective tests are discussed beginning on p. 45.

CHAPTERS 5 and 6 (pp. 74–76)

56. D The therapist would probably conclude that the patient is avoiding therapy (consciously or unconsciously). See p. 66.

57. A Necessary prerequisites to any therapy that will be successful in changing psychosexual orientation include relatively young age and motivation for change. The latter cannot be assessed while this patient is depressed. No single form of therapy has established success in changing psychosexual orientation (in contrast with associated anxiety, depression, or other emotional problems).

58. D In contrast with symptomatic relief (by suggestion, behavior therapy, or other techniques), psychoanalytic treatment seeks to eliminate or diminish the undesirable effects of unconscious conflicts (p. 65). This is more likely to be beneficial in neurotic disorders than in psychoses or personality disorders (p. 66). Prolonged and expensive treatment is inappropriate for the acute situational reaction, which generally responds promptly to other measures.

59. B Although aspects of all types of psychotherapy can be included in treating chronic ambulatory schizophrenia, the basic approach is long-term (not brief) *supportive psychotherapy* (pp. 67–68).

60. A Desensitization is one of the three main forms of behavior modification (behavior therapy) based on *learning theory*. It involves gradual systematic reduction of excessive (overlearned) avoidance re-

sponses. The other two major forms of behavior therapy are listed among the (incorrect) alternatives, namely, positive reinforcement (which involves shaping by successive approximations) and conditioned avoidance (which involves punishment of maladaptive behavior). See pp. 68–70.

61. A Occurrence of the behavior under conditions of nonreinforcement is necessary and sufficient for the extinction of a learned response, although there are many variables that affect the speed at which extinction occurs. Following a rest period there is often a "spontaneous recovery" of the response (at less than previous strength), so it is believed that total unlearning does not occur (p. 54).

62. D Punishment accompanied by a reward is likely to produce *conflict* rather than adaptive behavior. The other aspects of effective punishment are discussed on p. 57.

63. C Unconditional positive regard is one of the three principles of client-centered therapy (p. 68). The four forms of behavior therapy listed are discussed on pp. 68–70.

64. D See p. 67.

65. A A *negative reinforcer* is one that is undesirable (noxious or aversive), so that responses associated with its termination are strengthened. The latter situation is what is meant by *negative reinforcement* (p. 55). Choices B and C refer to punishment, and D would be described as nonreinforcement (which leads to extinction).

66. A Interpretation of transference and resistance continues to be a major tool of psychotherapies based on classical psychoanalysis. The first three alternatives are usually cited as discriminators between these methods (pp. 66–67).

67. A Certain patients are better able to accept interpretations of reality from peers in therapy groups than from authority figures in individual psychotherapy. This is particularly true of adolescents, delinquents, and those who tend to project unacceptable motives onto others. Group therapy is also indicated for those whose problems involve relationships with peers, although it will usually result in an initial increase in anxiety or disturbed behavior (p. 70).

68. A The various ways in which the patient-therapist relationship is used in the first three types of therapy listed are discussed in the corresponding sections of Chapter 6.

CHAPTER 7 (pp. 85–86)

69. B A healthy adult would normally have his first REM period about 90 minutes after falling asleep, whereas sleep onset REM is a common finding in *narcoleptics* (p. 84), and in patients who have recently *discontinued* regular use of REM- suppressing drugs. Barbiturates suppress REM sleep (p. 83), and REM sleep disorders have not been associated with nocturnal enuresis.

70. D Studies of pavor nocturnus have associated this phenomenon with *stages 3 and 4 of non-REM sleep* (p. 83).

71. D Dream reports are more frequent if the subject is awakened during REM sleep, but the notion that all dreaming occurs during the REM stage is no longer tenable (p. 82).

72. A Harley-Mason postulated a faulty metabolic pathway in the central nervous system as the cause of schizophrenia (the *transmethylation hypothesis*), which led to speculation that massive doses of nicotinic acid or multivitamins could be used to correct the metabolic error. Although anecdotal reports of dramatic cures persist, a number of extensive studies failed to show any benefit from this therapy except in the cases of patients who were clearly vitamin deficient, and a few studies found vitamin therapy inferior to use of a placebo. Nevertheless, the issue

is still debated in the literature, notably by Nobel laureate Linus Pauling and other advocates of an "orthomolecular" approach to psychiatric disorder. The drift hypothesis is discussed in Chapter 9, and the catecholamine hypothesis (of *affective disorders*) in Chapter 14.

73. C The division of an average night of sleep among the five stages listed is approximately as follows: 20% to 25% in REM sleep; 5% to 10% in stage 1; 50% in stage 2; and 20% divided between stages 3 and 4.

74. E LSD produces an *increase* in REM sleep (p. 83).

75. B The Klinefelter karyotype is XXY. The subject is anatomically male; some degree of mental retardation is frequent but not invariable (p. 80).

76. E The patient is anatomically female, although the genitals are infantile and the gonads are reduced to connective tissue streaks. One X chromosome is missing from some or all cells, resulting in a total count of 45. Mental retardation is sometimes found (p. 80).

77. D Huntington's chorea is the classic example of a trait transmitted by a single dominant gene with complete penetrance and little variation in expressivity (p. 77). It is therefore frequently used as an illustration of family pedigree studies.

78. E PKU is transmitted by a single pair of *recessive* genes (p. 77). The parents of affected individuals are usually heterozygous carriers and may themselves have diminished capacity to metabolize phenylalanine (since the gene is not *completely* recessive). Early detection and prompt therapeutic intervention (dietary modification) can prevent brain damage and resulting mental retardation.

79. C The "supermale" has XYY sex chromosomes. Such individuals are often found to be taller than average, and show mental retardation and/or aggressive behavior more frequently than normal XY males.

80. A The three forms of Down's syndrome are described on p. 80. Severe mental retardation is usual.

81. D Tuberous sclerosis (epiloia or Bourneville's disease) is transmitted by an autosomal-dominant gene having variable penetrance and expressivity (p. 77). New mutations are not infrequent. Intelligence may range from severe retardation to above normal; epilepsy, skin disorders, and nonmalignant tumors occur in some individuals.

82. B The two most convincing types of studies which control for the effects of environment have been comparison of concordance rates in monozygotic and dizygotic twins, and foster child (adoption) studies. Pedigree studies of schizophrenia have not been fruitful, and the major criticism of family expectancy studies has been their inability to separate hereditary from environmental effects.

83. A The first three choices are correct, but during REM sleep there is a marked *decrease* in muscle tension (p. 82).

84. C There is substantial evidence that intelligence is partially determined by heredity (the cumulative influence of multiple minor genes, or polygenic transmission). Borderline mental retardation (IQ 68 to 83) primarily represents the lower end of the normal distribution of intelligence in the population. Cerebral lipidoses and acute intermittent porphyria are believed to be transmitted by simple mendelian mechanisms (recessive and dominant, respectively). The genetic contribution to schizophrenic disorders is believed to result either from *several different* simple mendelian traits or from true polygenic transmission.

CHAPTER 8 (pp. 122–124)

85. B Synthetic antipsychotics *lower the seizure threshold* but they do have each of the other properties listed (with great varia-

tions in *intensity* among the drugs). See pp. 99–100.

86. B The best answer is *affective symptoms* (especially severe depression). See pp. 116 and 119–120.

87. D The two major groups of toxic symptoms resulting from lithium affect the *gastro-intestinal system* (e.g., diarrhea and vomiting), and the *central nervous system* (e.g., nystagmus and tremor) (p. 115). Lithium toxicity is intensely uncomfortable and most unlikely to produce euphoria; that latter is one sign of hypomania, which is an indication for lithium therapy.

88. D The answer is *reserpine* (p. 97). Protriptyline and tranylcypromine are antidepressants (TCA and MAOI respectively); lithium is an antimanic agent and does *not* cause depression; and meprobamate is a minor tranquilizer. Reserpine-induced depressions may be severe, and respond to tricyclic antidepressants (provided reserpine is discontinued), but ECT may be very dangerous until several drug-free weeks have elapsed (p. 117).

89. E Tardive dyskinesias are *chronic* extrapyramidal disorders characterized by *hyperactivity* (involuntary choreoathetoid movements) and thought to be a complication of long-term neuroleptic therapy. No universally effective treatment is yet known, but there is general agreement that anticholinergic medications exacerbate the symptoms (pp. 109–110).

90. D The term *antipsychotic* is usually reserved for drugs that ameliorate the functional psychotic symptoms of schizophrenia; however, minor tranquilizers may have some therapeutic value for similar symptoms in certain acute brain syndromes (p. 120). Although these drugs are commonly used as skeletal muscle relaxants, animal experiments have failed to adequately document this practice.

91. D This patient very likely has *akathisia*, an extrapyramidal side effect of the trifluo-

perazine. This syndrome (described on pp. 107–108) can be a difficult side effect to manage. If it is distressing (to the patient or other persons in his environment), relief may be obtained by decreasing neuroleptic dosage or prescribing anticholinergic medication — but akathisia is the EPS *least* likely to respond well to the latter alone. Akathisia often occurs because of rapidity of dosage increase rather than actual dosage. Treatment of acute EPS is discussed on pp. 108–109.

92. D *Paraldehyde* was formerly widely used in the treatment of withdrawal syndromes associated with alcohol, barbiturates, and other sedative-hypnotics. It is now rarely used because of its tendency to decompose easily into toxic substances and its disagreeable taste and odor. The latter is associated with its one significant advantage: it is excreted mainly through the lungs rather than the kidneys.

93. B Toxic psychoses caused by tricyclic antidepressants (and occasionally antipsychotics) resemble those associated with other *anticholinergic* drugs such as atropine. See p. 110 and also Chapter 12.

94. E *None* of the conditions listed is an absolute contraindication to ECT, although each may involve additional risks, which may be reduced by modification of the usual procedures (pp. 117–118). Lack of peripheral cholinesterase enzymes would cause *inability to metabolize succinylcholine* (and thus prolonged apnea).

95. B Several of the *hydrazine MAO inhibitors* were removed from clinical use because of this side effect, and it remains a serious problem with those still in use (p. 104). By contrast, the cholestatic jaundice associated with phenothiazines and tricyclic antidepressants is benign and readily reversible (provided the drug is discontinued).

96. D *Pigmentary retinopathy* is an idiosyncratic side effect of thioridazine, and

nearly all reported cases occurred with dosages exceeding 800 mg daily (p. 102).

97. D All three statements are true (pp. 117–118).

98. B Hyperarousal with tremors, psychosis, or seizures may follow abrupt termination of any sedative or minor tranquilizer (but *not* major tranquilizer, antidepressant, or opiate) that has been taken in high doses for a long period of time. The seizures may be fatal. See Chapter 12.

99. A *Agranulocytosis* is an extremely rare but invariably life-threatening side effect of certain drugs, including neuroleptics and tricyclic antidepressants (p. 111).

100. E Orthostatic hypotension is a nonspecific side effect of several psychotropic drugs in certain individuals and tends to persist with continuing dosage. Oculogyric crisis is an acute EPS (dystonic). Skin pigmentation changes are rare results of very long-term phenothiazine therapy that are caused by increased activity of MSH or precipitation of phenothiazine dye. Peripheral neuropathies are infrequent; the mechanism is unknown. Side effects of antipsychotics and tricyclic antidepressants are described on pp. 107–113.

101. B. Choices 1 and 3 are correct (p. 122). Amphetamines and other psychomotor stimulants usually rapidly exacerbate psychoses of all types, including involutional melancholia.

102. E. All the drugs listed affect the reticular activating system, but neuroleptics and minor tranquilizers are much more selective than barbiturates.

103. A Desirable effects of ECT include improvements (i.e., reduction) in depression and associated insomnia, anorexia, and weight loss. Undesirable (but not usually serious) side effects may include an acute brain syndrome with confusion and temporary amnesia (especially following bilateral treatments), increased anxiety (particularly if ECT is unmodified by pretreatment medications) and posttreatment head-aches, which are of brief duration and respond well to aspirin. The side effects of ECT are described on pp. 118–119.

104. D According to current usage the only absolute contraindication to lithium therapy is *inability to excrete lithium.* Serious cardiovascular disease is another major risk, but is considered a relative rather than an absolute contraindication. Lithium alters electrolyte storage and function, and the patient must be instructed to maintain adequate fluid and sodium intake, since hyponatremia potentiates toxic reactions from lithium (but is not a contraindication if there is adequate clinical supervision). Long-term use of lithium may compromise thyroid function, so preexisting dysfunction is another indication for especially careful clinical monitoring (pp. 114–115).

105. C Choices 2 and 4 are both true and may be important in the clinical management of certain patients (p. 121). However, meprobamate is considerably less expensive, and there is no evidence that it is less effective for short-term relief of anxiety.

106. E Each of the side effects listed is possible, and is generally independent of lithium dosage (p. 115).

107. D Anticholinergic drugs such as benztropine may ameliorate acute extrapyramidal disorders, including akathisia (pp. 108–109). However, the other three side effects listed result from the anticholinergic effects of chlorpromazine, and would therefore be exacerbated by additional anticholinergic medication (p. 112).

108. C Tolerance develops rapidly for the sedative effects of barbiturates, and at a slower rate for the antianxiety effects of all minor tranquilizers (p. 120). However, there is no evidence that tolerance is ever acquired for the *therapeutic effects* of antipsychotics or antidepressants, although patients do develop tolerance to most *side effects* of these drugs (p. 113).

109. **B** Neuroleptics potentiate most CNS depressants, *except for anticonvulsant effects,* which are antagonized, as are the antiparkinson effects of levodopa. Interactions of antipsychotics with other drugs are described on p. 100.

110. **A** The most important indication for TCAs is retarded depression (p. 105). Therapeutic response is usually gradual, and the painful affect itself may be the last symptom to improve; suicidal risk is often increased during the early stages of therapy (pp. 106–107). Although not usually used to treat *depression* in preadolescent children, imipramine and other TCAs are sometimes used in the treatment of childhood behavior disorders or enuresis (see Chap. 19).

111. **B** Microsomal enzyme induction, which alters the rate of metabolism of many drugs, is a significant disadvantage of barbiturates, glutethimide, and certain other sedative-hypnotic drugs, but does *not* occur with antipsychotics or benzodiazepines (p. 121).

CHAPTER 9 (pp. 136–137)

112. **B** The correct definition is B (p. 128). Choice A appears to be primary prevention, while C and D would involve tertiary prevention.

113. **D** A methadone maintenance program is not one of the five specific services required. In addition to the other four items listed, *community consultation* services are required (p. 127).

114. **A** Primary prevention is defined as efforts to lower the incidence (rate of new cases) of mental illness by counteracting the stressful social conditions involved in its genesis. Choice A most nearly fits this definition. Efforts toward early recognition and use of specific treatment modalities are related to *secondary* prevention (p. 128).

115. **A** The *lifetime expectancy* of requiring hospitalization for psychiatric treatment has long exceeded 10% (p. 131). Conservative estimates would be around 2% for *each* of the following diagnostic groups: organic brain syndromes, alcoholism and drug abuse, functional psychoses, depressive neuroses, and personality disorders.

116. **A** Ecological studies show a high frequency of certain disorders in the slums of large cities. Various cause-and-effect relationships have been proposed to account for this finding. One of these, the drift hypothesis, suggests that these disorders result in downward social mobility, accompanied by a tendency for these persons to migrate, or drift (geographically), into these areas (pp. 132–133).

117. **A** *Schizophrenia* continues to account for nearly half of all persons hospitalized for treatment in these facilities. (See Table 9-1 on p. 129).

118. **B** Community mental health centers serve persons of all ages within their catchment area (a specific geographic region having a population of about 100,000). There are no financial restrictions, and the local agency must conform with federal guidelines (p. 127).

119. **A** Epidemiological studies of global psychiatric impairment have consistently reported increased rates of disorder among the divorced (p. 131), the downwardly mobile (p. 135), the elderly (pp. 129–130), and urban groups (p. 132).

CHAPTER 10 (pp. 146–147)

120. **B** Testamentary capacity is the competency to make a valid will (p. 142).

121. **A** Laws governing admission to mental hospitals (commitment laws) usually do not directly affect other medical-legal issues such as criminal responsibility, competency to stand trial, competency to handle financial affairs, or testamentary capacity (p. 141). The various criteria employed in the determination of criminal responsibility are discussed on pp. 143–144

122. E Decisions regarding various types of competency, including testamentary capacity, are based on impairment of specific abilities (related to the act in question), and *not* on diagnostic labels.

123. A Specific mental abilities are required in connection with various types of competency. In general, the nature of these abilities is related to the nature of the act in question (e.g., to stand trial, enter into a contract, make a will, etc.). Adjudications of competency are based on these specific abilities and *not* on such broad criteria as choice 4. The criteria for competency to stand trial are discussed on p. 142.

124. A The first three choices are included in the M'Naghten test (p. 143). Choice 4 is known as the irresistible impulse test, which was formulated much later (p. 143).

125. E Only a minority of states still provide by law that incompetency is automatically inherent in *involuntary* psychiatric hospitalization (p. 141).

CHAPTER 11 (pp. 158–160)

126. C The symptoms listed are typical of *lead* toxicity (plumbism); treatment is by chelating agents such as dimercaprol (British antilewisite, or BAL) and calcium disodium edetate (p. 157).

127. D *Uremia* is a frequent complication of cardiovascular renal disease and invariably leads to some organic intellectual impairment (p. 156). Transfer to a psychiatric unit is usually contraindicated.

128. D The term *delirium* refers to a symptom complex (i.e., syndrome) in which the primary disturbance affects the sensorium. Delirium is an acute brain syndrome characterized by increased arousal and psychomotor activity, perceptual distortions (especially visual and tactile), and often extreme apprehension and anxiety and possibly unstable delusions. The cause usually originates outside the central nervous system (e.g., drug or poison intoxication, systemic infection, endocrine, metabolic, or nutritional disorders, etc.). See p. 150 and Table 11-1.

129. B Abrupt onset and sudden fluctuations in severity of symptoms are related to blood pressure and oxygen supply to the brain and are typical of cerebrovascular dementias (pp. 151–152). Of course, the arteriosclerotic process itself (in contrast with the organic brain syndrome it causes) has a gradual, insidious onset.

130. A The best answer is *Pick's disease* (p. 151). Generalized atrophy is more common in Alzheimer's disease and senile dementia (pp. 150–151), while Huntington's chorea affects the whole cortex and basal ganglia as well (p. 155).

131. E The triad described is characteristic of *Korsakoff's syndrome,* and may be accompanied by other signs of a chronic brain syndrome. Wernicke's syndrome is also associated with chronic alcoholism, but is an *acute,* life-threatening condition characterized by the triad of ataxia, clouding of consciousness, and ophthalmoplegia. Both are due to deficiencies of vitamin B complex, particularly thiamine (p. 153).

132. D Choice 4 is the definition of acute brain syndrome and is the only correct answer. The distinction is largely a theoretical one, since reversibility may be contingent on rapid and effective medical intervention. An acute brain syndrome may terminate in complete resolution, partial resolution with a residual chronic brain syndrome, or death (pp. 149–150).

133. A The first three tests are often helpful, but the MMPI has greatest validity for distinguishing neurotic from psychotic or character disorders, and is of little use for the problem mentioned. A detailed discussion of these topics is given in Chapter 4.

134. A The first three choices are correct (p. 155). Although inherited, the onset is usually in middle age and duration is prolonged for

5 to 20 years. Either neurological or psychiatric symptoms may predominate. "Functional" psychopathology (neurotic, psychotic, or behavioral) may be the most obvious early sign of any chronic brain syndrome having relatively slow onset (p. 150).

135. C According to DSM-II, Alzheimer's disease is a chronic brain syndrome with diffuse cortical atrophy having onset during the presenile period (i.e., before age 60). However, since it is identical with the pathological process resulting in senile dementia, age of onset remains the only basis for distinguishing between these two diagnoses, and many authorities now consider them interchangeable (p. 151).

136. A The first three choices are correct. Unlike barbiturates and some other drugs, antipsychotics are *not* contraindicated and may be helpful (p. 156).

137. B Treatment of bromism always includes giving chloride, and antipsychotics may be helpful to control delirium or other psychotic symptoms. Withdrawal from bromide does not involve seizures, so barbiturates are not indicated (pp. 157–158). Naloxone is an opiate antagonist and would have no effect in counteracting bromide toxicity.

138. B Although the term *dementia* refers to a syndrome, it is usually applied only when there are irreversible structural changes; the term *pseudodementia* would be a more accurate one for syndromes such as normal pressure hydrocephalus, which are reversed by therapeutic intervention. Dementia need not involve either psychotic symptoms or EEG abnormalities (p. 150 and Table 11-1).

139. A Pathological intoxication is a rare, idiosyncratic reaction to alcohol by certain predisposed individuals, and is correctly characterized by the first three choices. Duration ranges from minutes to days (p. 152).

140. A The first three choices are correct. Wernicke's encephalopathy is acute and life-threatening, with damage located in the midbrain (hemorrhages). Korsakoff's syndrome is chronic and associated with cortical damage and polyneuritis. Treatment of both should always include thiamine and other B vitamins (p. 153).

141 A GPI (dementia paralytica) occurs in about 5% of patients with untreated CNS syphilis. An Argyll-Robertson pupil is one that is responsive to accommodation effort, but not to light. Patients should always receive penicillin unless contraindicated (as by allergy), in which case other antibiotics or fever therapy may be indicated (p. 154).

142. C Visual or tactile hallucinations and illusions are usually suggestive of acute brain syndromes (toxic or otherwise), including most of the alcoholic psychoses. However, an exception is alcoholic hallucinosis in which, as in functional psychoses, auditory hallucinations in a clear sensorium predominate (p. 153).

143. C While any of the medications listed may carry some risk, a benzodiazepine (e.g., diazepam) or a sedating antihistamine (e.g., hydroxyzine) would be relatively safer than either a barbiturate (which more strongly potentiates the CNS depressant effects of alcohol) or an antipsychotic such as chlorpromazine (which is a strong potentiator, and may also produce severe hypotension). Benzodiazepines are poorly absorbed following intramuscular injections, so the preferred route of administration is either by mouth (if possible) or by slow intravenous injection.

144. A The characteristic symptoms of organic brain syndromes are impairment of orientation, memory, all intellectual processes, and judgment, together with lability or shallowness of affect. Differences between persons with identical brain dysfunction are attributable to their differing person-

alities and vulnerability, and may therefore include symptoms from the whole range of functional psychopathology (depressive, paranoid, neurotic, behavioral, etc.). Neologisms are suggestive of schizophrenia (which, however, may be precipitated or aggravated by an organic brain syndrome). Conversely, severe functional psychopathology may include any of the symptoms listed (pp. 149–150).

145. A Regression and increasing impairment during psychological testing or other intellectual tasks are characteristic of all organic brain syndromes. "Catastrophic anxiety" or agitation (e.g., weeping) are common when impairment is moderate and recognized by the patient. Confusion tends to be greater in darkness than when surroundings are well lighted.

CHAPTER 12 (pp. 173–174)

146. C The only false statement is C. Unlike earlier opiate antagonists, (e.g., pentazocine), naloxone has no agonist properties and is therefore nonaddicting. It does have the other properties listed. Treatment of an overdose by an addict may produce an abstinence syndrome but is life-saving (pp. 168–169).

147. B The correct answer is *acutely intoxicated.* Factors which modify individual response to alcohol, and the average blood levels corresponding to different stages of impairment, are discussed on pp. 166–167.

148. C Abrupt withdrawal of barbiturates is *contraindicated* if there is any possibility of physical dependence. Antipsychotic drugs such as chlorpromazine are relatively contraindicated because of their effects on the seizure threshold, temperature regulation, liver function, blood pressure, etc.; moreover, such drugs generally offer no advantages over adequate replacement therapy, for which most clinicians prefer a short-acting barbiturate. A few clinicians prefer to use the same drug, but

this is not a necessity. Benzodiazepines may not offer sufficient protection against seizures, and have the additional disadvantage of being eliminated very slowly. See p. 170 for a more complete discussion.

149. B The only correct answer is B. Withdrawal from amphetamines is accompanied by a period of hypersomnia and possible depression (p. 171).

150. A The correct answer is *methadone,* which is an opiate *agonist* used in substitution therapy (p. 169). Naloxone is an opioid *antagonist* that will precipitate or accentuate the opiate withdrawal syndrome (pp. 168–169).

151. C Withdrawal of most hypnotics, sedatives, and minor tranquilizers after prolonged use should be gradual (over 2 to 3 weeks), since abrupt withdrawal is likely to result in acute brain syndromes and epileptic seizures or status epilepticus, which may be fatal (p. 170). There is some variability across different drugs, and a few drugs have considerably lower potential for physical dependence than barbiturates, glutethimide, and meprobamate. Gradual withdrawal of opiates is the usual practice, since abrupt withdrawal (cold turkey) is unpleasant, but the opiate abstinence syndrome is not life-threatening except when there are certain coincidental physical problems (p. 169). Abrupt withdrawal of amphetamines is followed by prolonged sleep and depression, sometimes with suicidal behavior, so close observation is often important (p. 171).

152. C Choices 2 and 4 are correct; all these factors are discussed on pp. 166–167.

153. A This syndrome is called *amphetamine psychosis* or *cocaine psychosis,* and is associated with the CNS sympathomimetics and related drugs (amphetamines, cocaine, methylphenidate, phenmetrazine, etc.). Treatment is the same as for paranoid schizophrenia (especially antipsychotic drugs, which may be needed for a

prolonged time after illicit drug ingestion has stopped) except that psychosocial therapies should be directed at the drug abuse (p. 171). Jimsonweed produces a toxic confusional syndrome associated with anticholinergic drugs (p. 172).

154. C Naloxone is an opiate antagonist, and is also effective against synthetic opioids, so choices 2 and 4 are correct (pp. 168–169).

155. D Antipsychotics have therapeutic advantages in the treatment of toxic syndromes produced by dopaminergic agonists such as amphetamines. Intoxication by LSD or other psychedelics is usually best treated by psychological means and a relatively safe nonspecific sedative such as a benzodiazepine. Antipsychotics potentiate the effects of CNS depressants such as alcohol, and have their own anticholinergic action which would be additively superimposed on the toxic effects of atropine and similar drugs; they are therefore *contraindicated* in such syndromes.

CHAPTER 13 (pp. 187–189)

156. E Schizophrenics may experience all types of hallucinations, but the most frequent is *auditory.*

157. E The first four alternatives are Bleuler's primary symptoms, often referred to as defects in the "four A's." They are discussed on p. 175.

158. A The unfavorable sign is *emotional blunting;* a chronic course is probable, with gradual onset at an early age. However, prominent depression involves high risk of suicide in schizo-affective disorders.

159. A Schizophrenias are a group of disorders characterized by disturbances in thinking, mood, and behavior. The thought disorder is usually regarded as primary, and other manifestations as secondary (p. 176). However, this answer may be regarded as controversial by some psychiatrists.

160. B The average age at first psychiatric admission for schizophrenia is slightly under 25 years for males and slightly over 25 years for females, but the average for both sexes combined is probably still over 25 years. Since the availability of antipsychotic drugs, discharge rates have increased, as have readmission rates at other ages, but duration of stay in hospital (for each admission and lifetime total) has greatly decreased.

161. B The correct answer is *hebephrenic schizophrenia.* Labile and inappropriate affect may be observed in several other forms, but is most common and most enduring in the hebephrenic type. The subtypes of schizophrenia are described on pp. 176–178.

162. C The correct answer is *paranoid schizophrenia.* Other forms that are frequently diagnosed include schizo-affective schizophrenia, acute schizophrenic episode (schizophreniform psychosis), and chronic undifferentiated schizophrenia. The diagnoses of hebephrenic and simple subtypes are now rare.

163. A This is a characteristic feature of *simple schizophrenia* (rarely diagnosed).

164. D The answer is *schizo-affective schizophrenia* (also called *schizo-affective psychosis*), which is a combination of schizophrenic thought disorder with prominent affective disorder (depression or elation); appropriate treatment should be directed at both components.

165. E These symptoms are most characteristic of *catatonic schizophrenia.*

166. A The answer is *simple schizophrenia.* The other forms are likely to have a more rapid onset with grossly abnormal thinking, affect, and behavior.

167. D The highest risk of suicide occurs in the *schizo-affective* subtype.

168. B The description is characteristic of *hebephrenic schizophrenia.*

169. E All four statistics are in agreement with data currently available. It is generally

believed that no *single-gene* hypothesis can account for such statistics, and therefore most current speculation involves either (1) *genetic heterogeneity* (multiple single-gene mechanisms, which produce different subgroups of schizophrenias), or (2) *polygenic transmission* (i.e., the hypothesis that hereditary predisposition to schizophrenia is a continuously variable characteristic attributable to the cumulative effects of multiple minor genes at many different loci). The genetic transmission of schizophrenia is discussed on pp. 178–180 and also in Chapter 7.

170. E   Choices 1 and 3 represent paranoid personality traits, whereas 2 and 4 represent overt behaviors that may result from paranoid ideation (pp. 186–187).

171. A   Choices 1, 2, and 3 are correct. Obsessive-compulsive personality traits would suggest a more favorable prognosis than either paranoid or schizoid traits.

172. E   All four choices are correct. The process-reactive continuum of schizophrenias is discussed on p. 178.

173. C   Regressive behavior and delusional thinking are found in a variety of mental disorders. Neologisms are considered by many as practically pathognomonic of schizophrenia, and catatonic stupor with mutism and waxy flexibility is most frequently indicative of schizophrenia. However, an organic brain syndrome may precipitate or exacerbate any form of "functional" psychopathology, including schizophrenia, as discussed in Chapter 11.

174. D   Choice 4 is correct. Antipsychotic medications at adequate dosage constitute a major part of therapy, as does protection of the patient, his family, and society if there is a possibility of suicidal, assaultive, or homicidal behavior. Delusions are defined as fixed false beliefs that are maintained in spite of logical arguments and contrary evidence, and it is rarely useful to confront delusional patients as sug-

gested by choice 2. Paranoid patients may interpret such behavior as persecutory and include the therapist in the delusional system.

175. A   The definitions of these diagnostic labels emphasize items 1 and 3, although schizophrenics, rarely, may have logically systematized delusions. Paranoid schizophrenia rarely has onset after age 40, and paranoid state rarely before that age. Any paranoid patient may have affective disturbance (euphoria, depression, anxiety, fear, etc.) associated with his delusional beliefs.

CHAPTER 14 (pp. 204–206)

176. C   There is usually a clear relationship between affect and thought content in patients with affective disorders, but not in schizophrenics. Manics are more responsive to external stimuli than schizophrenics, and may experience hallucinations and delusions (pp. 193–194).

177. E   Paranoid delusions include delusions of reference, persecution, active or passive influence, and grandeur, and are not incompatible with any psychotic diagnosis. The different types of delusions are defined in Chapter 2.

178. D   If all forms of adult psychopathology are included, and the tabulation covers all types of hospitals and clinics, males are affected at least as frequently as females. However, females have consistently been reported in higher numbers than males for neuroses, affective psychoses, and paranoid states.

179. D   The answer is *obsessive-compulsive* (p. 192).

180. C   The best answer is C. The most significant losses usually involve dearly loved persons for whom there may be ambivalent or conflicting feelings (e.g., love and anger). Since the hostile feelings are unacceptable if recognized, they are defended against by the mechanisms of

retroflexion and *introjection,* resulting in lowered self-esteem, guilt, a desire for punishment, and ultimately depression. This concept is discussed on p. 198, and the defense mechanisms are defined in Chapter 1.

181. E The best descriptive label is *hypomania* (p. 193).

182. D There is usually *not* a family history of unipolar or bipolar affective disorders, and there may be a family history of schizophrenic disorder (p. 192). Somatic complaints are quite common and may be the initial reason for seeking medical assistance; in advanced cases these complaints become increasingly bizarre and of delusional intensity. There is high risk of suicide, but generally a good response to antidepressant medication and especially to ECT. It should be noted that intellectual impairment, as reflected by IQ test scores or mental status examination, may be prominent in involutional melancholia, but that such symptoms are *functional* and therefore disappear when the depression is alleviated.

183. A Lithium salts are considered the best treatment for acute mania, but require 1 to 2 weeks for maximal therapeutic effect. If the situation is urgent (because of hyperactivity, etc.), or if lithium is considered too dangerous, either antipsychotic drugs or electroconvulsive therapy may be effective on at least a temporary basis. Benzodiazepines (e.g., diazepam or chlordiazepoxide), barbiturates, and other sedatives are not effective except for producing sleep or profound sedation.

184. E All are correct. Choices 1 and 3 are discussed on p. 198, and choices 2 and 4 on p. 194.

185. A The first three choices are frequent in mania; hallucinations and delusions are less frequent, usually being seen only in very advanced cases (pp. 193–194).

186. A Lindemann's findings are summarized on

pp. 191–192; choice 4 is one of his examples of *pathological grief.*

187. A Statistics about base rates of mental illnesses must always be interpreted cautiously, since they may be distorted by factors such as the following: whether first hospital admissions, all hospital admissions, or both inpatients and outpatients are tabulated; diagnostic uncertainty or bias; differences in diagnostic practices related to region, type of hospital, or type of patient (e.g., socioeconomic status); and which types of hospitals are included. However, it appears likely that the first three choices are correct, and that females outnumber males in affective disorders (but not in schizophrenias, where the sexes are equally affected).

188. B ECT remains superior to drug therapy for psychotic depression (although it is not always the initial treatment of choice). Lithium is the best treatment for acute mania, but ECT is an option that should not be overlooked if lithium cannot be used or an emergency exists. A true paranoid state would be unlikely to significantly benefit from ECT. Treatment of affective disorders is discussed on pp. 203–204, and also in Chapter 8.

189. E All of these symptoms are frequently but not invariably present in depression, and are not the only manifestations of these disorders. See the Beck Depression Inventory on pp. 195–197.

190. E Manifestations of depression in children and adolescents may differ from those in adults, and will be discussed more fully in Chapter 19.

CHAPTER 15 (pp. 217–218)

191. D Current theories emphasize anxiety as the common denominator of all neurotic symptoms; the form of symptoms is determined by the defense mechanisms employed by the ego to ensure continuing exclusion from awareness of the painful

memories or forbidden impulses producing the anxiety. Choice E is false; choices A, B, and C apply to certain other disorders in addition to neuroses.

192. A There is general agreement that hysterical paralyses and anesthesias have been less frequently diagnosed since World War II than previously, although there has been an increase in other forms of conversion disorder and neuroses of all other types.

193. C The principal forms of conversion hysteria are described on p. 211. Reflexes are within normal limits, and the plantar response is flexor. Hysterical epileptiform seizures are typically not accompanied by physical injury, tongue-biting, incontinence, or subsequent amnesia; movements are usually described as disorganized writhing and thrashing rather than rhythmic clonus, although duration may be prolonged and the patient may *appear* completely unresponsive to stimuli.

194. A *Primary gain* refers to *internal* (intrapsychic) advantages derived from the symptoms (continuing exclusion from consciousness of painful conflicts, memories, or impulses) and is involved in *precipitation* of the neurosis. *Secondary gain* refers to *external* advantages obtained while ill, and is an important factor in *perpetuation* of the symptoms (p. 211).

195. E Gross motor hysteria is believed to be *decreasing* in frequency, but is developed and maintained under circumstances involving reinforcement of disability and other secondary gains.

196. E All of the alternatives are true. The dynamics of phobic disorders are discussed on p. 210.

197. A The answer is *conversion hysteria,* in which the patient often displays a remarkable lack of distress despite the disabling nature of his symptoms (*la belle indifférence,* p. 211). In neurotic depressions the anxiety is usually a prominent complaint.

198. E The only correct answer is *psychotic depression.* Delusional thinking is characteristic of psychosis and *not* neurosis. Delusions involving helplessness, worthlessness, sinfulness, punishment, or bizarre somatic changes are typical of depressive psychoses, as is early morning awakening and greatly reduced energy level. Such disorders were described in Chapter 14, and must always be differentiated from neurotic disorders.

199. A The first three choices are correct. Secondary gain consists of the *external* benefit derived from any illness, in contrast with the primary gain of a neurosis, which consists of relief from emotional conflict and freedom from anxiety accomplished by a defense mechanism or symptom (p. 211).

200. A The first three choices are correct (p. 211). The term *compensation neurosis* refers to a conversion disorder in which the secondary gain includes monetary compensation for disability.

201. C Pain is a common form of conversion hysteria. In the case described, there may be emotional conflict over ambivalent feelings toward the deceased father, leading to a pathological form of grief (symptom imitation) which helps to keep the conflict repressed (primary gain). Ganser's syndrome is a pseudopsychotic *syndrome of approximate answers* that may be due to malingering or hysteria, and is usually found in prisoners awaiting trial.

202. E Neurotic symptoms are believed to be manifestations of anxiety or fear and are produced by the ego's use of various defense mechanisms in order to maintain repression of the true source from conscious awareness. They are ubiquitous, and may be seen in persons of all ages and diagnoses. The definition of neurotic illness is therefore a matter of degree, depending on the frequency and extent of impaired functioning produced by such symptoms (which are frequently activated

or exacerbated by all forms of functional psychosis and organic brain syndromes).

203. E All choices are correct. Anxiety neurosis is described on pp. 209–210.

204. E All choices are correct. The four forms of hysterical conversion symptoms are described on p. 211. Local trauma or atrophy may be observed and result from involuntary movements, prolonged muscle contracture, or disuse of muscles. A lump in the throat *(globus hystericus)* is one of the classical hysterical manifestations.

205. E The dynamics of obsessive-compulsive disorders are described on p. 210. Repression is a common denominator of all defense mechanisms and neurotic symptoms (see Chap. 1).

CHAPTER 16 (pp. 229–230)

206. A The answer is *easy fatigability,* which is characteristic of the asthenic personality and of depression, but *not* of hysteria (p. 222).

207. D The answer is *multiple personality,* a rare type of hysterical dissociative disorder (p. 211). The schizoid personality is described on p. 221.

208. B The answer is *avoidance of competition,* which is a schizoid personality trait. The cyclothymic personality is described on pp. 221–222.

209. A Projection is typical of the *paranoid personality* (p. 221).

210. C This is characteristic of both. The nature of the delinquent behavior is not the basis for distinguishing antisocial personality from dyssocial behavior.

211. A This is true of antisocial personality. The dyssocial person typically has a functional superego that corresponds to the subculture with which he identifies but is viewed as deviant by the larger society in which he lives.

212. A The true sociopath is incapable of significant enduring loyalty to any moral code, person, or group. The dyssocial person

does manifest such loyalties, and this constitutes the primary distinction between the two types.

213. C Personality disorders are distinguished from neurosis by a relative absence of persistent excessive anxiety, and from psychosis by relatively normal capacity for reality testing. The behavior patterns are usually already evident during adolescence and change little throughout life, and motivation for therapeutic assistance in effecting change is usually low (p. 221)

214. E Johnson and Szurek's views on the development of antisocial personality are outlined on p. 226.

215. A The first three choices are correct. Choice 4 is true of the antisocial personality, but persons with neurotic personality types are usually excessively concerned with how others feel about them (in spite of frequent behaviors that invite rejection).

CHAPTER 17 (pp. 238–239)

216. D The best answer is *anxiety* (or fear or panic).

217. A The recommended answer is 5%. The vast majority of cases have a major psychogenic component.

218. B Physicians tend to reinforce overconcern and disability when they undertake extensive somatic investigations with minimal feedback of negative findings to the patient. They also reinforce an inappropriate belief in exclusively somatic pathology and denial of emotional factors when they disregard the latter and adopt a solely somatic approach to therapy.

219. C The answer is *supportive psychotherapy,* including environmental manipulation (p. 238). Patients with psychophysiological disorders have dependency problems, limited facility of expression, and other interpersonal traits that make most of them unsuitable for group therapy, and they need more support than psychoanalysis offers. Antianxiety medication

is most effective in relieving short-term (situational) anxiety and may be helpful to peptic ulcer patients in such circumstances.

220. D   All three choices are true. Rheumatoid arthritis is discussed on pp. 237–238.

221. E   Penile erection and ejaculation are controlled by the autonomic nervous system. By definition, this rules out a diagnosis of hysteria (which requires that the affected function be under voluntary control). Choices A, B, C, and D may or may not be true, but are unrelated to the definition of psychophysiological disorder (p. 233).

222. C   Peptic ulcer (p. 235) and obsessive-compulsive neurosis are more frequent in the higher socioeconomic classes, while obesity (p. 236) and antisocial personality are more frequent in the lower classes.

223. C   Higher than average gastric acid secretions are believed to be a necessary predisposing factor, but life stresses also play a causative role in duodenal ulcer disease (p. 235).

224. A   Migraine headaches are usually *unilateral,* and are frequently accompanied by nausea and visual disturbances. The prevailing affect-equivalent is thought to be anger, and there is a strong familial tendency (p. 238).

225. A   The first three choices are correct (p. 233). Secondary gain (external advantages from being ill) may occur in any illness, including psychophysiological disorders.

CHAPTER 18 (pp. 257–258)

226. E   The answer is the *squeeze technique,* described on p. 248. Masters and Johnson report success in treating 97% of premature ejaculation cases in this manner (p. 249).

227. A   Transsexualism is *the desire to be transformed into the opposite sex* (p. 253).

228. A   The question is assumed to refer to therapy for change of psychosexual orientation (not for change in homosexual performance). *Relatively young age* and *motivation for change* are necessary prerequisites to any other favorable factors.

No single form of therapy has established success in changing psychosexual orientation, in contrast with altering associated anxiety, depression, and other emotional problems. (Also see question 57, Chapter 6.)

229. E   The typical exhibitionist is *lonely, shy, and insecure,* but none of the other attributes listed are true (pp. 253–254).

230. C   Hampson and associates have provided evidence that adult gender role (psychological sex) is determined more strongly by *assigned sex and rearing* than by any other factor (p. 256).

CHAPTER 19 (pp. 282–285)

231. C   The best answer is *juvenile delinquency,* although this is not really a perfect answer. Juvenile delinquency and adult antisocial behavior may result from superego "lacunae," or blind spots, for a few specific types of deviant behavior. Such lacunae develop when parents have covertly, nonverbally, and often unwittingly reinforced behaviors that they ostensibly forbid. However, some juvenile delinquents have a generalized weakness of superego, and others have a very adequate superego that merely happens to have been supplied with deviant values by a subculture (p. 275). Infantile autism and childhood schizophrenia involve severe *ego* defects. Anaclitic depression occurs very early, before much superego development could be expected. Neurotic patients tend to have an unduly *strong* superego.

232. E   The best answer is "none of the above." All psychoses tend to be regressive. Reaction to stimulants in psychosis is variable but in general they are not considered helpful at any age (although some children with minimal brain dysfunction with psychotic features may improve). Choice C is incorrect; exogenous situational factors appear relatively more important in functional psychoses of adult life. Psychoses

at any age often leave residual impairment, and this is especially true in childhood.

233. E   The best answer is E. A secondary, less important benefit may be increased reliability. Consent of one parent or legal guardian is sufficient for treatment. C alludes to a rather uncommon occurrence that the interviewer should keep in the back of his mind as a possibility, and D represents a common myth.

234. C   The correct answer is *fear*. Usually a response to a highly frustrating home environment, the overwhelming fear is supplemented by feelings of worthlessness and discouragement.

235. E   Most childhood psychiatric problems are either more frequent in males or found in both sexes in approximately equal proportions.

236. D   The description given is typical of normal adolescence, and contains no evidence of psychopathology. Family therapy is not indicated unless there is great conflict or danger of decompensation.

237. E   Kanner's original observation that autism is an upper- or middle-class phenomenon has been vindicated after some suspicion that it was an artifact of recognition and diagnosis. There is no correlation between family history of schizophrenia and autism, which is one of the reasons for distinguishing autism from schizophrenia. Though parents of autistic children have normal intelligence, some authors state that 80% of autistic children are mentally retarded in addition to being autistic. Racial or ethnic factors have not been implicated.

238. B   The correct answer is *Harlow's monkey studies*. In addition to the effects of maternal deprivation, these studies have shown the importance of tactile stimulation as a component of mothering, and also the importance of peer contact to sexual and social development. Maternal deprivation is not ordinarily considered an important part of the etiology of child-

hood autism (by Kanner or others). Jean Piaget studied *normal* cognitive development. "Little Hans" was concerned partly with the results of hysterical mothering and partly with a common childhood phobia. The identity crisis commonly occurs during adolescence and has no documented relationship to earlier maternal deprivation.

239. E   Choices A, B, C, and D are all false. An IQ of 80 would technically fall into the questionable category of borderline mental retardation, but this diagnosis would not be justified with only this information. IQ scores cannot be interpreted without knowing what test was used and in what context. An 8-year-old child with an IQ of 80 would have a mental age of 6.4 years. Some such children are able to progress through school with no special assistance, although understandably they would tend to earn grades in the lower half of their class. Each child needs individual assessment regarding need for special tutoring. By the age of 8 years IQ testing has very good predictive value *in regard to academic success*. It is not as good at any age for predicting career success, athletic prowess, creativity, artistic talent, or common sense.

240. B   Paranoid delusions, rare in childhood, would be a sign of psychosis rather than adjustment reaction. Childhood disturbances of eating habits, sleeping, bowel and bladder function, and other vegetative functions are often symptomatic of adjustment reaction. Likewise, regressive phenomena or delay in the normal maturational phasing may be symptomatic of adjustment reaction, although they may also be symptomatic of other physical, medical, or surgical problems (p. 276).

241. A   The correct answer is *separation anxiety* (p. 277). Far from being mentally retarded, school phobics are often above average in IQ. Hyperkinetic children

appear to have no higher incidence of school phobia than other children — they are more likely to be suspended or expelled than to refuse to go. School phobics usually do very well academically in spite of much absenteeism. Anxiety about being away from the mother (occasionally the father) seems to be at the core of the child's fear of leaving home. There is often fear of harm coming to the mother, which may be related to oversubmissive maternal anxiety about winning the child's approval.

242. C The only answer that is not wrong as worded is C. While it is very helpful to interview child and parents together (to see the interaction), it is also advisable to see the child alone for part of the time, even if only to see what happens when he is separated from the parents. While it is desirable for the child to bring up topics by himself, important areas should not be neglected merely because he fails to bring them up. Rewarding the child by social approval facilitates the interview, but the tangible bribe implied in D does not seem appropriate. While some implication of confidentiality is desirable, absolute secrecy should not be promised even to an adolescent, let alone a 6-year-old child. Principles and techniques of child psychiatric interviews are discussed on pp. 265–267.

243. D Anorexia nervosa involves great variation in nutritional intake, and may include episodes of overeating (bulimia), vomiting (which may be self-induced), pica, and a history of obesity. There is denial of illness, of disability, of painful affect, and of unacceptable motivation (e.g., aggressive or sexual). Physical activity is often *increased* except in extreme cachexia (p. 281).

244. D Conversion of anxiety, anger, depression, or other feelings into physical symptoms typically involves voluntary muscles or

sensation. By contrast, psychophysiological disorders involve the autonomic nervous system with much subjective distress. Drug experimentation would likely cause more generalized symptoms not localized to one arm. Adjustment reaction or stress disturbance should not be diagnosed when a more specifically descriptive diagnosis is possible (p. 276). An intracranial neoplasm seems unlikely to cause weakness in one arm with no other findings.

245. D Answer A refers to *Leo Kanner,* B to *H. F. Harlow,* C to *Erik Erikson,* and E to *Anna Freud.* Piaget called himself a "genetic epistemologist" because he studied children's developing ability to perceive and learn. He described a developmental phenomenon of cognitive dynamic equilibrium: The child at any stage perceives, knows, and thinks in age-appropriate schemas. New information is changed to fit these schemas as it is taken in; at the same time, it changes the schemas. The process as described by Piaget is reminiscent of the biological process of assimilating food, although he did not push that analogy. His four main stages of cognitive development are shown in Table 19-1 (p. 261).

246. E Practically any stress or change from the familiar can cause transient regression in a toddler, and supportive understanding from an adult is helpful in these circumstances.

247. A The first choice of medication as an adjunct to treatment should usually be a stimulant, such as dextroamphetamine or methylphenidate, but neuroleptics such as chlorpromazine are sometimes used when the stimulants are not helpful. Barbiturates may actually make the hyperactive symptoms worse (p. 273).

248. B The tendency for females to attempt suicide more often but succeed less often is true for all ages, including adolescence.

Suicide ranks about third among causes of death during adolescence. Successful suicide is more frequent among those with *higher* intelligence and socioeconomic status.

249. B The first and third answers are correct, and the other two choices are *contraindicated.* The unknown can be terrifying, especially when associated with adult concern that children can always sense (even when adults attempt to conceal it). Uncertainty and ignorance leave the child at the mercy of his own fantasies, which are usually worse than the reality. Even adults often believe that something "too terrible to talk about" is much worse than something that can be calmly discussed. Sedation of children often works paradoxically, making them more frightened and raising fears of losing control. Even necessary narcotics are often experienced by children as unpleasant or "weird." When such medication is tolerated well, this is usually because of good psychological support from the hospital staff.

250. E Depression in a child or adolescent can be manifested not only by adultlike tears, sadness, self-blame, and suicidal behavior, but also by antisocial or unruly acting out. All four choices are therefore correct.

251. E All choices are correct (p. 270).

252. B Removal from school, either temporary or permanent, is *contraindicated* in school phobia; one of the interventions required is insistence that the child attend school regularly while treatment proceeds. School phobia often masquerades as physical symptoms occurring on school days, so that such children are usually brought to the pediatrician or family doctor before anyone thinks of consulting a psychiatrist. In more difficult cases, antidepressant medication has been reported helpful, but this is usually not initially indicated (p. 277).

253. D By definition an adjustment reaction involves a reaction to some stress, which can occur at any age and in either the presence or absence of organic problems In fact, a child with an organic problem is more likely to have adjustment reactic because of his increased vulnerability (p. 276).

254. A Although it is always *possible* for parent to modify the constitutional temperame of a child, it is not always *easy* (p. 262).

255. E All choices are correct. Parental overind gence and overprotection may delay the development of speech by making it un- necessary for the child to ask for what h wants.

CHAPTER 20 (pp. 296–297)

256. C Severe retardation is usually due to brai pathology that is environmental in origi There are many types involving predispc tion inherited by simple mendelian mecl nisms, although each is infrequent, and close relatives usually have normal intell gence. By contrast, mild retardation is usually familial, and is believed to have ፡ substantial genetic component transmitt by multiple minor genes with cumulativ effects (i.e., *polygenic* transmission) ratł than by simple mendelian mechanisms (p. 289).

257. D PKU is due to a single pair of recessive genes and is amenable to treatment. Parents are usually heterozygous carriers who have reduced capacity to metaboliz phenylalanine (i.e., the gene is not *completely* recessive) but do not have gross PKU (p. 292).

258. C The answer is *rubella* (p. 290). Congenit syphilis was formerly another major cau: of mental retardation, but it is now rela- tively rare.

259. A The correct answer is *Tay-Sachs disease* (p. 291). Gaucher's disease and Nieman Pick disease are also associated with this genetic-ethnic background, but most other disorders of fat metabolism are no

260. C Most come from impoverished families, and there is an unduly high frequency of mental retardation among parents and siblings, partly attributable to *polygenic* inheritance and partly to psychosocial (environmental) deprivation. The typical IQ score is 50 to 70, and they lack verbal skills. They do worst of all in classroom situations, but may adapt well elsewhere (p. 295).

261. A Severe retardation is contrasted with mild retardation on p. 289.

262. C See p. 294. There is no delay in ossification. Dry, pale, coarse skin would be more typical of a hypothyroid cretin.

263. A The first three choices are correct (p. 291). Wilson's disease is a disorder of copper metabolism (p. 292).

264. A Eczema and seizures are each present in about one-third of all cases. The musty odor of the urine was the basis for the original discovery of the disease, and the best-known diagnostic test consists of adding ferric chloride to the urine to produce a green color (p. 292).

265. A The first three choices are correct (p. 293); choice 4 is more suggestive of *Turner's syndrome.*

266. A The first three choices are correct (p. 293). The disease is transmitted by an autosomal-dominant gene with reduced penetrance and variable expressivity.

267. E Mental retardation is defined as subaverage intellectual functioning that originates in the developmental period and is associated with impairment of adaptive behavior (p. 287). Onset and hence prevention may be postnatal in some cases.

268. D Most mentally retarded persons do not require institutional treatment, and the large number of monogenic varieties are each relatively rare. Mild retardation is about eight times as frequent as the more severe forms, and is usually not attributable to birth trauma, infection, or metabolic errors (p. 289).

269. A Mental retardation is identified more often in males than females because of associated behavioral problems (e.g., sexual or aggressive). There is a strong correlation between intelligence and social class, associated with a higher frequency of retardation in inner city areas.

270. C It is a truism that all phenotypic characteristics involve interaction between genetic and environmental factors, but examination questions are rarely looking for this type of insight. Down's syndrome and Klinefelter's syndrome result from chromosomal anomalies and are primarily genetically determined (although special training and education may substantially increase intellectual function). In galactosemia and PKU the development of mental retardation requires *both* a specific genetic predisposition and postnatal exposure to certain environmental (nutritional) agents.

Index